TECHNICAL COLLEGE OF THE LOWCOUNTRY
LEARNING RESOURCES CENTER
POST OFFICE BOX 1288
BEAUFORT, SOUTH CAROLINA 29901-1288

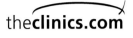

theclinics.com

PSYCHIATRIC CLINICS
OF NORTH AMERICA

Schizophrenia: A Complex Disease Necessitating Complex Care

GUEST EDITORS
Peter F. Buckley, MD and
Erick L. Messias, MD, MPH, PhD

September 2007 • Volume 30 • Number 3

SAUNDERS

An Imprint of Elsevier, Inc.
PHILADELPHIA   LONDON   TORONTO   MONTREAL   SYDNEY   TOKYO

W.B. SAUNDERS COMPANY
A Division of Elsevier Inc.

1600 John F. Kennedy Boulevard • Suite 1800 • Philadelphia, PA 19103-2899

http://www.theclinics.com

PSYCHIATRIC CLINICS OF NORTH AMERICA	**Volume 30, Number 3**
September 2007	**ISSN 0193-953X**
Editor: Sarah E. Barth	**ISBN-13: 978-1-4160-5116-9**
	ISBN-10: 1-4160-5116-3

Copyright © 2007 Elsevier Inc. All rights reserved. No part of this publication may be reproduced or transmitted in any form or by any means, electronic or mechanical, including photocopy, recording, or any information retrieval system, without written permission from the Publisher.

Single photocopies of single articles may be made for personal use as allowed by national copyright laws. Permission of the Publisher and payment of a fee is required for all other photocopying, including multiple or systematic copying, copying for advertising or promotional purposes, resale, and all forms of document delivery. Special rates are available for educational institutions that wish to make photocopies for non-profit educational classroom use. Permissions may be sought directly from Elsevier's Global Rights Department in Oxford, UK: phone 215-239-3804 or +44 (0) 1865 843830, fax +44 (0) 1865 853333, e-mail: healthpermissions@elsevier.com. Requests may also be completed on-line via the Elsevier homepage (http://www.elsevier.com/permissions). In the USA, users may clear permissions and make payments through the Copyright Clearance Center, Inc., 222 Rosewood Drive, Danvers, MA 01923, USA; phone: (978) 750-8400, fax: (978) 750-4744, and in the UK through the Copyright Licensing Agency Rapid Clearance Service (CLARCS), 90 Tottenham Court Road, London W1P 0LP, UK; phone: (+44) 171 436 5931; fax: (+44) 171 436 3986. Other countries may have a local reprographic rights agency for payments.

Reprints. For copies of 100 or more, of articles in this publication, please contact the Commercial Reprints Department, Elsevier Inc., 360 Park Avenue South, New York, New York 10010-1710. Tel.: (212) 633-3813, Fax: (212) 462-1935, e-mail: reprints@elsevier.com.

The ideas and opinions expressed in *Psychiatric Clinics of North America* do not necessarily reflect those of the Publisher. The Publisher does not assume any responsibility for any injury and/or damage to persons or property arising out of or related to any use of the material contained in this periodical. The reader is advised to check the appropriate medical literature and the product information currently provided by the manufacturer of each drug to be administered, to verify the dosage, the method and duration of administration, or contraindications. It is the responsibility of the treating physician or other health care professional, relying on independent experience and knowledge of the patient, to determine drug dosages and the best treatment for the patient. Mention of any product in this issue should not be construed as endorsement by the contributors, editors, or the Publisher of the product or manufacturers' claims.

Psychiatric Clinics of North America (ISSN 0193-953X) is published quarterly by Elsevier Inc., 360 Park Avenue South, New York, NY 10010-1710. Months of issue are March, June, September, and December. Business and Editorial Offices: 1600 John F. Kennedy Blvd., Suite 1800, Philadelphia, PA 19103-2899. Customer Service Office: 6277 Sea Harbor Drive, Orlando, FL 32887-4800 Periodicals postage paid at New York, NY and additional mailing offices. Subscription prices are $194.00 per year (US individuals), $329.00 per year (US institutions), $97.00 per year (US students/residents), $232.00 per year (Canadian individuals), $400.00 per year (Canadian Institutions), $270.00 per year (foreign individuals), $400.00 per year (foreign institutions), and $135.00 per year (international & Canadian students/residents). Foreign air speed delivery is included in all *Clinics'* subscription prices. All prices are subject to change without notice. **POSTMASTER:** Send address changes to *Psychiatric Clinics of North America*, Elsevier Periodicals Customer Service, 6277 Sea Harbor Drive, Orlando, FL 32887-4800. Customer Service: 1-800-654-2452 (US). From outside of the US, call 1-407-345-4000.

Psychiatric Clinics of North America is covered in *Index Medicus, Current Contents/Social and Behavioral Sciences, Social Science Citation Index, Embase/Excerpta Medica,* and PsycINFO.

Printed in the United States of America.

PSYCHIATRIC CLINICS
OF NORTH AMERICA

ELSEVIER
SAUNDERS

Schizophrenia: A Complex Disease Necessitating Complex Care

GUEST EDITORS

PETER F. BUCKLEY, MD, Professor and Chairman, Department of Psychiatry and Health Behavior, Medical College of Georgia, Augusta, Georgia

ERICK L. MESSIAS, MD, MPH, PhD, Associate Professor, Department of Psychiatry and Health Behavior, Medical College of Georgia, Augusta, Georgia

CONTRIBUTORS

DOUGLAS L. BOGGS, PharmD, MS, Research Fellow, Maryland Psychiatric Research Center, University of Maryland School of Medicine, Baltimore, Maryland

PETER F. BUCKLEY, MD, Professor and Chairman, Department of Psychiatry and Health Behavior, Medical College of Georgia, Augusta, Georgia

MATTHEW J. BYERLY, MD, Assistant Professor, Department of Psychiatry, The University of Texas Southwestern Medical Center at Dallas, Dallas, Texas

CHUAN-YU CHEN, PhD, Assistant Investigator, Division of Mental Health and Substance Abuse Research, National Health Research Institutes, Taipei, Taiwan

ROBERT R. CONLEY, MD, Professor of Psychiatry and Chief, Treatment Research Program, Maryland Psychiatric Research Center, University of Maryland School of Medicine, Baltimore, Maryland

AIDEN P. CORVIN, MRCPsych, PhD, Senior Lecturer in Psychiatry, Department of Psychiatry, Trinity Centre for Health Sciences, Trinity College, St. James's Hospital, Dublin, Ireland

NANCY H. COVELL, PhD, Assistant Professor, Division of Health Services Research, Department of Psychiatry, Mount Sinai School of Medicine, New York, New York; and Research Division, Department of Mental Health and Addiction Services, Hartford, Connecticut

LARRY DAVIDSON, PhD, Associate Professor of Psychology in Psychiatry; and Director of Program for Recovery and Community Health, Department of Psychiatry, Yale University, New Haven, Connecticut

GARY DONOHOE, DClinPsych, Lecturer in Clinical Psychology, Department of Psychiatry, Trinity Centre for Health Sciences, Trinity College, St. James's Hospital, Dublin, Ireland

WILLIAM W. EATON, PhD, Professor and Chair, Department of Mental Health, Johns Hopkins Bloomberg School of Public Health, Baltimore, Maryland

HELIO ELKIS, MD, PhD, Associate Professor and Chairman; and Director, Schizophrenia Program (Projesq), Department and Institute of Psychiatry, University of São Paulo Medical School (FMUSP), São Paulo, Brazil

SUSAN M. ESSOCK, PhD, Department of Psychiatry, College of Physicians and Surgeons, Columbia University; and Director, Department of Mental Health Services and Policy Research, New York State Psychiatric Institute, New York, New York

GARETH FENLEY, Certified Peer Specialist, Department of Psychiatry and Health Behavior, Medical College of Georgia, Augusta, Georgia

ADRIANA FOSTER, MD, Assistant Professor of Psychiatry, Department of Psychiatry and Health Behavior, Medical College of Georgia, Augusta, Georgia

LARRY FRICKS, Director, Appalachian Consulting Group, Incorporated, Cleveland, Georgia

MICHAEL GILL, MRCPsych, MD, EMBO Young Investigator and Professor of Psychiatry, Department of Psychiatry, Trinity Centre for Health Sciences, Trinity College, St. James's Hospital, Dublin, Ireland

JODI M. GONZALEZ, PhD, Assistant Professor, Department of Psychiatry, Division of Mood & Anxiety Disorders, University of Texas Health Science Center at San Antonio, San Antonio, Texas

MICHAEL GRODY, MD, Psychiatric Resident, The Zucker Hillside Hospital, North Shore-Long Island Jewish Health System, Glen Oaks, New York

PHILIP D. HARVEY, PhD, Department of Psychiatry, Mt. Sinai School of Medicine, New York, New York

LEIGHTON Y. HUEY, MD, Birnbaum/Blum Professor, Chair, and Training Director, Department of Psychiatry, University of Connecticut School of Medicine, Farmington, Connecticut; and Board Member, The Annapolis Coalition on the Behavioral Health Workforce, Cincinnati, Ohio

DEANNA L. KELLY, PharmD, BCPP, Associate Professor of Psychiatry, Maryland Psychiatric Research Center, University of Maryland School of Medicine, Baltimore, Maryland

ANZALEE KHAN, MS, Department of Psychiatry, New York University, and Manhattan Psychiatric Center, New York, New York

BRIAN KIRKPATRICK, MD, Department of Psychiatry and Health Behavior, Medical College of Georgia, Augusta, Georgia

HARRIET P. LEFLEY, PhD, Member, National Alliance on Mental Illness Scientific Council; Member, Curriculum and Training Committee, Member, Consumer and Family Subcommittee, The Annapolis Coalition on the Behavioral Health Workforce; and Professor, Department of Psychiatry and Behavioral Sciences, University of Miami Miller School of Medicine, Miami, Florida

EMMELINE LESCOUFLAIR, MD, Research Scientist, Department of Psychiatry, The University of Texas Southwestern Medical Center at Dallas, Dallas, Texas

J.P. LINDENMAYER, MD, Department of Psychiatry, New York University, and Manhattan Psychiatric Center, New York, New York

P. ALEX MABE, PhD, Professor and Director of Psychology Residency Training, Department of Psychiatry and Health Behavior, Medical College of Georgia, Augusta, Georgia

ERICK L. MESSIAS, MD, MPH, PhD, Associate Professor, Department of Psychiatry and Health Behavior, Medical College of Georgia, Augusta, Georgia

ALEXANDER L. MILLER, MD, Auler Professor and Chief, Division of Schizophrenia and Related Disorders, Department of Psychiatry, The University of Texas Health Science Center at San Antonio, San Antonio, Texas

DEL D. MILLER, PharmD, MD, Professor of Psychiatry, University of Iowa, Carver College of Medicine, Psychiatry Research, Iowa City, Iowa

KEVIN J. MITCHELL, PhD, Lecturer in Genetics, Smurfit Institute of Genetics, Trinity College, Dublin, Ireland

TROY A. MOORE, PharmD, MS, Research Fellow, Division of Schizophrenia and Related Disorders, Department of Psychiatry, The University of Texas Health Science Center at San Antonio, San Antonio, Texas

PAUL A. NAKONEZNY, PhD, Assistant Professor, Department of Biostatistics & Clinical Science, The University of Texas Southwestern Medical Center at Dallas, Dallas, Texas

COLM M.P. O'TUATHAIGH, PhD, Research Fellow in Neuroscience, Molecular & Cellular Therapeutics, Royal College of Surgeons in Ireland, Dublin, Ireland

SCOTT A. PEEBLES, PhD, Postdoctoral Fellow, Department of Psychiatry and Health Behavior, Medical College of Georgia, Augusta, Georgia

DAVID L. SHERN, PhD, National Steering Committee Member, The Annapolis Coalition on the Behavioral Health Workforce, Cincinnati, Ohio; and President and CEO, Mental Health America (formerly The National Health Association), Alexandria, Virginia

DAWN I. VELLIGAN, PhD, Professor, Department of Psychiatry; and Co-Chief, Division of Schizophrenia and Related Disorders, University of Texas Health Science Center at San Antonio, San Antonio, Texas

JOHN L. WADDINGTON, PhD, DSc, Professor of Neuroscience, Molecular & Cellular Therapeutics, Royal College of Surgeons in Ireland, Dublin; and Cavan-Monaghan Mental Health Service, St. Davnet's Hospital, Monaghan, Ireland

CYNTHIA A. WAINSCOTT, BA, Member, Consumer and Family Subcommittee, The Annapolis Coalition on the Behavioral Health Workforce; and Immediate Past Chair, Mental Health America, Cartersville, Georgia

PETER J. WEIDEN, MD, Director, Psychosis Program, Department of Psychiatry, University of Illinois Medical Center, Chicago, Illinois

Schizophrenia: A Complex Disease Necessitating Complex Care

methods of investigating potential candidate genes. It focuses next on the most prominent current candidate genes and describes (1) evidence for their association with schizophrenia and research into the function of each gene; (2) investigation of the clinical phenotypes and endophenotypes associated with each gene, at the levels of psychopathologic, neurocognitive, electrophysiologic, neuroimaging, and neuropathologic findings; and (3) research into the ethologic, cognitive, social, and psychopharmacologic phenotype of mutants with targeted deletion of each gene. It examines gene–gene and gene–environment interactions. Finally, it looks at future directions for research.

This article examines real-world antipsychotic use in the treatment of schizophrenia by comparing real-world prescribing with medication algorithms and guidelines, by evaluating the evidence underlying recommendations and guidelines, and by examining the roles of side effects and medication adherence in real-world prescribing decisions.

Emergent pharmacogenetic studies indicate that the efficacy of antipsychotic medications in schizophrenia may be predicted through genetic analysis. There also is evidence that the side-effect profiles of second-generation antipsychotic medications and their propensity to cause weight gain, glucose and lipid abnormalities, and tardive dyskinesia may be predicted by pharmacogenetic analysis in this patient population. In the future, this targeted approach with the choice of antipsychotic medication based on the likelihood of clinical response and development of side effects in light of a particular patient's genetic status may gain hold as new treatments are developed with even fewer side effects.

For individuals who have schizophrenia, adherence to medication is often poor, and stopping medication often has serious consequences. This article provides an update on recent literature regarding the frequency, clinical and social impact, and clinical correlates of nonadherence to antipsychotic medication in schizophrenia. The authors then review published trials of interventions to improve adherence in schizophrenia.

Coronary heart disease (CHD) is a major cause of mortality in people who have schizophrenia, and it is caused by many factors relating to lifestyle choices, antipsychotic treatment, and other medical comorbidities. This article focuses on modifiable risk factors such as cigarette smoking, diabetes, hyperlipidemia, hypertension, and the metabolic syndrome, all of which occur more frequently in patients who have schizophrenia than in the general population. Although treatment of risk factors for CHD is still far from ideal, all attempts should be made to strive for wellness to improve patients' long-term outcomes.

"First-episode schizophrenia" is a clinical and research term that often is used to emphasize the special issues that arise when working with this patient population. The notion that schizophrenia has an inexorable downhill course or is a deteriorating illness is being challenged by more sophisticated understanding of what happens before the initial episode and new understanding of the interactions between biologic vulnerabilities and specific environmental risk during adolescence and early adulthood, such as marijuana use. While the incidence rate of "first-episode" will make this a relatively small percentage of a usual clinical caseload, it is a critically important time for the future course of the illness. The hope is that proper management during this critical period will favorably influence the long-term trajectory of outcome for this individual patient. A growing body of evidence suggests that certain approaches and interventions are more helpful than others, such as understanding of the overwhelming nature of the experience to patients and families, aiming to achieve a full and broad pharmacologic response to initial antipsychotic therapy, while also being on the lookout for vulnerability and extreme sensitivity to side effects, and to anticipate a high likelihood of premature medication discontinuation. Clinicians and treatment services should try to identify "first-episode" patients in time to be able to anticipate and address these issues.

This article opens with a brief history of pharmacologic treatment of schizophrenia. It then discusses the definition and treatment of treatment-resistant schizophrenia, with particular attention to clinical, biological and neuroimaging correlates, as well as the best treatment options, including the use of clozapine in patients who meet the definition of treatment-resistant schizophrenia.

PSYCHIATRIC CLINICS
OF NORTH AMERICA

ELSEVIER
SAUNDERS

THE CLINICS ARE NOW AVAILABLE ONLINE!

Access your subscription at:
http://www.theclinics.com

Preface

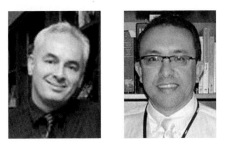

Peter F. Buckley, MD
Erick L. Messias, MD, MPH, PhD

Guest Editors

S ince the last issue of the *Psychiatric Clinics of North America* devoted to
schizophrenia 4 years ago, knowledge on the various aspects of the disease has grown tremendously. The whole concept of schizophrenia itself
has become much more sophisticated and its care provisions are more comprehensive and challenging. As such, this new issue on schizophrenia, entitled
"Schizophrenia: A Complex Disease Necessitating Complex Care" encompasses a broad range of important and relevant issues, realizing the goal of
translating current research to the everyday practice of psychiatry. From epidemiology to a variety of perspectives in psychopharmacology and the recovery
perspective, this issue provides a view of the state-of-the-art in schizophrenia research and treatment.

Though the epidemiology of schizophrenia provides clues about etiology
and risk factors, it has also generated myths that have perpetuated misconceptions about the disease. After completing a review of recent epidemiologic findings, Messias and colleagues discuss the epidemiologic myths of schizophrenia,
such as the universal incidence, and the equal gender risk in schizophrenia.

An intrinsic problem in clinical research of schizophrenia is how to measure
and quantify psychopathology—especially in schizophrenia, where many domains of symptoms occur together. The article by Lindenmayer and colleagues
critically reviews some of the available assessment tools of these domains together with other associated syndromes. The instruments chosen cover the
broad range of psychopathology seen in patients with schizophrenia, including
areas such as negative symptoms and functional disability, areas that are gaining prominence in research.

0193-953X/07/$ – see front matter
doi:10.1016/j.psc.2007.05.002

© 2007 Elsevier Inc. All rights reserved.
psych.theclinics.com

Substantial progress—in part owing to recent refinements in human genetics and neuroimaging—has been made in unraveling the genetic underpinnings of clinical aspects of schizophrenia. The extent of genetic findings, their etiopathologic and functional significance, and putative clinical correlates are reviewed in the article by Waddington and Gill devoted to functional genomics.

Despite the growing use of second-generation antipsychotics and the mounting evidence from clinical trials, there is still a gap between data and real-world practices regarding these medications. Moore and colleagues revisit this issue by comparing real-world prescription of antipsychotics with medication algorithms and guidelines.

Foster and colleagues tackle the emerging knowledge base regarding pharmacogenetic studies on antipsychotic medication, both from the perspective of efficacy and side effect development. There are significant findings in terms of the association between dopamine and serotonin receptor genes and response to antipsychotic treatment. Furthermore, the genetic makeup of individuals also seems to be related to the incidence and magnitude of side effects, such as weight gain and tardive dyskinesia.

One of the main challenges in treating schizophrenia is to make sure the patient is compliant with the treatment recommendations, and especially that they take their medication. After reviewing the prevalence and correlates of medication adherence in schizophrenia, Byerly and colleagues provide a review of interventions to address this issue. There are psychosocial and pharmacologic approaches to adherence, both of which are reviewed in this article.

As our knowledge about medical comorbidities in schizophrenia has improved, so has our responsibility to prevent, detect, and manage chronic conditions such as diabetes, the metabolic syndrome, hypertension, coronary heart disease, and respiratory disorders in this population. The article by Kelly and colleagues describes the advances in the knowledge about medical comorbidities in schizophrenia, focusing on coronary heart disease and its modifiable risk factors.

When treating persons with schizophrenia, those in their first break—the "first episode" patients—are in a critically important time for the future of the course of the illness. Weiden and colleagues provide a thorough review of the findings regarding correlates and treatment options for first-episode patients. The article notes that not all interventions are made equal, and that there are optimal approaches to maximize outcomes at this crucial moment.

Despite the advent of a variety of treatment options, the thorny issue of treatment-resistant schizophrenia (TRS) continues to challenge clinicians, and this topic is reviewed by Elkis. In this review, the different concepts and definitions of TRS are presented, and the clinical and biologic correlates are revised. The article concludes with a review of the evidence regarding treatment options for TRS.

Huey and other members of the Annapolis coalition discuss the historical concepts of schizophrenia and their impact in patients and their families. This article provides an overview of the current understanding of the role of families in treatment and recovery.

Finally, surveying the recovery movement and its applications in schizophrenia, Peebles and colleagues conclude that the model is a philosophical guide for treatment provisions to better serve those with severe and persistent mental disorders. The authors exemplify the power of this model in system transformation by studying the innovative peer support concept.

Schizophrenia, once epitomized as the sacred symbol of psychiatry, remains a formidable clinical challenge and is a target for multidisciplinary research efforts, from genomics and proteinomics to psychosocial service research. We strove to compile a rich and representative sample of both the clinical issues and the current research findings into one issue. We thank the authors for their care and effort in making this collection of articles a relevant, original, and well-crafted issue on the state-of-the-art of schizophrenia research.

Peter F. Buckley, MD
Erick L. Messias, MD, MPH, PhD
Department of Psychiatry and Health Behavior
Medical College of Georgia
997 St. Sebastian Way
Augusta, GA 30912

E-mail addresses: pbuckley@mcg.edu
emessias@mcg.edu

Epidemiology of Schizophrenia: Review of Findings and Myths

Erick L. Messias, MD, MPH, PhD[a],*, Chuan-Yu Chen, PhD[b], William W. Eaton, PhD[c]

[a]Department of Psychiatry and Health Behavior, Medical College of Georgia, 1515 Pope Avenue, Augusta, GA 30912, USA
[b]Division of Mental Health and Substance Abuse Research, National Health Research Institutes, Fl. 5, Campus 2, No. 309, Sung-Te Road, Taipei 110, Taiwan
[c]Department of Mental Health, Johns Hopkins Bloomberg School of Public Health, 624 North Broadway, Room 850, Baltimore, MD 21205, USA

The epidemiology of schizophrenia has progressed from descriptive accounts to a surge in analytic epidemiologic findings over the last 2 decades. This article reviews the epidemiology of schizophrenia, concentrating on the results that are most credible methodologically and consistent across studies and focusing particularly on the most recent developments. The authors also comment on some misconceptions regarding schizophrenia epidemiology, specifically pointing to widespread misinterpretations of evidence regarding the incidence of schizophrenia and the gender ratio of the disease.

DESCRIPTIVE EPIDEMIOLOGY: PREVALENCE AND INCIDENCE OF SCHIZOPHRENIA

Prevalence

The point prevalence of a disease is the proportion of the population that has the disorder at a point in time. The point prevalence of schizophrenia is about 5/1000 in the population. The estimate depends on the age distribution of the population: for example, if persons too young to be at risk are included in the denominator, the estimates will be lower. Table 1 presents findings from areas in which credible estimates of both prevalence and incidence are available. The prevalence in Table 1 ranges from 2.7/1000 to 8.3/1000, and this range would not be affected greatly if several dozen other studies, available from prior reviews, were included [1]. Lifetime prevalence has been estimated by surveys of examinations by medically trained persons; the resulting estimates do not different widely from those shown in Table 1 [1].

*Corresponding author. E-mail address: emessias@mcg.edu (E.L. Messias).

0193-953X/07/$ – see front matter
doi:10.1016/j.psc.2007.04.007
© 2007 Elsevier Inc. All rights reserved.
psych.theclinics.com

Table 1
Prevalence and incidence of schizophrenia per 1000 population

Area	Date	Author	Age in years	Prevalence Type	Rate	Incidence
Denmark	1977	Nielsen	15 +	Lifetime	2.7	
	1972	Munk-Jorgensen	All	Annual		0.12
Baltimore, Maryland, USA	1963	Wing	All	1 year	7	
	1963	Warthen	All	Annual		0.7
Camberwell, England	1963	Wing	15+	One year	4.4	
	1971	Hailey	All	Annual		0.11
Ireland	1973	Walsh	15+	Point	8.3	
	1986	World Health Organization	15–54	Annual		0.22
Portogruaro, Italy	1982–1989	de Salvia et al			2.7	
	1989	de Salvia et al		Annual		0.19
Hampstead, England	1991–1995	Jeffreys et al			5.1	
	1991–1995	McNaught et al		Annual		0.21

Data from Eaton WW. Epidemiology of schizophrenia. Epidemiol Rev 1985;7:105–26; Eaton WW. Update on the epidemiology of schizophrenia. Epidemiol Rev 1991;13:320–28; with additions from McNaught AS, Jeffreys SE, Harvey CA, et al. The Hampstead Schizophrenia Survey 1991. II: Incidence and migration in inner London. Br J Psychiatry 1997;170:307–11; Jeffreys SE, Harvey CA, McNaught AS, et al. The Hampstead Schizophrenia Survey 1991. I: Prevalence and service use comparisons in an inner London health authority, 1986–1991. Br J Psychiatry 1997;170:301–6; and de Salvia D, Barbato A, Salvo P, et al. Prevalence and incidence of schizophrenic disorders in Portogruaro. An Italian case register study. J Nerv Ment Dis 1993;181(5):275–82.

Incidence

The incidence of schizophrenia is about 0.20/1000/year. The incidences presented are all estimated for 1 year, making the comparison somewhat tighter. The range in annual incidence in Table 1 is from 0.11/1000/year to 0.70/1000/year, and this range would not be affected greatly if several dozen other studies, reviewed elsewhere, were included [2,3]. The presentation of prevalence and incidence figures from the same areas in juxtaposition shows that the point prevalence usually is more than 10 times the annual incidence, indicating the chronic nature of the disorder.

There is considerable variation in incidence rates around the world, as shown in Fig. 1. The dark bars represent the World Health Organization study of incidence, which reveals a smaller variation, presumably resulting from the standardization of method [4]. That study suggested to some that there was little or no variation in schizophrenia around the world, which

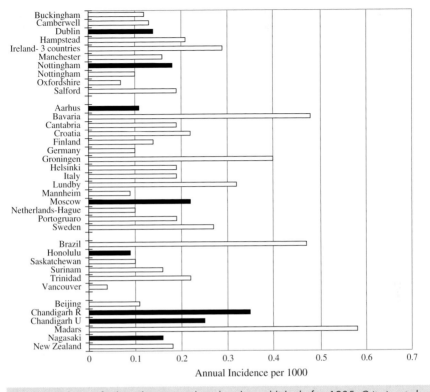

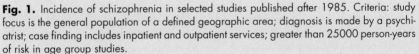

Fig. 1. Incidence of schizophrenia in selected studies published after 1985. Criteria: study focus is the general population of a defined geographic area; diagnosis is made by a psychiatrist; case finding includes inpatient and outpatient services; greater than 25000 person-years of risk in age group studies.

would make schizophrenia a very unusual disease indeed. Fig. 1 shows variation greater than one order of magnitude, from a low estimate in Vancouver of 0.04/1000/year to a high estimate in Madras of 0.58/1000/year. Both the Vancouver [5] and Madras [6] studies were carefully done, and their estimates are credible.

The force of morbidity for schizophrenia peaks in young adulthood. The age of onset varies between men and women, with males tending to have a younger onset [7]. The peak incidence for males and females is in the decade between the ages of 15 and 24 years. The peak for young adults is more marked for males, and women have a second peak in the years between the ages of 55 and 64 years. Evidence suggests that males have higher lifetime risk of schizophrenia; two meta-analysis addressing that issue show that males have about a 30% to 40% higher lifetime risk of developing schizophrenia [8,9].

ANALYTIC EPIDEMIOLOGY: NATURAL HISTORY AND RISK FACTORS

Natural History

Onset

The onset of schizophrenia is varied. In the classic long-term follow-up study by Ciompi [10], about 50% had an acute onset, and 50% had a long prodrome. The intensive study of prodrome by Hafner and colleagues [11] suggests that onset of negative symptoms tends to occur about 5 years before the initial psychotic episode, with onset of positive symptoms much closer to the first hospitalization.

Childhood developmental abnormalities

Many long-term follow-up studies, both retrospective and prospective, suggest that a variety of signs, symptoms, conditions, and behaviors are associated with an increased risk for schizophrenia, but none has adequate strength or uniqueness to be useful in prediction. Earlier work on groups at high-risk has shown that offspring of schizophrenic parents were more likely than the offspring of controls to have a lower IQ, poor attention skills, thought disorder–like symptoms, poor social adjustment, and psychiatric symptoms [11–13]. Although several concerns have been raised regarding the generalizability of high-risk findings to nonfamilial forms of schizophrenia, recent longitudinal studies conducted in the United Kingdom, Sweden, Finland, and New Zealand have provided evidence that individuals who have schizophrenia differ from their peers, even in early childhood, in a variety of developmental markers, such as the age of attaining developmental milestones [14–16], levels of cognitive functioning [17,18], educational achievement [14,19–21], neurologic and motor development [22–24], social competence [20,25], and psychologic disturbances [25]. More recent evidence also suggests the association with low IQ is specific to schizophrenia, because it was not found in bipolar disorder [26]. There seem to be no common causal paths linking these developmental markers with schizophrenia [27]. Indeed, individuals who later develop schizophrenia or related disorders already may have experienced a general or pan-developmental impairment early in their childhood. Prospectively collected data from the 1972–1973 birth cohort in New Zealand showed that schizophrenic subjects may have suffered significant deficits in neuromotor, language, and cognitive development in the first decade of their lives [21]. The compelling evidence linking an array of childhood developmental abnormalities and schizophrenia echoes the hypothesis that schizophrenia is a neurodevelopmental disorder for which causes may be traced to a defect in the early brain development [28–31].

Course

The symptomatic course of schizophrenia is varied. In Ciompi's classic study [10], about half the subjects had an undulating course, with partial or full remissions followed by recurrences, in an unpredictable pattern. About one third had relatively chronic, unremitting course with poor outcome. A small minority in that study had a steady pattern of recovery with good outcome. Follow-up studies that are not strictly prospective, such as the study by Ciompi [10], can be deceptive, because there is a tendency to focus on a residue of chronic cases, making the disorder seem more chronic than it actually is. Fig. 2 shows data on time to rehospitalization for a cohort of schizophrenic patients in Denmark. The proportion remaining in the community without rehospitalization is shown on the vertical axis, and time is on the horizontal axis. After the initial hospitalization, about 25% are not rehospitalized even after 15 years. For the subgroup of the cohort with 10 hospitalizations, more than 90% are rehospitalized within 3 years following the tenth episode. Although reoccurrence of episodes might reinforce the illness (the so-called "schubweis [stepwise] process"), or hospitalization itself might be damaging [32], it seems more likely the cohort sorts itself into those who have tendency for greater or less chronicity of disorder. This process may lead clinicians and others to overestimate the chronicity of the disorder, because they see individuals in the bottom curve of Fig. 2 about 15 times as often as individuals in the top curve [33]. For this reason, the natural history of schizophrenia is best studied with cohorts of first onsets [34].

Outcome

For the most part, predictors of outcome for schizophrenia remain elusive. In a review of 13 prospective studies of the course of illness in first-onset cohorts, negative symptoms predicted poor outcome in four studies, and gradual onset, typical of negative symptoms as noted previously, predicted poor outcome in several studies [34]. There is variation in the course of schizophrenia around the world, with better prognosis in so-called "developing" countries. Table 2 shows a summary of data from the 1979 World Health Organization study

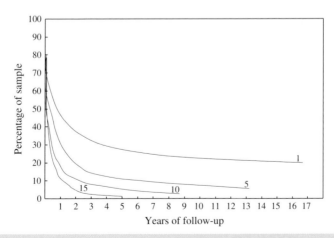

Fig. 2. Community survival in schizophrenia in patients who have had 1, 5, 10, or 15 hospital discharges. *From* Mortensen PB, Eaton WW. Predictors for readmission risk in schizophrenia. Psychol Med 1994;24:223–32; Reprinted with permission from Cambridge University Press.

Table 2
World Health Organization follow-up of schizophrenia

Location	Sample Size	No Symptoms (%)	Chronic Psychosis (%)
Developed countries			
London, England	50	6	40
Aarhus, Denmark	64	5	14
Moscow, Russia	66	17	21
Washington, DC, USA	65	6	23
	51	3	23
Developing countries			
Agra, India	73	42	10
Cali, Colombia	91	11	21
Ibadan, Nigeria	68	34	10

Data from Leff J, Sartorius N, Jablensky A, et al. The International Pilot Study of Schizophrenia: five-year follow-up findings. Psychol Med. 1992;22(1):131–45.

on this issue [35], with the columns at the far right extracted by the authors from the publication of Leff and colleagues [36]. Schizophrenic persons in developing countries are less likely than those in the developed countries to have been chronically psychotic over the period of follow-up and are more likely to have no residual symptoms after 5 years. This result remains to be explained. It could be that schizophrenia in developing countries includes a subset with better prognosis because of the risk factor structure in those areas, such as higher mortality of compromised fetuses. Another interpretation is that the environment of recovery in the developed world is more pernicious, involving harsher economic competition, a greater degree of stigma, and smaller family networks to share the burden of care for persons who have schizophrenia.

The course of schizophrenia, from early prodrome through to later outcome, is influenced by social variables, including socioeconomic position and marital status [37]. Even 20 years before diagnosis, an individual who eventually is diagnosed as having schizophrenia is more likely to be unmarried than other members of his or her age cohort (relative odds, 4). The relative odds of being single, as compared with those never diagnosed as having schizophrenia, peak at the time of admission, at more than 15, and remain high for decades afterward. The effect is greater for males, possibly because their earlier onset occurs during the years when marriages are most likely to be formed. Likewise, the individual who eventually is diagnosed as having schizophrenia is more likely than others in his or her age cohort to be unemployed many years earlier than the first diagnosis of schizophrenia and many years afterward. Although there is extensive literature on the relationship of low socioeconomic position to risk for schizophrenia [38,39], it seems likely that the association results from the effects of the insidious onset on the individual's ability to compete in the job market. Recent studies from Scandinavia suggest that, if anything, the parents of persons who have schizophrenia are likely to come from a higher, not a lower, social position [40].

Risk Factors

The genetics of schizophrenia, including family history as a risk factor, are beyond the scope of a general review on the epidemiology of schizophrenia. This section presents risk factors that have been reported in several credible studies and for which it is fairly clear that the risk factor was present before the onset of schizophrenia.

Season of birth

For a long time it has been known that individuals who have schizophrenia are more likely to be born in the winter, and the results have been reported from the samples in both the Northern and Southern hemispheres. The relative risk is small, on the order of a 10% increase for those born in the winter versus summer, but it has been replicated many times [41,42]. One possible explanation is that the second trimester of pregnancy occurs in the height of the influenza season and that maternal infections during that period raise th risk for schizophrenia in the offspring. Another explanation offered by a recent study suggests that the seasonal effects may increase one's risk of schizophrenia by the interaction with genetic vulnerability [43].

Birth complications

The finding regarding season of birth suggests that something about pregnancy and birth might be awry in individuals who later develop schizophrenia. Case-control studies on this issue have been available for decades, but the generally positive findings were clouded by the possibility that the mother's recall was biased. In the last 15 years many studies have reported a relative odds of about 2 for those with one or another sort of birth complication, and several meta-analyses on this topic exist [44–46]. Later analyses have begun to specify the individual type of birth complication, with the hope of elucidating the causal mechanism. A recent meta-analytic review of this literature categorizes the types of birth complications as (1) complications of pregnancy (bleeding, diabetes, rhesus incompatibility, pre-eclampsia); (2) abnormal fetal growth and development: (low birth weight, congenital malformations, reduced head circumference), and (3) complications of delivery (uterine atony, asphyxia, emergency cesarean section) [22]. The review concludes that the investigations into specific mechanisms need to move now from the epidemiologic perspective to include a combination of disciplines and approaches. The complications variously suggest malnutrition [47], extreme prematurity, and hypoxia or ischemia [30,48–50] as possible causes.

Parental age

The association between advanced parental age and a higher risk of schizophrenia was first proposed in the mid-twentieth century and has gained extensive scientific attention in recent years. Based on the family background data of 1000 patients in hospitals in Ontario, Canada, Gregory [51] reported that parents of patients who had schizophrenia were, on average, 2 to 3 years older than the parents of persons in the patients' age cohort who did not have schizophrenia . Subsequent investigations showed inconsistent findings [52,53], however, and it was argued that the observed higher risk in schizophrenia associated with older maternal age might be largely confounded by raised paternal age [52,54]. Recently, several population-based epidemiologic studies in Demark, Israel, Sweden, and the United States have provided stronger evidence regarding the role of paternal age in schizophrenia [9,55–59]. A population-based birth cohort study from in Israel found that the relative risk of schizophrenia rose monotonically in each 5-year group of paternal age, with a maximum relative risk of 2.96 (95% confidence interval, 1.60–5.47) in the group aged 55 years or older in comparison with a paternal age of 20 to 24 years. Additionally, once paternal age is statistically adjusted, maternal age is no longer a significant predictor of schizophrenia. The evidence from one nested case-control study indicates that the increased risk for schizophrenia related to paternal age is generally greater in women [58]. In addition, current population-based cohort research suggests that the increased risk of schizophrenia related to advancing paternal age seems significant only among those without a family history of schizophrenia, indicating the possibility that de novo mutations accumulate in sperm [60].

Infections and the immune system
A series of ecologic studies suggests that persons whose mothers were in their second trimester of pregnancy during an influenza epidemic are at higher risk for developing schizophrenia [59,61–63]. Infection during pregnancy as a risk factor is consistent with the neurodevelopmental theory of schizophrenia [29,64]. Later studies, which are more convincing, include individual assessment of infection, either by comparison of antibodies in adults who have schizophrenia and in normal individuals [65], or even more convincing prospective studies in which the infection can be determined to have occurred during the pregnancy. There is consistent evidence that individuals who have antibodies to *Toxoplasmosis gondii* have higher prevalence of schizophrenia [66]. One study suggests a relative risk of 5.2 for individuals with documented infection by the rubella virus during fetal development [67]. Another prospective study found higher risk for psychosis in individuals whose mothers had higher levels of antibodies to Herpes simplex virus [68]. A study in Brazil compared individuals who had meningitis during the 1971 to 1974 epidemic with their siblings who did not have meningitis and found that that the prevalence of psychosis, and specifically schizophrenia, was five times higher in those who had meningitis. The finding is intriguing because the average age of infection with meningitis was 26 months, much later than prenatal infection [69]. If this finding is replicated, it will have important implications for the neurodevelopmental theory of schizophrenia.

Autoimmune diseases
A relatively small but consistent literature indicates that persons who have schizophrenia have unusual resistance or susceptibility to autoimmune diseases. Studies have consistently shown that individuals who have schizophrenia

are somehow less likely to have rheumatoid arthritis [70]. Although medications for schizophrenia may be protective for rheumatoid arthritis in some unknown way, some of the studies were conducted before neuroleptic medications were available. Other physiologic consequences of schizophrenia may be protective, or a single gene may raise the risk for the one disorder and give protection against the other. A single small study suggests that mothers of individuals who have schizophrenia have a lower risk for rheumatoid arthritis, but the study's size and quality are not convincing [71]. It is intriguing, in this regard, that case control studies have shown that persons taking nonsteroidal anti-inflammatory medications, which primarily treat arthritis, may be protected from dementia [72,73].

Other autoimmune disorders have been linked to schizophrenia, including thyroid disorders [74], type 1 diabetes [75], and celiac disease [76]. Currently the evidence is strongest for thyroid disorders and celiac disease. In a study from the Danish population registries, persons whose parents had celiac disease were three times as likely to be diagnosed later as having schizophrenia. Celiac disease is an immune reaction to wheat gluten. One possible explanation is that the increased permeability of the intestine brought about by celiac disease increases the level of antigen exposure, thereby increasing the risk of autoimmune response. It also is possible that gluten proteins are broken down into psychoactive peptides [77].

The results linking schizophrenia to autoimmune disease are paralleled by the clinical and laboratory study of autoimmune processes in schizophrenia. There apparently are abnormalities of the immune system in schizophrenia, but it is not clear whether these are causal or a consequence of schizophrenia or its treatment [78]. It is possible that a single weakness in the immune system in persons who have schizophrenia explains both the data on infections and the results in autoimmune disorders, but this possibility remains to be proven [79]. Meanwhile, there are ongoing clinical trials of anti-inflammatory [80] and antibiotic [81] agents for schizophrenia.

Ethnicity

Ethnic status is a relatively easily identified individual characteristic that indicates a shared history with others. Markers of ethnic status include race, country of origin, and religion. Country of origin has proven to be a consistent risk factor for schizophrenia in the United Kingdom and the Netherlands. In the United Kingdom, those immigrating from Africa or the Caribbean and their second-generation offspring have rates of schizophrenia up to 10 times higher than those in the general population [82]. Because immigrant groups who do not have black skin do not have higher rates, and because the second generation is affected, the stresses of immigration are unlikely to be causative. Because rates in the countries of origin are not elevated, it is unlikely that a genetic difference between races is causative. The cause seems to be the psychologic conditions associated with being black in England or being from Surinam in Holland. It could be discrimination or a more subtle form of difficulty associated with planning one's life when the future is as uncertain, as it is for racial groups at the structural bottom of society [83,84].

Cannabis use

Numerous case-control studies show that persons who have schizophrenia are more likely to have taken, or be using, cannabis [85]. Recently prospective studies in Sweden, the Netherlands, New Zealand, and Israel have shown that the risk for developing schizophrenia is 2 to 25 times higher in persons who have used cannabis [86–89]. Individuals in the premorbid phase of schizophrenia might be responding to initial, mild symptoms of schizophrenia by using drugs, even though these studies have attempted to control for premorbid conditions. On the other hand, it could be that cannabis precipitates, or even causes, an episode of schizophrenia [90–95].

Urban residence

In the 1930s Faris and Dunham [96] showed that, although the addresses of first admissions for manic depressive illness were distributed more or less randomly throughout Chicago, admissions for schizophrenia tended to come from the center of the city, with rates decreasing as one moves outward into zones of transition, working class, and family neighborhoods. This and other similar findings [97] were interpreted as reflecting the tendency for individuals who would develop schizophrenia to move into the city. Later studies from Europe, however, were strictly prospective, with the cohort defined in late adolescence, well before onset [98], or even at birth [99]. The relative risk of developing schizophrenia is about two to four times higher for those born in urban areas. The difficulty lies in identifying the plausible biologic process associated with urban residence. It could include differences in the physical environment, such as the higher concentration of lead in the soil and air in cities; differences in the cultural environment, such as the expectation that one will leave the family of origin and define a new life plan [83]; differences in birth practices, such as breastfeeding [100]; crowding, which might permit spread of infections [101] as discussed later; differences in the manner in which animals are, or are not, brought into the household [102]; and a host of other factors [103].

MYTHS IN SCHIZOPHRENIA EPIDEMIOLOGY

In recent years reviews have led to a reconsideration of some aspects of schizophrenia epidemiology that are widely cited but poorly supported by evidence [104]. The first is the notion that schizophrenia has universal incidence across cultures and countries. The second is the belief that schizophrenia distributes itself equality in males and females. Taken together these beliefs could be conceptualized as (1) schizophrenia is an equalitarian disorder, and (2) schizophrenia is an exceptional disorder [104]. It is puzzling that these two interrelated beliefs are usually cited as evidence for a biologic origin of the disease, when most diseases in medicine do vary across cultures, countries, and gender.

As seen in Table 1 and Fig. 1, the incidence of schizophrenia varies significantly across countries. Another study found the incidence of schizophrenia varying significantly, with a median value of 15.2 per 100,000 population and with a range of 7.7 to 43 [8]. A review of available data from 31 studies estimates the median male: female ratio to be 1:4 [104]. Two independent meta-analyses, with some overlap in study sampling, have shown men to be at increased risk of developing schizophrenia [8,9].

DISCUSSION

What has been accomplished over the last several decades, and what are prospects for future progress? Even as late as 25 years ago, the epidemiology of schizophrenia was nearly a blank page. There was even argument about the value of the concept itself. The only risk factors that seemed strong and consistent were lower social class and a family history of schizophrenia. Since then there has been considerable progress delineating a more-or-less consistent picture of the descriptive epidemiology and the natural history of schizophrenia. Research in analytic epidemiology has generated a series of heretofore-unsuspected risk factors, as described previously. In general, the risk factors have been considered in the context of theories about how schizophrenia actually might develop in the psychologic and physiologic life of the individual—even if the linkage is sometimes speculative. These developments are healthy.

In the future there will be concerted efforts to study risk factors in combination. This process has begun already. For example, Mortensen and colleagues [105] have studied the combined effects of season of birth, urbanization of birthplace, and family history of schizophrenia. The combination is informative in evaluating the importance of the risk factors. Although the relative risk for urban birth is much smaller than the risk associated with having a parent who has schizophrenia, the importance of urban birth is greater, because a much larger proportion of the population is born in urban areas than to parents who have schizophrenia—the situation of relative versus population-attributable risk [105]. If the causal path connected to urban birth could be identified, the prospects for prevention would be much stronger.

The combination of risk factors will facilitate prospective studies of high-risk individuals for whom the high risk is not simply the result of family history, as in earlier high-risk studies. Furthermore, combination of risk factors will raise the positive predictive value of the risk formulation to the point that it may be ethically feasible to approach individuals, identify the risk, and begin efforts to protect them from the catastrophic effects of the first episode of schizophrenia. Such studies have begun, albeit very cautiously [106–108]. In general, epidemiologic research has built a strong knowledge base over the past quarter century, and this knowledge base will continue to contribute to public health efforts at prevention of schizophrenia in the coming decades.

References

[1] Eaton W, Chen C-Y. Epidemiology. In: Lieberman J, Stroup T, Perkins DO, editors. The American Psychiatric Publishing Textbook of Schizophrenia. Washington, DC: American Psychiatric Publishing; 2006.

[2] Eaton WW. Update on the epidemiology of schizophrenia. Epidemiol Rev 1991;13:320–8.

[3] Eaton W. Evidence for universality and uniformity of schizophrenia around the world: assessment and implications. Darmstadt (Germany): Steinkopf; 1999.

[4] Sartorius N, Jablensky A, Korten A, et al. Early manifestations and first-contact incidence of schizophrenia in different cultures. A preliminary report on the initial evaluation phase of the WHO Collaborative Study on Determinants of Outcome of Severe Mental Disorders. Psychol Med 1986;16(4):909–28.

[5] Beiser M, Erickson D, Fleming JA, et al. Establishing the onset of psychotic illness. Am J Psychiatry 1993;150(9):1349–54.

[6] Rajkummar S. Incidence of schizophrenia in an urban community in Madras. Indian J Psychiat 1993;35:18–21.

[7] Munk-Jorgensen P. First-admission rates and marital status of schizophrenics. Acta Psychiatr Scand 1987;76:210–6.

[8] McGrath J, Saha S, Welham J, et al. A systematic review of the incidence of schizophrenia: the distribution of rates and the influence of sex, urbanicity, migrant status and methodology. BMC Med 2004;2:13.

[9] Aleman A, Kahn RS, Selten JP. Sex differences in the risk of schizophrenia: evidence from meta-analysis. Arch Gen Psychiatry 2003;60(6):565–71.

[10] Ciompi L. Catamnestic long-term study on the course of life and aging of schizophrenics. Schizophr Bull 1980;6(4):606–18.

[11] Hafner H, Maurer K, Loffler W. Onset and prodromal phase as determinants of the course. In: Gattaz WF, Hafner H, editors. Search for the causes of schizophrenia, vol. IV: balance of the century. Darmstadt (Germany): Steinkopf Springer; 1999. p. 35–58.

[12] Tarrant CJ, Jones PB. Precursors to schizophrenia: do biological markers have specificity? Can J Psychiatr 1999;44(4):335–49.

[13] Niemi LT, Suvisaari JM, Tuulio-Henriksson A, et al. Childhood developmental abnormalities in schizophrenia: evidence from high-risk studies. Schizophr Res 2003;60(2–3):239–58.

[14] Jones P, Rodgers B, Murray R, et al. Child development risk factors for adult schizophrenia in the British 1946 birth cohort. Lancet 1994;344(8934):1398–402.

[15] Jones P. The early origins of schizophrenia. Br Med Bull 1997;53(1):135–55.

[16] Isohanni M, Jones PB, Moilanen K, et al. Early developmental milestones in adult schizophrenia and other psychoses. A 31-year follow-up of the northern Finland 1966 birth cohort. Schizophr Res 2001;52(1–2):1–19.

[17] Gunnell D, Harrison G, Rasmussen F, et al. Associations between premorbid intellectual performance, early-life exposures and early-onset schizophrenia. Cohort study. Br J Psychiatry 2002;181:298–305.

[18] David AS, Malmberg A, Brandt L, et al. IQ and risk for schizophrenia: a population-based cohort study. Psychol Med 1997;27(6):1311–23.

[19] Isohanni I, Jarvelin MR, Nieminen P, et al. School performance as a predictor of psychiatric hospitalization in adult life. A 28-year follow-up in the northern Finland 1966 birth cohort. Psychol Med 1998;28(4):967–74.

[20] Done DJ, Crow TJ, Johnstone EC, et al. Childhood antecedents of schizophrenia and affective illness: social adjustment at ages 7 and 11. BMJ 1994;309(6956):699–703.

[21] Cannon TD, Rosso IM, Bearden CE, et al. A prospective cohort study of neurodevelopmental processes in the genesis and epigenesis of schizophrenia. Dev Psychopathol 1999;11(3):467–85.

[22] Leask SJ, Done DJ, Crow TJ. Adult psychosis, common childhood infections and neurological soft signs in a national birth cohort. Br J Psychiatry 2002;181:387–92.

[23] Cannon M, Jones PB, Murray RM. Obstetric complications and schizophrenia: historical and meta-analytic review. Am J psychiatry 2002;159(7):1080–92.

[24] Cannon M, Jones P, Huttunen MO, et al. School performance in Finnish children and later development of schizophrenia: a population-based longitudinal study. Arch Gen Psychiatry 1999;56(5):457–63.

[25] Malmberg A, Lewis G, David A, et al. Premorbid adjustment and personality in people with schizophrenia. Br J Psychiatry 1998;172:308–13 [discussion: 314–305].

[26] Zammit S, Allebeck P, David AS, et al. A longitudinal study of premorbid IQ score and risk of developing schizophrenia, bipolar disorder, severe depression, and other nonaffective psychoses. Arch Gen Psychiatry 2004;61(4):354–60.

[27] Jones PB, Tarrant CJ. Specificity of developmental precursors to schizophrenia and affective disorders. Schizophr Res 1999;39(2):121–5 [discussion: 161].

[28] Weinberger DR. From neuropathology to neurodevelopment. Lancet 1995;346(8974): 552–7.

[29] Murray RM, Lewis SW. Is schizophrenia a neurodevelopmental disorder? BMJ 1987;295(6600):681–2.

[30] Isohanni M, Murray GK, Jokelainen J, et al. The persistence of developmental markers in childhood and adolescence and risk for schizophrenic psychoses in adult life. A 34-year follow-up of the Northern Finland 1966 birth cohort. Schizophr Res 2004;71(2–3): 213–25.

[31] Isohanni M, Lauronen E, Moilanen K, et al. Predictors of schizophrenia: evidence from the northern Finland 1966 birth cohort and other sources. Br J Psychiatry 2005;48:s4–7.

[32] Eaton WW Jr. Mental hospitalization as a reinforcement process. Am Sociol Rev 1974;39(2):252–60.

[33] Cohen P, Cohen J. The Clinician's Illusion. Arch Gen Psychiatry 1984;41:1178–82.

[34] Ram R, Bromet EJ, Eaton WW, et al. The natural course of schizophrenia: a review of first-admission studies. Schizophr Bull 1992;18(2):185–207.

[35] World Health Organization: Schizophrenia: An International Follow-up Study. New York, Wiley, 1979.

[36] Leff J, Sartorius N, Jablensky A, et al. The International Pilot Study of Schizophrenia: five-year follow-up findings. Psychol Med 1992;22(1):131–45.

[37] Agerbo E, Byrne M, Eaton WW, et al. Marital and labor market status in the long run in schizophrenia. Arch Gen Psychiatry 2004;61(1):28–33.

[38] Dohrenwend BP, Levav I, Shrout PE, et al. Socioeconomic status and psychiatric disorders: the causation-selection issue. Science 1992;255(5047):946–52.

[39] 1854 Comission on Lunacy. Report on Insanity and Idiocy in Massachusetts. Boston: Harvard University Press; 1971.

[40] Byrne M, Agerbo E, Eaton WW, et al. Parental socio-economic status and risk of first admission with schizophrenia- a Danish national register based study. Social psychiatry and psychiatric epidemiology 2004;39(2):87–96.

[41] Davies G, Welham J, Chant D, et al. A systematic review and meta-analysis of Northern hemisphere season of birth studies in schizophrenia. Schizophr Bull 2003;29(3):587–93.

[42] Torrey EF, Miller J, Rawlings R, et al. Seasonality of births in schizophrenia and bipolar disorder: a review of the literature. Schizophr Res 1997;28(1):1–38.

[43] Carrion-Baralt JR, Smith CJ, Rossy-Fullana E, et al. Seasonality effects on schizophrenic births in multiplex families in a tropical island. Psychiatry Res 2006;142(1):93–7.

[44] Verdoux H, Geddes JR, Takei N, et al. Obstetric complications and age at onset in schizophrenia: an international collaborative meta-analysis of individual patient data. Am J psychiatry 1997;154(9):1220–7.

[45] Geddes JR, Verdoux H, Takei N, et al. Schizophrenia and complications of pregnancy and labor: an individual patient data meta-analysis. Schizophr Bull 1999;25(3):413–23.

[46] Geddes JR, Lawrie SM. Obstetric complications and schizophrenia: a meta-analysis. Br J Psychiatry 1995;167(6):786–93.

[47] Susser ES, Lin SP. Schizophrenia after prenatal exposure to the Dutch Hunger Winter of 1944-1945. Archives of general psychiatry 1992;49(12):983–8.

[48] Zornberg GL, Buka SL, Tsuang MT. Hypoxic-ischemia-related fetal/neonatal complications and risk of schizophrenia and other nonaffective psychoses: a 19-year longitudinal study. Am J Psychiatry 2000;157(2):196–202.

[49] Rosso IM, Cannon TD, Huttunen T, et al. Obstetric risk factors for early-onset schizophrenia in a Finnish birth cohort. Am J Psychiatry 2000;157(5):801–7.

[50] Dalman C, Allebeck P, Cullberg J, et al. Obstetric complications and the risk of schizophrenia: a longitudinal study of a national birth cohort. Archives of general psychiatry 1999;56(3):234–40.

[51] Gregory I. Factors influencing first admission rates to Canadian mental hospitals: III; an analysis by education, marital status, country of birth, religion, and rural-urban residence, 1950-1952. Canadian Journal of psychiatry 1959;4:133–51.

[52] Hare EH, Moran PA. Raised parental age in psychiatric patients: evidence for the constitutional hypothesis. Br J Psychiatry 1979;134:169–77.

[53] Granville-Grossman KL. Parental age and schizophrenia. Br J Psychiatry 1966;112(490):899–905.

[54] Kinnell HG. Parental age in schizophrenia. Br J Psychiatry 1983;142:204.

[55] Zammit S, Allebeck P, Dalman C, et al. Paternal age and risk for schizophrenia. Br J Psychiatry 2003;183:405–8.

[56] Malaspina D, Harlap S, Fennig S, et al. Advancing paternal age and the risk of schizophrenia. Archives of general psychiatry 2001;58(4):361–7.

[57] Dalman C, Allebeck P. Paternal age and schizophrenia: further support for an association. The American journal of psychiatry 2002;159(9):1591–2.

[58] Byrne M, Agerbo E, Ewald H, et al. Parental age and risk of schizophrenia: a case-control study. Archives of general psychiatry 2003;60(7):673–8.

[59] Brown AS, Schaefer CA, Wyatt RJ, et al. Paternal age and risk of schizophrenia in adult offspring. The American journal of psychiatry 2002;159(9):1528–33.

[60] Sipos A, Rasmussen F, Harrison G, et al. Paternal age and schizophrenia: a population based cohort study. BMJ (Clinical research ed 2004;329(7474):1070.

[61] Munk-Jorgensen P, Ewald H. Epidemiology in neurobiological research: exemplified by the influenza-schizophrenia theory. Br J Psychiatry 2004;40(Suppl):S30–2.

[62] Mednick S, Machon RA, Huttunen MO, et al. Adult schizophrenia following prenatal exposure to an influenza epidemic. Arch Gen Psychiatry 1988;45:189–92.

[63] Brown AS, Begg MD, Gravenstein S, et al. Serologic evidence of prenatal influenza in the etiology of schizophrenia. Arch Gen Psychiatry 2004;61(8):774–80.

[64] Weinberger DR. Implications of normal brain development for the pathogenesis of schizophrenia. Archives of general psychiatry 1987;44(7):660–9.

[65] Yolken RH, Torrey EF. Viruses, schizophrenia, and bipolar disorder. Clin Microbiol Rev 1995;8(1):131–45.

[66] Torrey EF, Yolken RH. Toxoplasma gondii and schizophrenia. Emerging Infect Dis 2003;9(11):1375–80.

[67] Brown AS, Cohen P, Greenwald S, et al. Nonaffective psychosis after prenatal exposure to rubella. The American journal of psychiatry 2000;157(3):438–43.

[68] Buka SL, Tsuang MT, Torrey EF, et al. Maternal infections and subsequent psychosis among offspring. Archives of general psychiatry 2001;58(11):1032–7.

[69] Gattaz WF, Abrahao AL, Foccacia R. Childhood meningitis, brain maturation and the risk of psychosis. European archives of psychiatry and clinical neuroscience 2004;254(1):23–6.

[70] Eaton WW, Hayward C, Ram R. Schizophrenia and rheumatoid arthritis: a review. Schizophr Res 1992;6(3):181–92.

[71] McLaughin D. Racial and sex differences in length of hospitalization of schizophrenics. Honolulu (Hawaii); 1977.

[72] in 't Veld BA, Launer LJ, Breteler MM, et al. Pharmacologic agents associated with a preventive effect on Alzheimer's disease: a review of the epidemiologic evidence. Epidemiol Rev 2002;24(2):248–68.

[73] Etminan M, Gill S, Samii A. Effect of non-steroidal anti-inflammatory drugs on risk of Alzheimer's disease: systematic review and meta-analysis of observational studies. BMJ (Clinical research ed 2003;327(7407):128.

[74] DeLisi LE, Boccio AM, Riordan H, et al. Familial thyroid disease and delayed language development in first admission patients with schizophrenia. Psychiatry Res 1991;38(1): 39–50.

[75] Wright P, Sham PC, Gilvarry CM, et al. Autoimmune diseases in the pedigrees of schizophrenic and control subjects. Schizophr Res 1996;20(3):261–7.

[76] Eaton W, Mortensen PB, Agerbo E, et al. Coeliac disease and schizophrenia: population based case control study with linkage of Danish national registers. BMJ (Clinical research ed 2004;328(7437):438–9.

[77] Dohan FC. Hypothesis: genes and neuroactive peptides from food as cause of schizophrenia. Advances in biochemical psychopharmacology 1980;22:535–48.

[78] Ganguli R, Brar JS, Rabin BS. Immune abnormalities in schizophrenia: evidence for the autoimmune hypothesis. Harvard review of psychiatry 1994;2(2):70–83.

[79] Rothermundt M, Arolt V, Bayer TA. Review of immunological and immunopathological findings in schizophrenia. Brain, Behavior, and Immunity 2001;15(4):319–39.

[80] Muller N, Riedel M, Scheppach C, et al. Beneficial antipsychotic effects of celecoxib add-on therapy compared to risperidone alone in schizophrenia. The American journal of psychiatry 2002;159(6):1029–34.

[81] Dickerson FB, Boronow JJ, Stallings CR, et al. Reduction of symptoms by valacyclovir in cytomegalovirus-seropositive individuals with schizophrenia. The American journal of psychiatry 2003;160(12):2234–6.

[82] Eaton W, Harrison G. Ethnic disadvantage and schizophrenia. Acta Psychiatr Scand Suppl 2000;(407):38–43.

[83] Eaton W, Harrison G. Life chances, life planning, and schizophrenia: a review and interpretation of research on social deprivation. International Journal of Mental Health 2001;30:58–81.

[84] Leao TS, Sundquist J, Frank G, et al. Incidence of schizophrenia or other psychoses in first- and second-generation immigrants: a national cohort study. The Journal of nervous and mental disease 2006;194(1):27–33.

[85] Hall W, Degenhardt L. Cannabis use and psychosis: a review of clinical and epidemiological evidence. The Australian and New Zealand journal of psychiatry 2000;34(1): 26–34.

[86] Zammit S, Allebeck P, Andreasson S, et al. Self reported cannabis use as a risk factor for schizophrenia in Swedish conscripts of 1969: historical cohort study. BMJ (Clinical research ed 2002;325(7374):1199.

[87] Weiser M, Reichenberg A, Rabinowitz J, et al. Self-reported drug abuse in male adolescents with behavioral disturbances, and follow-up for future schizophrenia. Biol Psychiatry 2003;54(6):655–60.

[88] van Os J, Bak M, Hanssen M, et al. Cannabis use and psychosis: a longitudinal population-based study. American journal of epidemiology 2002;156(4):319–27.

[89] Arseneault L, Cannon M, Poulton R, et al. Cannabis use in adolescence and risk for adult psychosis: longitudinal prospective study. BMJ 2002;325(7374):1212–3.

[90] Veen ND, Selten JP, van der Tweel I, et al. Cannabis use and age at onset of schizophrenia. The American journal of psychiatry 2004;161(3):501–6.

[91] Henquet C, Murray R, Linszen D, et al. The environment and schizophrenia: the role of cannabis use. Schizophr Bull 2005;31(3):608–12.

[92] Degenhardt L, Hall W. Is cannabis use a contributory cause of psychosis? Canadian journal of psychiatry 2006;51(9):556–65.

[93] Caspi A, Moffitt TE, Cannon M, et al. Moderation of the effect of adolescent-onset cannabis use on adult psychosis by a functional polymorphism in the catechol-O-methyltransferase gene: longitudinal evidence of a gene X environment interaction. Biol Psychiatry 2005;57(10):1117–27.

[94] Barnes TR, Mutsatsa SH, Hutton SB, et al. Comorbid substance use and age at onset of schizophrenia. Br J Psychiatry 2006;188:237–42.

[95] Arendt M, Rosenberg R, Foldager L, et al. Cannabis-induced psychosis and subsequent schizophrenia-spectrum disorders: follow-up study of 535 incident cases. Br J Psychiatry 2005;187:510–5.

[96] Faris RE, Dunham W. Mental disorders in urban areas. Chicago: University of Chicago Press, 1939.

[97] Eaton WW. Residence, social class, and schizophrenia. Journal of health and social behavior 1974;15(4):289–99.

[98] Lewis G, David A, Andreasson S, et al. Schizophrenia and city life. Lancet 1992; 340(8812):137–40.

[99] Marcelis M, Navarro-Mateu F, Murray R, et al. Urbanization and psychosis: a study of 1942–1978 birth cohorts in The Netherlands. Psychol Med 1998;28(4):871–9.

[100] McCreadie RG. The Nithsdale Schizophrenia Surveys. 16. Breast-feeding and schizophrenia: preliminary results and hypotheses. Br J Psychiatry 1997;170:334–7.

[101] Torrey EF, Yolken RH. At issue: is household crowding a risk factor for schizophrenia and bipolar disorder? Schizophr Bull 1998;24(3):321–4.

[102] Torrey EF, Yolken RH. Could schizophrenia be a viral zoonosis transmitted from house cats? Schizophr Bull 1995;21(2):167–71.

[103] van Os J, Krabbendam L, Myin-Germeys I, et al. The schizophrenia enviroment. Current opinion in psychiatry 2005;18(2):141–5.

[104] McGrath JJ. Myths and plain truths about schizophrenia epidemiology–the NAPE lecture 2004. Acta Psychiatr Scand 2005;111(1):4–11.

[105] Mortensen PB, Pedersen CB, Westergaard T, et al. Familial and non-familial risk factors for schizophrenia: a population-based study. N Engl J Med 1999;340:603–8.

[106] Woods SW, Breier A, Zipursky RB, et al. Randomized trial of olanzapine versus placebo in the symptomatic acute treatment of the schizophrenic prodrome. Biological Psychiatry 2003;54(4):453–64.

[107] Tsuang MT, Stone WS, Seidman LJ, et al. Treatment of nonpsychotic relatives of patients with schizophrenia: four case studies. Biological Psychiatry 1999;45(11):1412–8.

[108] McGorry P, Mihaloppoulos C. EPPIC: an evolving system of early detection and optimal management. Schizophrenia Bulletin 1996;22:305–26.

Schizophrenia: Measurements of Psychopathology

J.P. Lindenmayer, MD[a], Philip D. Harvey, PhD[b],*,
Anzalee Khan, MS[a], Brian Kirkpatrick, MD[c]

[a]Department of Psychiatry, New York University, and Manhattan Psychiatric Center, New York, NY, USA
[b]Department of Psychiatry, Mt. Sinai School of Medicine, New York, NY, USA
[c]Department of Psychiatry and Health Behavior, Medical College of Georgia, Augusta, GA, USA

A key problem in schizophrenia research is how to assess the effects of treatment interventions given the spectrum of schizophrenia symptoms and patients' functioning. Measuring symptoms is complex, because these symptoms cover a wide variety of psychopathologic domains. The commonly recognized domains are the positive, negative, cognitive, excitement, and depression domains. This article critically reviews some of the available assessment tools of these domains together with other associated syndromes. The instruments discussed cover the broad range of psychopathology found in patients who have schizophrenia.

A growing number of scales have been introduced, and there is often a question as to which rating scales to use in an individual clinical situation. This article reviews the most commonly used psychopathology rating scales in an attempt to aid clinicians and researchers. In particular, it focuses on two areas of assessment in which the field is changing rapidly: the assessment of function, and negative symptoms.

ASSESSMENT RATING SCALES

Although there is substantial agreement among clinicians and researchers about the symptom domains that should be assessed in patients who have schizophrenia, there are important differences concerning the conceptualization of how to group symptoms into particular constructs. A number of studies have examined the symptom presentation of large samples of patients with schizophrenia using factor analysis with newer symptom scales. This process has resulted in a number of enlarged syndromal models of schizophrenia.

Factor analyses based on the Scale for the Assessment of Positive Symptoms (SAPS) and the SANS have suggested a clustering of schizophrenia symptoms into three factors [1–3]: (1) positive or psychotic cluster (hallucinations,

*Corresponding author. E-mail address: philipdharvey1@cs.com (P.D. Harvey).

0193-953X/07/$ – see front matter
doi:10.1016/j.psc.2007.04.005
© 2007 Elsevier Inc. All rights reserved.
psych.theclinics.com

delusions, catatonic symptoms); (2) negative cluster (anhedonia, avolition, poverty of speech, blunted affect); and (3) disorganization cluster (disorganized speech, inappropriate affect, bizarre behavior). Using the Positive and Negative Syndrome Scale (PANSS), researchers Peralta and colleagues [3], Lindenmayer and colleagues [4–6], Marder and colleagues [7], White and colleagues [8], and Toomey and colleagues [9] have proposed a five-factor model of schizophrenia, consisting of (1) a positive factor (delusions, hallucinatory behavior, grandiosity, unusual thought content, suspiciousness/persecution), (2) a negative factor (blunted affect, emotional withdrawal, poor rapport, passive/apathetic social withdrawal, lack of spontaneity, active social avoidance), (3) an excitement factor (excitement, hostility, uncooperativeness, poor impulse control), (4) a cognitive (or disorganization) factor (conceptual disorganization, difficulty with abstract thinking, disorientation, poor attention, preoccupation), and (5) a depression/anxiety factor (anxiety, guilt feelings, tension, and depression) [10–13]. This model has proved to be very robust across various illness phases, cross-culturally, and longitudinally and to be stable after antipsychotic treatments.

The following sections review clinical assessment tools for four of these domains together with assessment methods for other associated syndromes.

MEASUREMENT OF POSITIVE SYMPTOMS
The Brief Psychiatric Rating Scale
The Brief Psychiatric Rating Scale (BPRS) is an 18-item scale measuring positive symptoms, general psychopathology, and affective symptoms [14]. The BPRS is a clinician-rated tool and is designed to assess the severity of psychopathology and its change. The BPRS initially was designed to produce a total score indicating an overall level of psychiatric symptoms that can be used to assess changes resulting from treatment. The items cover a broad range of symptoms that are seen commonly in psychosis, including hallucinations, delusions, and disorganization, as well as mood disturbances that also may accompany relapse (eg, hostility, anxiety, and depression).

The BPRS originally consisted of 16 items [14]; the addition of two items created the traditional or standard 18-item version [15–18] that is the most widely used version. An expanded 24-item version [19,20] was introduced later. The 16 original items of the BPRS include somatic concern, anxiety, emotional withdrawal, conceptual disorganization, guilt feelings, tension, mannerisms and posturing, grandiosity, depressive mood, hostility, suspiciousness, hallucinatory behavior, motor retardation, uncooperativeness, unusual thought content, and blunted affect. Two additional items, excitement and disorientation, were added later [15]. Items on the BPRS are rated on a seven-point ordinal scale, ranging from "not present" (1) to "extremely severe" (7). Ratings on the BPRS scale are based on observation of the patient and verbal reporting by the patient [21]. The BPRS is rated after a brief (20–30 minute), nonstructured interview. To enhance the reliability of the BPRS, versions of the scale accompanied by operational definitions of severity levels (anchor points) have been developed [19,22–25].

Psychometric characteristics

In a large number of studies, the BPRS showed good reliability coefficients both for total score and for individual items [26]. Lower reliability coefficients have been reported with less experienced raters [27,28]. Hedlund and Vieweg [26] reviewed published studies assessing the BPRS interrater reliability and found Pearson correlations for the total pathology score were 0.80 or greater for 10 of 13 studies. McGorry and colleagues [24] reported needing more than 30 joint rating sessions to achieve consistently reliable scores among seven psychiatrists for an Intraclass Correlation Coefficient (ICC) of 0.80. Gabbard and colleagues [23] found reliability improved for 15 of the 18 items when they moved from the original anchors to anchors with detailed descriptors. Concurrent validity is demonstrated in treatment trials by comparable changes observed in other assessment measures such as the Clinical Global Impressions (CGI) and the Hamilton Rating Scale for Depression [28,29].

Clinical implications

Although its psychometric properties in terms of reliability, validity, and sensitivity have been examined extensively, the clinical implications of BPRS scores are not always clear. For example, it has never been analyzed what the clinical meaning of the severity of illness of a patient with a BPRS total score of 50 or 90 represents. In addition, the definition of a clinically significant improvement in score is not yet agreed on; however, reductions of at least 20% [30–33], 30% [34–36], 40% [37], or 50% [38] of the initial BPRS score have been used as a cutoff to define response.

The BPRS is among the most researched instruments used in psychiatry and is familiar to clinicians and researchers whose work involves symptom scores and changes. The BPRS also has been shown to be sensitive to change and thus may be used to rate treatment response. The BPRS, however, is limited in scope by its focus primarily on positive symptoms and general psychopathology. Despite its moderately high correlation with the Scale for the Assessment of Negative Symptoms (SANS) [39], it does not focus on negative symptoms. As a result, it needs to be used in combination with a negative symptom assessment tool if negative symptomatology is to be captured. Challenges also arise in scoring the BPRS: its interpretation can be ambiguous because symptoms can be scored in several ways (eg, on a scale of 0 to 6 or on a scale of 1 to 7); this dual scoring method must be considered when interpreting scores. Additionally, the nonlinearity of the 1-to-7 scale can complicate the interpretation and appreciation of changes over time, particularly in regard to response rates. Finally, the lack of descriptive clinical anchoring points opens the BPRS to a certain degree of subjectivity.

Scale for the Assessment of Positive Symptoms

Andreasen and colleagues [40] developed the SAPS and the SANS, which consist of 35 and 29 items, respectively. The SAPS is designed to assess positive and disorganization symptoms, including hallucinations, delusions, bizarre behaviors, and formal thought disorder. The SANS is described further in the section on negative symptom scales.

The SAPS groups positive symptoms into five subscales of symptoms (hallucinations, delusions, bizarre behavior, positive formal thought disorder, and inappropriate affect) with 30 individual items. The items are scored on a six-point Likert type scale ranging from 0 (the symptom is absent) to 5 (the symptom is present in a severe form). A subscale score for each domain is obtained by summing each of the items in that domain; the range of possible scores in a domain depends on the number of items in the domain. For example, the sum of four global domain scores produces a summary score (scored from 0 to 20), and the sum of the 30 individual items produces a composite score (scored from 0 to 150). Andreasen [41] recommends using a summary score as a measure of the overall severity of positive and negative symptom severity. Higher scores represent more severe impairments. The SAPS takes approximately 30 minutes to administer. The time frame for rating this measure can vary from within the past week for patients in treatment for an acute episode to the past 6 months for patients who have chronic, clinically stable illness. It is recommended that ratings be made by trained raters (preferably psychiatric clinicians) on the basis of a standard clinical interview, behaviors observed during the interview, a review of clinical material, and information from the subject's family and caregivers. The SAPS and SANS are copyrighted and are available from the authors. A semistructured diagnostic interview is embedded in the comprehensive assessment of symptoms and history [42].

Psychometric characteristics
The interrater reliability of the SAPS summary score has been reported as 0.84 [43] in a sample of patients with schizophrenia. The ICC for SAPS domain scores was fair to excellent, ranging from 0.50 to 0.91. Many studies have examined the internal consistency of the SAPS and the SANS [40,44,45] with similar Cronbach alpha ranges. Andreasen and Grove [46] showed that the internal consistency of the SAPS and SANS produces Cronbach alphas for the SAPS of 0.48, reflecting positive and disorganization symptoms. The internal consistency for the SANS produced Cronbach alphas of 0.86, showing high internal consistency and suggesting no disparate constructs as seen with the SAPS.

Kay and colleagues [47] in a sample of 82 schizophrenic patients reported correlations of 0.77 ($P < .001$) between the positive syndrome score on the PANSS and the summary score of the SAPS and between the negative syndrome score on the PANSS and the summary score of the SANS.

Clinical implications
The SAPS and the SANS have been used in numerous clinical trials to assess the psychopathology of schizophrenia. Because of their extensiveness, it may be difficult to administer them as part of a routine clinical interview. A potential advantage of the SAPS and the SANS in clinical settings is that the global rating includes the impact of the symptom on patient functioning. As demonstrated in

numerous studies, both measures have good concurrent validity and provide consistent and valid results as assessed by the concurrent administration of other assessment tools. The SAPS and the SANS are commonly used in conjunction with the BPRS, particularly in clinical research studies. On the other hand, the SAPS and the SANS have been criticized for their complexity and for the need for thorough rater training to achieve satisfactory interrater reliability.

The Positive and Negative Syndrome Scale

Kay and colleagues [48] developed the PANSS consisting of three subscales measuring seven positive, seven negative, and 16 general psychopathology symptoms. This 30-item scale has demonstrated reliable psychometric properties in clinical trials of subjects with schizophrenia in assessing symptoms and their change throughout the course of treatment [4,6,47,49–52]. It was conceived as an operationalized, treatment-sensitive instrument that provides balanced representation of positive and negative symptoms and gauges their relationship to one another and to global psychopathology. The PANSS includes 18 items from the BPRS and 12 additional items from the Psychopathology Rating Schedule [53]. The authors' goal was to develop a rating scale that improved on the BPRS by including negative items that are clinically important in schizophrenia.

Items on the PANSS are scored from 1 (absent) to 7 (extreme). The PANSS should be administered by personnel trained in psychiatric interview techniques and with experience working with persons with schizophrenia. It takes approximately 30 to 40 minutes to complete. It was developed with a comprehensive anchoring system to improve the reliability of ratings. The three subscales contain the following individual items:

- Positive symptoms: delusions, conceptual disorganization, hallucinatory behavior, excitement, grandiosity, suspiciousness/persecution, hostility
- Negative symptoms: blunted affect, emotional withdrawal, poor rapport, passive/apathetic social withdrawal, difficulty in abstract thinking, lack of spontaneity and flow of conversation, stereotyped thinking
- General psychopathology symptoms: somatic concern, anxiety, guilt feelings, tension, mannerism and posturing, depression, motor retardation, uncooperativeness, unusual thought content, disorientation, poor attention, lack of judgment and insight, disturbance and volition, poor impulse control, preoccupation, active social avoidance.

The time frame for rating the PANSS is generally within the past week before the rating. A semistructured interview for the PANSS called the SCI-PANSS [54] has been developed to guide interviewers through specific questions to elicit the information required to evaluate the presence and severity of symptoms evaluated by the PANSS. The items of the PANSS are summed to determine scores on the three subscales (positive, negative, and general psychopathology) and the total scores (the sum of all three subscales). The potential range of scores on the positive and negative scales is 7 to 49, with a score of

7 indicating no symptoms. The potential range of scores on the general psycho-pathology scale is 16 to 112.

The PANSS has been adapted for children and adolescents age 6 to 16 years who have severe psychiatric illness. This scale is referred to as the "Kiddie PANSS" [55].

Psychometric characteristics
A number of studies have established good-to-excellent reliability with the PANSS. Bell and colleagues [49] examined the interrater reliability of the PANSS in a sample of 56 patients who had *Diagnostic and Statistical Manual of Mental Disorders edition 3, revised (DSM IIIR)* diagnoses of schizophrenia or schiz-oaffective disorder. On the items that constitute the positive syndrome scale, ICCs ranged from 0.81 to 0.93. For the negative syndrome items, ICCs ranged from 0.63 to 0.90. The ICCs of the general psychopathology scales ranged from 0.54 to 0.92. Most other studies have ICCs within the range observed by Bell and colleagues [49].

Review of five studies involving the PANSS provided "evidence of its crite-rion-related validity with antecedent, genealogical, and concurrent measures, its predictive validity, its drug sensitivity, and its utility for both typological and dimensional assessment" [48].

Clinical implications
The PANSS provides an objective and reliable assessment of common symp-toms in patients who have schizophrenia and other psychotic disorders. It may be used in clinical settings to assess severity of symptoms, to delineate and describe target symptoms, and to quantify severity of relapse. In particular, the PANSS has been used in many pharmacologic and nonpharmacologic trials and is potentially useful in a clinical setting to monitor response to treatment in-terventions. It covers positive and negative symptoms associated with schizo-phrenia, as well as other symptoms (eg, aggression, thought disturbance, depression). In addition, the clinical descriptors provided for each item improve reliability. The PANSS has also a well-established factor structure and test–retest reliability and is considered an improvement on the BPRS, addressing broader psychopathology and with greater reliability Because the PANSS is a comprehen-sive tool and includes 30 items, it requires a long interview with the patient (30–40 minutes). The typical duration of patient interviews in clinical practice may be insufficient to allow administration of the PANSS. Additionally, the PANSS is based in part on subjective patient reporting, because the assessment of some items is based on patients' perceptions of their experiences in the previous week; patients' views might be influenced by their experience of previous inter-views, and results might be subjectively influenced.

MEASUREMENT OF NEGATIVE SYMPTOMS
The Scale for the Assessment of Negative Symptoms
The SANS includes five areas of negative symptoms [40]. Scoring of items is based on a six-point scale from 0 (not present) to 5 (severe). The SANS assesses

five symptom complexes to obtain clinical ratings of negative symptoms in patients who have schizophrenia.

The SANS symptom complexes include affective blunting, alogia (impoverished thinking), avolition/apathy, anhedonia/asociality, and disturbance of attention. The final symptom complex seems to have less obvious relevance to negative symptoms than the other four complexes. Ratings are made on each negative symptom cluster after consideration has been given to each of the items contained within the various complex scores. There are item descriptions and anchor-point descriptions given for each score.

Psychometric characteristics
It was found that the average ICC for all items on the SANS was 0.52, ranging from 0.28 to 0.74. The average ICC for the global ratings on the SANS was 0.51, and for specific items it was 0.53 [43]. Two of the global ratings on the SANS (affective flattening and attentional impairment) had ICCs of less than 0.40, which is rather low. The ICC for the SANS summary score (total of global ratings) was 0.60, and for the composite score (total specific symptom ratings) it was 0.68. In the same study [43] the SAPS was compared with items of the PANSS positive syndrome scale. The average ICC for all items was 0.52 with a range from −0.01 to 0.91. The average ICC of the global items was higher (0.75) than that of more specific items (0.62). For each of the subscales except bizarre behavior, the global rating had an interrater reliability as high or higher than any rating of a specific symptom. Fenton and McGlashan [56] report a mean correlation of 0.82 between several measures of negative symptoms, including the negative syndrome scale of the PANSS and the SANS, but the specific correlation between these two instruments is not reported.

Although the SAPS and SANS aim to assess specific positive and negative schizophrenia symptoms, respectively, the SANS may not be adapted to measure secondary negative symptoms. Both instruments are predominantly research instruments.

The Negative Symptom Assessment

The Negative Symptoms Assessment (NSA) is a reliable six-point rating scale consisting of 16 items evaluating behaviors commonly associated with negative symptoms [57,58]. The NSA uses a semistructured interview and defined anchor points to characterize a wide range of negative symptoms. It assesses the domains of communication, emotion/affect, social involvement, motivation, and retardation. The rules for rating the NSA specify that scores do not necessarily imply psychopathology or etiology. The rater should be aware of outside sources of information (eg, family members, care givers) and contradictory information should use best clinical judgment in assigning the rating. Information also is elicited by observation of behaviors during the interview, which takes approximately 20 to 30 minutes to complete.

The reference time frame for the NSA is similar to that for the PANSS, that is, the previous 7 days for relevant items. The severity scores of the behavior being assessed range from 1 to 6 points:

1. Not reduced or absent as compared with a healthy young human
2. Minimally reduced, significance is questionable
3. Mildly reduced (might only be noted as reduced by a trained rater, but the rater notes a definite reduction)
4. Moderately reduced (its reduction should be obvious to an untrained rater)
5. Markedly reduced (this behavior is easily observable and definitely interferes with the subject's functioning)
6. Severely reduced or entirely absent (it is glaring and markedly interferes with functioning)

The anchor points for rating the NSA should be used as guides. No set of anchors could possibly describe or be applicable to all persons.

Psychometric characteristics
Interrater reliability for the NSA yielded scores ranging from 0.79 to 0.93. High concurrent validity was found between NSA total scores, BPRS withdrawal scores, and SANS total scores. Construct validity was assessed using correlations obtained by factor analysis of the NSA with the total and global scores on the NSA, which were highly correlated, suggesting that the scale reflected the concept of negative symptoms [57]. Factor analysis of the original 26-item NSA produced seven factors: affect/emotion, external involvement, retardation, personal presentation, thinking, interpersonal interest, and blocking.

Clinical implications
To measure negative symptoms in clinical practice, the assessment tool must be short, intuitive for the clinician to use, and easy to rate with clear anchors but still retain sensitivity to detect changes in negative symptoms. For example in clinical practice it may be useful to use just 4 of the 16 items of the NSA to augment simple intuitive approaches to assessing the negative symptoms [59,60]. These four items are: reduced range of emotions, reduced interests, reduced social drive, and restricted speech quantity.

MEASURING GLOBAL PSYCHOPATHOLOGY
The Clinical Global Impressions Scale
The CGI scale is a clinician's rating of the subject's illness and is based on the overall clinical impression by an experienced rater. The goal of the CGI is to allow the clinician to rate the severity of illness and its change over time, taking into account the patient's clinical condition [61]. This scale includes two separate measures: (1) severity of illness (assessment of patient's current symptom severity, referred to here as CGI-Severity) and (2) global improvement (comparison of the patient's baseline condition with his/her current condition.

The CGI has been used widely in clinical research, especially in clinical trials concerning psychotropic treatments for schizophrenia, bipolar disorder [62], and anxiety [63]. It has a strong appeal for use as a simple scale for clinical practice as well.

CGI-Severity is rated on a seven-point scale from 1 (normal) to 7 (extremely ill); the CGI-Improvement is rated on a seven-point scale from 1 (very much improved) to 7 (very much worse). The CGI-Severity measure requires the clinician to rate the severity of the patient's illness at the time of assessment relative to the clinician's past experience with patients who have the same diagnosis as normal (not at all ill), borderline mentally ill, mildly ill, moderately ill, markedly ill, severely ill, or extremely ill.

The CGI-Improvement measure requires the clinician to rate how much the patient's illness has improved or worsened relative to a baseline state (eg, very much improved, much improved, moderately improved, minimally improved, no change, minimally worse, moderately worse, much worse, or very much worse). It is recommended that the rater use all available sources of information about the subject's behavior.

In general, the CGI-Severity scale is completed once before treatment and the CGI-Improvement is completed at least once after completion of a treatment trial. More frequent ratings to follow change may be desirable. The scale takes about 1 to 2 minutes to score after the clinical interview.

Psychometric characteristics
The authors believe the first study to demonstrate and document the interrater and test–retest reliability of the CGI was conducted by Dahlke and colleagues [64,65]. This study revealed relatively good reliability scores for CGI-Severity ratings but not for the CGI-Improvement ratings. A later study by Weitkunat and colleagues [66] also found the CGI-Improvement measure to have unimpressive test–retest reliability. Both studies clearly indicated a need for improved CGI guidelines and assessment criteria to strengthen the reliability of the ratings. Beneke and Rasmus [67] examined the reliability and clinical concepts of scores and normality of the CGI items in 175 patients who had schizophrenia, depression, and anxiety from 8-week clinical trials. Scores on the global improvement and therapeutic effects subscales were highly correlated (r = 0.90), but there was only a moderate correlation (r = −0.47 to −0.66) between changes in the CGI-Severity and CGI-Improvement subscales.

Dahlke and colleagues [64] found relatively good reliability for the CGI-Severity ratings (0.66) for physicians and low reliability (0.41) for nursing staff. The CGI-Improvement rating, however, showed low reliability of 0.51 for physicians and 0.35 for nursing staff. Haro and colleagues [68] developed a CGI-Severity and a CGI-Improvement scale for Schizophrenia.

Clinical implications
The CGI scale is one of the most widely used outcome measures and has proven to be a robust measure of efficacy in drug-treatment trials. The scale

is clinically understandable, simple to use, and sensitive to change. The scale of severity of illness is based on the rater's subjective views of symptom severity, which can vary between raters and make consistent interpretation of CGI scores problematic in practice. A number of weaknesses could explain this possible lack of validity of the CGI: there is no specific interviewer guide, and whereas most other symptoms scales have fairly clear and specific response options, and the response format used in the CGI to assess change or severity of illness is more likely to be ambiguous (what is the definition of a patient who is "severely ill"?). Although the CGI scale can be administered quickly, it is paramount, particularly for the CGI-Improvement scale, for the rater to know the patient. If a clinical history is not available, the tool cannot be used.

MEASURES FOR DEPRESSION AND SUICIDAL IDEATION
Calgary Depression Scale for Schizophrenia
The Calgary Depression Scale for Schizophrenia (CDSS) is a nine-item scale designed to estimate the severity of depression in patients who have schizophrenia [69]. It has been found to be superior to the Hamilton Depression Rating Scale, the Montgomery-Asberg Depression Rating Scale, and other depression scales for patients with schizophrenia [70–74].

The CDSS is a semistandardized observer rating scale consisting of nine items, each graded on a four-point Likert type scale (0, absent; 1, mild; 2, moderate; 3, severe). The sum score is derived by adding the point scores of all nine items. The CDSS is sensitive to change and contains a guided interview for the rater to follow. Of the nine items of the CDSS, eight are structured questions, and one is observer rated.

The general rules for rating require that the interviewer clearly identify the past week as the reference time frame and determine during the interview the severity of relevant behaviors (using a range and specifically including worst), the frequency of the relevant behaviors, and whether the pattern of the behaviors is stable, worsening, improving, or indeterminate. When making the final ratings, the interviewer also should identify the anchors that reflect the range of behaviors captured during the interview. Administration of the CDSS takes 15 to 20 minutes. It is designed to be used primarily by clinicians who have prior experience evaluating and treating patients who have schizophrenia. The CDSS has been developed specifically to assess the level of depression in schizophrenia. It has been evaluated extensively in both relapsed and remitted patients and seems to be sensitive to change.

Psychometric characteristics
The CDSS has excellent psychometric properties of internal consistency, interrater reliability, sensitivity, and specificity [75–78]. Reports on discriminant and convergent validity have been reported in a large number of studies [78–80]. In most settings CDSS total scores show only low-to-modest overlap with positive and negative symptoms and no substantial correlation with

extrapyramidal symptoms during acute schizophrenia [75,81–86]. In chronic illness states the overlap between positive and depressive symptoms seems somewhat higher [87].

The nine items of the CDSS comprise a highly sensitive, one-dimensional scale with high internal consistency in healthy subjects corroborating findings in schizophrenic samples [70,75,76,88,89]. The CDSS showed high interrater reliability (ICC = 0.89). The internal consistency ranged from Cronbach alphas of 0.70 to 0.90 [90].

Clinical implications

An advantage of the CDSS is its brevity and therefore its clinical utility in non-research settings. It has fewer factors and less overlap with positive and negative symptoms than the Hamilton Depression Scale, both at the time of relapse and at the time of remission. An experienced rater should develop adequate interrater reliability within 5 practice interviews.

The InterSePT Scale for Suicidal Thinking

The InterSePT Scale for Suicidal Thinking (ISST) is a semi-structured 12-item instrument for the assessment of current suicidal ideation in patients who have schizophrenia and schizoaffective disorders [91]. Before the development of the ISST, there were a few attempts to develop instruments that measure suicidal ideation specifically geared to patients who have schizophrenia. Most instruments are risk-assessment tools, which provide only a limited evaluation of current suicidal ideation and are unlikely to show change with treatment [92]. Further, most available suicidal ideation scales have been developed for patients who have mood disorders [93,94]. The goals of the ISST are to assess suicidal ideation in patients who have schizophrenia, to implement appropriate clinical interventions, and to assess the effects of these interventions on suicidal thinking. In addition, a reliable measure of current suicidal ideation may be a more measurable target of pharmacotherapy than overall suicidality, which is a more heterogeneous and multidimensional phenomenon.

The ISST takes approximately 20 minutes to complete. It was derived from the Scale for Suicide Ideation, a 19-item scale, which has been validated and has proven reliable in a depressed population [93] but not in patients who have schizophrenia. Each of the 12 items is rated on three levels of increasing intensity (0, 1, or 2). The total score is computed by adding scores for the 12 individual items. It quantifies the current conscious and overtly expressed suicidal thinking in schizophrenic patients by canvassing various suicidal thoughts and wishes.

The ISST scale contains semistructured questions for the patient for each item. The questions and instructions for the use of the scale are located on the measure and do not require a separate manual. Information for rating is obtained from the direct interview with the patient and from all available information about the patient as obtained from medical records, family, caregiver, and the patient's doctor.

Psychometric characteristics

The ICC for the total ISST score was 0.90, and mean weighted item kappa coefficients ranged from 0.66 to 0.92 [91]. Internal reliability (Cronbach alpha) was high, ranging from 0.67 to 0.89 for the individual items, and the overall Cronbach alpha coefficient for all items was 0.88. The ISST total score was highly correlated with the CGI-Suicidality score (r = 0.86; $P<$.0001). ISST total scores significantly differentiated the different levels of CGI-Suicidality score.

Clinical implications

The ISST has been used in a number of clinical trials to assess suicidal ideations in patients with schizophrenia and schizoaffective disorders. In addition, the ISST has been used in studies as an anchor with which to compare newer instruments [95]. In clinical practice, the ISST, although extremely valuable, is underused in the evaluation of suicidal symptoms in schizophrenia and schizoaffective disorder. Furthermore, it should be noted that this assessment tool relies heavily on the clinical interviewing skills and expertise of the assessment rater.

THE MEASUREMENT OF DISORGANIZATION OF THOUGHT

Formal thought disorder is a multifaceted construct that encompasses a diverse set of thinking disturbances, including loose and indirect associations, overly abstract or concrete responses, illogicality, inappropriate intrusion of personal material, and unusual word usage [96]. Careful listening to patients' word productions and sentence construction allows the assessment of thought disorder. Difficulty in abstract thinking and concrete thinking can be measured with proverb interpretations and similarities. Proverb interpretation challenges the individual's ability in abstract symbolic thinking, in shifting of sets, and in the ability to generalize. The task of establishing similarities reveals difficulties in classification and categorization. Object-sorting tasks can be used to assess overinclusion; an overinclusive reply would include too many or unsuitable items within a group of items. Thought disorder is related directly to disordered language functioning and is a reflection of poor neurocognitive functioning.

The Assessment of Thought, Language and Communication (TLC) scale offers a clinical rating for a series of different types of thought disorders. The SAPS [40], the SANS [40], and the PANSS [48] provide some measures of thought disorder. Additionally, the BPRS conceptual disorganization item has been used to assess formal thought disorder [97].

Scale for the Assessment of Thought, Language and Communication

One of the most widely used instruments for assessing formal thought disorder has been the TLC scale, devised by Andreasen. Subsets of TLC items are incorporated in the positive thought disorder subscale of the SAPS and in the alogia subscale of the SANS. The 18-item TLC scale provides concise definitions of many aspects of thought disorder and was designed to provide the user with specific definitions and quantitative ratings for 18 subtypes of aberrant language. These subtypes cover the broad range of communication deviance displayed by schizophrenic patients.

The TLC contains 18 items including one global item score. Both the global score and the scores of each item (poverty of speech, poverty of content of speech, pressure of speech, distractibility, tangentiality, derailment, incoherence, illogicality, clanging, neologisms, word approximations, circumstantiality, loss of goal, perseveration, echolalia, blocking, stilted speech, self-reference) are used to assess thought disorder. Administering the scale takes approximately 30 minutes. It is recommended that the TLC be administered by a trained clinician who is familiar with the patient.

Psychometric characteristics
A review by Andreasen and Grove [46] documented the reliability and validity of the scale. Interrater reliability ranged from 0.35 to 0.80 (weighted kappa) on 18 items of thought disorder and one global item. Although the BPRS thought disorder cluster was significantly related to the global rating of thought disorder on the TLC (r = 0.71), only half of the variance in thought disorder measured by the TLC was accounted for by the BPRS factor. Thus, this study supports Andreasen's contention that the TLC is a reliable instrument and suggests that the instrument may provide significant information about thinking disorders.

Clinical implications
The TLC scale is widely used to assess thought disorder with good reliability, particularly in research studies examining thought disorder or thought disturbances in schizophrenia. Because of the need for careful training and because of the extensiveness of the measure, however, it has limited use for clinical practice.

ASSESSMENT OF FUNCTIONAL DISABILITY
The *DSM* diagnostic criteria for schizophrenia require a decline in functioning from a higher, better level. Functional disability in schizophrenia is responsible for the majority of the cost of the illness, in that multiple domains of everyday functional outcome are impaired in schizophrenia. Rates of competitive employment are under 20%, and, even in supported employment, job tenure lasts only a few months on average, with as many as 50% of patients who attain work having unsatisfactory job terminations [98–100]. Patients achieve lower educational levels than would be expected by socioeconomic status and other demographic variables [101]. A variety of deficits are observed in independent living skills including the abilities related to using public transportation, cooking, finding and caring for living quarters, money management, and medication adherence [102–105]. Some chronic patients even manifest substantial impairments in basic activities of daily living [106], and the major medical morbidity associated with schizophrenia is at least partly the result of reduced ability of

schizophrenia patients to seek health care, particularly preventive care, spontaneously.

As many as two thirds of patients who have schizophrenia are unable to fulfill basic social roles (eg, as a spouse, parent, or worker), even when psychotic symptoms are in remission. Most patients have significant impairments in social relationships; they often are isolated, and when they do interact with others, they have difficulty maintaining appropriate conversations, expressing their needs and feelings, achieving social goals, or developing close relationships. The social networks of patients who have schizophrenia are smaller than those of healthy individuals [101,107]. Premorbid social competence is among the best predictors of long-term outcome, either because poor premorbid adjustment is a marker of a more pernicious form of illness or because social competence is a coping skill that helps the individual achieve goals and avoid stress, or for both reasons. These multiple domains of impairment combine to make schizophrenia among the top disabling conditions worldwide for young adults, according to the World Health Organization [108,109]. Although psychiatry has been successful in treating the positive symptoms of schizophrenia, not much progress has been made in treating the major role impairments associated with the disorder.

For treatment to be successful, valid assessments of functional disability are needed. There are surprising challenges in this area. In particular, the method used to obtain information on functional deficits seems to be related to the success with which the deficits can be measured. Multiple factors affect functional disability, and these factors must be assessed along with the deficits in everyday functional performance.

The Competence/Performance Distinction

Critical to any attempt to measure disability accurately is the separation of assessment domains into what the person can do and what the person actually does. This separation, referred to as the "competence/performance distinction," is critical for comprehensive understanding of functional disability [110], because functional capacity does not overlap completely with real-world performance. This disparity in ability and performance may result from the characteristics of the individuals and from other environmental factors.

Among the personal characteristics that may influence real-world performance, beyond the influence of functional capacity, are confidence, motivation, willingness to take risks, and the ability to self-evaluate and self-monitor. Self-evaluation has been shown to be particularly impaired in people who have schizophrenia [111,112]. An overestimation of skills can lead to a person's attempting excessively challenging tasks, whereas an underestimation can lead to unwillingness to make efforts in situations where success might occur.

Methods for Assessment of Functional Disability

Multiple instruments are available for assessing a variety of outcome domains, including indices of competence and real-world outcomes. It is important to separate the content domains of outcome and potential disability, which include social, vocational, self-care, and independent living, from the methods used to assess these domains. Assessment methods include global rating scales designed to be rated on the basis of all available information, self-reporting instruments, direct observation of behavior, informant reports, and performance-based measures of functional skills.

Each of these methods has strengths and weaknesses. Self-reporting is useful because only the person being assessed has access to many behaviors. Direct observation allows the assessor to develop highly objective and reliable coding systems. Informant reports avoid many of the potential response biases in other methods, and contrasting reports from different informants may provide a broad-brush picture of variance in performance in different settings. Performance-based measures eliminate the possibility of response biases and can be adjusted to capture highly specific features of functional skills. As for limitations, self-reporting in patients who have schizophrenia is particularly biased, for several reasons. Direct observation is not useful for many behaviors, and for patients who are socially isolated and unemployed, the frequency of the target adaptive behaviors of interest is quite low. Many people who have schizophrenia lack good informants, and the amount of their contact with the patients can be quite variable. Performance-based measures of capacity require evidence of concurrent validity and, as noted previously, other influences on everyday performance can reduce the relationship between competence and performance to a substantial degree. Finally, in performance-based measures, the subject must participate actively in the assessment process, and poor motivation or uncooperativeness could lead to low scores.

The Limitations of Self-Reporting of Functional Disability in Schizophrenia

It has long been known that people who have schizophrenia manifest reduced awareness of the presence and significance of their psychotic symptoms [113]. Despite this finding, many rating scales for functional outcomes are designed to collect self-reported information from people who have schizophrenia about their functioning, including self-evaluation of social functioning and complex features of occupational and everyday living skills. Several recent studies have suggested that this method may be a problematic way to assess functioning. For instance, McKibbin and colleagues [114] found that the correlation between self-reported illness burden and self-reported disability was quite substantial, but neither of these self reports correlated with either the patient's neuropsychologic performance or performance on a measure of functional capacity. Keefe and colleagues [115] found that correlation between self-reported cognitive deficits and performance on a neuropsychologic assessment was .04 in a sample of schizophrenia patients. In contrast, an informant rating of cognitive impairment, provided by someone who was unaware of the patient's neuropsychologic performance, was correlated .40 with neuropsychologic performance. The single largest correlate of neuropsychologic performance was the performance-based measure of functional capacity. In another study [116], patients who had schizophrenia and their case managers were asked to complete the same rating scale for everyday functioning, and the patients also underwent an assessment of neuropsychologic and functional capacity. For every domain of functioning examined, the case manager's reports and the patient's reports were poorly correlated, and only in the area of personal care (activities of daily living) were the correlations even statistically significant. When correlations between case manager and self reports, neuropsychologic performance, and functional capacity were calculated, the case manger report was more strongly correlated with the external validators for every functional domain.

These data suggest that self reports by people who have schizophrenia are less reliable than the reports of specific informants,. On the surface these findings also suggest that requiring reports from informed observers, such as psychiatric case managers or caregiver relatives, would be a more appropriate strategy. Caregivers' ratings have advantages over self-reporting measures in that the caregivers' insight, memory, and assessment may be more accurate than that of the patient. Moreover, these assessments, if done by family members, allow the rating of behaviors that treatment providers rarely have opportunity to observe. Caregiver-rated scales and information provided by caregivers can be problematic, however, because different observers base their responses on different behavioral samples, spend differing amounts of time with the subject, and may have different standards for appropriate performance. These differences among caregivers can create considerable variability in measurement. Moreover, as many as one third to one half of patients are not able to name a person who can supply this type of information [117].

One exception to the lack of appropriate informants may be patients who live in supervised residences, such as locked board-and-care homes, nursing homes, or long-stay psychiatric hospitals. Several studies have reported high levels of interrater reliability and convergent validity with these ratings on scales designed for institutionalized patients [106,118]. Even those ratings can be flawed, however, and it cannot be assumed that because the staff knows the patient well that they will generate valid ratings. Bowie and colleagues [119] found that clinical staff ratings and clinical researcher ratings of the same patients in nursing home care were very poorly correlated. Because the clinical researcher's ratings of disability were more strongly correlated with neuropsychologic performance than the ratings of the clinical staff, it can be assumed that the researcher ratings had greater validity.

Suggestions for Assessment of Functional Disability

It is important to measure both potential and achievement in patients who have schizophrenia. The authors suggest that researchers should consider how best to measure disability and reduction of disability directly. There are several means for doing so, and performance-based measures of functional capacity in the domains of social, vocational, and everyday living skills may be critical for accurate assessment of potential. Whenever possible, multiple sources of information should be considered in the assessment of everyday disability. The research reviewed previously suggests that clinicians who have extensive contact with patients, such as case managers, are among the best sources for these reports. At the same time, relatives can provide perspectives on patient behavior that may not be available to outpatient clinicians. Finally, reliance on self-reporting alone by people who have schizophrenia is a strategy with many flaws. The extremely low correlation between self-reported disability and other indices of disability such as observer ratings and performance-based measures, even in areas that would be considered quite objective and measurable (eg, hours worked during a week), suggests that the information collected from uncorroborated self reports may not be useful. Feasible performance-based measures have been developed, and normative standards are being published to make these assessments applicable in clinical practice. At the same time, not all these methods would be directly accessible to practicing psychiatrists.

In the interim, there are several suggestions. Vocational rehabilitation assessment provides excellent information on occupational and everyday living skills. Careful direct observation of patient's social skills provides excellent information about social competence, because the way that a patient communicates and interacts has considerable influence on the way that he or she is perceived by other members of the community. Obtaining as much information as possible from multiple sources will provide wide-ranging information about a patient's competencies, and areas of inconsistency between observers or over time with the same rater may provide valid information regarding variability in behavior across situations and over time.

THE ASSESSMENT OF NEGATIVE SYMPTOMS
Dimensional Assessment
The term "negative symptoms" refers to the absence or decrease of normal behaviors. A Consensus Development Conference sponsored by the US National Institute of Mental Health concluded that negative symptoms include blunted affect, poverty of speech, asociality, anhedonia, and avolition [120]. Rating scales for negative symptoms usually include measures of blunted affect, poverty of speech, and some variety of social dysfunction. These scales, however, may vary substantially with regard to other items and domains. The scores on these scales are the basis for conclusions about the efficacy of treatments for negative symptoms. Therefore careful consideration is warranted to understand what treatment studies can and cannot tell about the treatment of negative symptoms.

This discussion concentrates on the two most widely used negative symptom rating scales, the negative syndrome scale of the PANSS [48] and the SANS [40]. Several aspects of these scales have been discussed previously. Both include measures of blunted affect and poverty of speech, and there is some similarity between other SANS subscales and PANSS items as well (Table 1). This apparent similarity conceals important differences. For

Table 1
Item overlap in the Positive and Negative Syndrome Scale (PANSS) and the Scale for the Assessment of Negative Symptoms (SANS)

PANSS Negative Syndrome Scale Items	SANS Subscales
Blunted affect	Affective flattening or blunting
Lack of spontaneity and flow of conversation	Alogia
Passive/apathetic social withdrawal	Anhedonia/asociality
	Avolition/apathy
Difficulty in abstract thinking	Attention
Stereotyped thinking	
Emotional withdrawal	
Poor rapport	

instance, poverty of content of speech is part of the SANS alogia subscale, but no similar item is present in the PANSS. Similarly, the SANS attention subscale is not the same as the difficulty in abstract thinking and stereotyped thinking items found in the PANSS. This item (Poor Attention) is found in the PANSS in the General Psychopathology Subscale. A fairly high correlation has been found between SANS and PANSS total scores [43], but the reason for this correlation, given the differences in scale items, is not clear. Perhaps negative symptoms include items broader than the items in either of these scales, and so the many items on these scales truly co-vary. It may be, however, that there is a halo effect within each scale, so that scores on the blunted affect and poverty of speech items heavily influence the ratings on the other items in these scales. That is, much of the agreement across the scales may result from the presence of blunted affect and poverty on both. Another anomaly of these scales is that there is not a high degree of agreement when they are used to classify individual patients as having a negative symptom syndrome (ie, high versus low negative symptoms) [39,56] despite the high correlation between their total scores.

Two consensus development groups have commented on an important shortcoming of the performance of these scales in the context of treatment trials, namely the problem of "pseudospecificity." The items in these scales are liable to change as depression and psychotic symptoms change. (A more detailed discussion of this issue can be found in [121].) Because depressive symptoms tend to improve as psychotic symptoms improve during recovery from an acute exacerbation of psychosis, negative symptom scale ratings are likely to improve with recovery as well, simply because of the improvements in these other symptoms. Thus, in the context of a treatment trial with an antipsychotic, a change in a negative symptom may be secondary to these other changes. More generally, even outside the context of improvement in a clinical trial, negative symptom scores may often reflect impairments caused by depression, anxiety, psychotic confusion, suspicious withdrawal, distracting hallucinations, and other problems.

These negative symptoms have been referred to as "secondary" negative symptoms.

The apathetic, unemotional patient is the patient that typically comes to mind in discussions of negative symptoms. Kraepelin [122] described this patient's impairment as "a weakening of . . . the mainsprings of volition." Because of the pseudospecificity problem, however—that is, because of the impact of depression, psychotic symptoms, and other potential confounders on negative symptom rating scales—these scales measure something much broader. Therefore, it usually is not possible to know from the results of a trial stating that a treatment has efficacy for negative symptoms, whether there is improvement in the apathy syndrome found in schizophrenia, because the change in rating scale scores may result from improvement in other symptoms. If the trial has a specific study design, the conclusion that the apathy syndrome has improved is more certain. Such a trial needs to study clinically stable patients with relatively minimal psychotic, depressive symptoms and extrapyramidal symptoms who exhibit negative symptoms despite antipsychotic treatment [120,121,123]. In this way, changes in psychotic and depressive symptoms cannot confound the change in negative symptoms.

In an effort to minimize the problem of secondary negative symptoms that are caused by psychotic and depressive symptoms, and to make other improvements in the rating of negative symptoms, the NIMH is sponsoring a project to develop a new negative symptom rating scale. This scale will include items for the five symptom areas noted previously, namely, blunted affect, poverty of speech, asociality, anhedonia, and avolition.

Categorical Assessment

Another approach to the study of negative symptoms is to make a diagnosis, separating unemotional, apathetic patients whose negative symptoms are stable and not caused by psychotic symptoms, depression, or other dysphoria from patients whose negative symptoms are likely to be secondary to these factors. This approach is not based on a change measure, although it could be used to determine who would enter treatment trials for negative symptoms and thereby facilitate the study design, outlined previously, that could be used to determine efficacy for "true" negative symptoms.

Research on deficit/nondeficit categorization [124] has been based on this approach of diagnosing patients who have schizophrenia with true or primary negative symptoms [125] (ie, those whose negative symptoms are not caused by psychotic symptoms, depression, or other problems) from patients whose symptoms are caused by these other problems. The group with primary or idiopathic negative symptoms are said to have "deficit schizophrenia"; schizophrenics patients who do not have primary negative symptoms are termed "nondeficit." Deficit and nondeficit groups have been shown to differ in signs and symptoms (other than negative symptoms), course of illness, biologic correlates, treatment response, and etiologic factors [126–128]. There is evidence that the negative symptoms of the deficit group are refractory to treatment with clozapine, olanzapine, and psychosocial treatment [129–131]. Improvement of the negative symptoms of this group would be the acid test for efficacious treatment of negative symptoms.

References

[1] Andreasen NC, Arndt S, Miller D, et al. Correlational studies of the Scale for the Assessment of Negative Symptoms and the Scale for the Assessment of Positive Symptoms: an overview and update. Psychopathology 1995;28(1):7–17.

[2] Liddle PF. The symptoms of chronic schizophrenia. A re-examination of the positive-negative dichotomy. Br J Psychiatry 1987;151:145–51.

[3] Peralta V, de Leon J, Cuesta MJ. Are there more than two syndromes in schizophrenia? A critique of the positive-negative dichotomy. Br J Psychiatry 1992;161:335–43.

[4] Lindenmayer JP, Bernstein-Hyman R, Grochowski S. Five-factor model of schizophrenia. Initial validation. J Nerv Ment Dis 1994;182(11):631–8.

[5] Lindenmayer JP, Brown E, Baker RW, et al. A multisite, multimodel evaluation of the factorial structure of the Positive and Negative Syndrome Scale. J Nerv Ment Dis 180(11):723–8.

[6] Lindenmayer JP, Bernstein-Hyman R, Grochowski S, et al. Psychopathology of schizophrenia: initial validation of a 5-factor model. Psychopathology 1995;28(1):22–31.

[7] Marder SR, Davis JM, Chouinard G. The effects of risperidone on the five dimensions of schizophrenia derived by factor analysis: combined results of the North American trials. J Clin Psychiatry 1997;58(12):538–46 [Erratum in: J Clin Psychiatry 1998;59(4):200].

[8] White L, Harvey PD, Opler L, et al. Empirical assessment of the factorial structure of clinical symptoms in schizophrenia. A multisite, multimodel evaluation of the factorial structure of the Positive and Negative Syndrome Scale. The PANSS Study Group. Psychopathology 1997;30(5):263–74.

[9] Toomey R, Kremen WS, Simpson JC, et al. Revisiting the factor structure for positive and negative symptoms: evidence from a large heterogeneous group of psychiatric patients. Am J Psychiatry 1997;154(3):371–7.

[10] Tuominen K, Lonnqvist J, Addington D, et al. The Schizophrenia Suicide Risk Scale (SSRS): development and initial validation. Schizophr Res 2001;47(2–3):199–213.

[11] Woerner MG, Mannuzza S, Kane JM. Anchoring the BPRS: an aid to improved reliability. Psychopharmacol Bull 1998;24:112–7.

[12] Young RC, Biggs JT, Ziegler VE, et al. A rating scale for mania: reliability, validity and sensitivity. Br J Psychiatry 1978;133:429–35.

[13] Yudofsky SC, Silver JM, Jackson W, et al. Overt Aggression Scale: preliminary results. J Neuropsychiatry Clin Neurosci 1986;3(2):S52–6.

[14] Overall JE, Gorham DR. The Brief Psychiatric Rating Scale. Psychol Rep 1962;10: 790–812.

[15] Overall JE. In: Pichot, editor. Psychological measurements in psychopharmacology, modern problems of pharmacopsychiatry, vol. 7. Basel (Switzerland): S Karger; 1974. p. 67–78.

[16] Peralta V, Cuesta MJ. How many and which are the psychopathological dimensions in schizophrenia? Issues influencing their ascertainment. Schizophr Res 2001; 30;49(3):269–85.

[17] Peralta V, de Leon J, Cuesta MJ. Are there more than two syndromes in schizophrenia? A critique of the positive-negative dichotomy. Br J Psychiatry 1987;161:335–43.

[18] Petterson U, Fyro B, Sedvall G. A new scale for the longitudinal rating of manic states. Acta Psychiatr Scand 1973;49(3):248–56.

[19] Lukoff D, Liberman RP, Nuechterlein KH. Symptom monitoring in the rehabilitation of schizophrenic patients. Schizophr Bull 1986;12:578–602.

[20] Lykouras L, Oulis P, Psarros K, et al. Five-factor model of schizophrenic psychopathology: how valid is it? Eur Arch Psychiatry Clin Neurosci 2000;250(2):93–100.

[21] Sajatovic M, Bingham CR, Garver D, et al. An assessment of clinical practice of clozapine therapy for veterans. Psychiatric Svcs 2000;51(5):669–71.

[22] Bech P, Kastrup M, Raraelsen OJ. Mini-compendium of rating scales for states of anxiety, depression, mania, and schizophrenia with corresponding DSM-III syndromes. Acta Psychiatr Scand 1986;83(Suppl 326):7–37.

[23] Gabbard GO, Coyne L, Kennedy LL, et al. Inter-rater reliability in the use of the Brief Psychiatric Rating Scale. Bull Menninger Clin 1987;51:519–31.

[24] McGorry PD, Goodwin RJ, Stuart GW. The development, use, and reliability of the Brief Psychiatric Rating Scale (nursing modification)—an assessment procedure for the nursing team in clinical and research settings. Compr Psychiatry 1988;29:575–87.

[25] Woerner MG, Mannuzza S, Kane JM. Anchoring the BPRS: an aid to improved reliability. Psychopharmacol Bull 1988;24(1):112–7.

[26] Bech P, Malt VF, Dencker SJ, et al. Scales for assessment of diagnosis and severity of mental disorders. Acta Psychiatr Scand 1993;87(Suppl 372):35–40.

[27] Andersen J, Larsen JK, Schultz V, et al. The Brief Psychiatric Rating Scale. Dimension of schizophrenia—reliability and construct validity. Psychopathology 1989;22: 168–76.

[28] Hedlund JL, Vieweg BW. The Brief Psychiatric Rating Scale (BPRS): a comprehensive review. Journal of Operational Psychiatry 1980;11:48–65.

[29] Faustman WO. Brief Psychiatric Rating Scale. In: Maruish ME, editor. The use of psychological testing for treatment planning and outcome assessment. Hillsdale (NJ); 1994. p. 371–401.

[30] Kane JM, Honigfeld G, Singer J, et al. Clozapine for the treatment-resistant schizophrenic. A double-blind comparison with chlorpromazine. Arch Gen Psychiatry 1988;45:789–96.

[31] Marder SR, Meibach RC. Risperidone in the treatment of schizophrenia. Am J Psychiatry 1994;151:825–35.

[32] Mass R, Schoemig T, Hitschfeld K, et al. Psychopathological syndromes of schizophrenia: evaluation of the dimensional structure of the Positive and Negative Syndrome Scale. Schizophr Bull 2000;26:167–77.

[33] McGlashan TH, Fenton WS. The positive-negative distinction in schizophrenia. Review of natural history validators. Arch Gen Psychiatry 1992;49(1):63–72.

[34] Arvanitis LA, Miller BG, Seroquel Trial 13 Study Group. Multiple fixed doses of 'Seroquel' (quetiapine) in patients with acute exacerbation of schizophrenia: a comparison with haloperidol and placebo. Biol Psychiatry 1997;42:233–46.

[35] Small JG, Hirsch SR, Arvanitis LA, et al. Quetiapine in patients with schizophrenia. A high- and low-dose comparison with placebo. Arch Gen Psychiatry 1997;54:549–57.

[36] Sorgi P, Ratey J, Knoedler DW, et al. Rating aggression in the clinical setting. A retrospective adaptation of the Overt Aggression Scale: preliminary results. J Neuropsychiatry Clin Neurosci 1991;3(2):S52–6.

[37] Beasley CM, Tollefson GD, Tran P, et al. Olanzapine versus haloperidol and placebo. Acute phase results of the American double-blind olanzapine trial. Neuropsychopharmacology 1996;14:111–23.

[38] Peuskens J, Link CGG. A comparison of quetiapine and chlorpromazine in the treatment of schizophrenia. Acta Psychiatr Scand 1997;96:265–73.

[39] Gur RE, Mozley PD, Resnick SM, et al. Relations among clinical scales in schizophrenia. Am J Psychiatry 1991;148(4):472–8.

[40] Andreasen NC. Negative symptoms in schizophrenia. Definition and reliability. Arch Gen Psychiatry 1982;39(7):784–8.

[41] Andreasen NC. The Scale for Assessment of Positive Symptoms. Iowa City (IA): University of Iowa; 1984.

[42] Andreasen NC, Flaum M, Arndt S. The Comprehensive Assessment of Symptoms and History (CASH): an instrument for assessing psychopathology and diagnosis. Arch Gen Psychiarty 1992;49:615–23.

[43] Norman RM, Malla AK, Cortese L, et al. A study of the interrelationship between and comparative interrater reliability of the SAPS, SANS and PANSS. Schizophr Res 1996;19(1): 73–85.

[44] Andreasen NC. The scale for assessment of negative symptoms. Iowa City (IA): University of Iowa; 1984.

[45] Mueser KT, Sayers SL, Schooler NR, et al. A multisite investigation of the reliability of the Scale for the Assessment of Negative Symptoms. Am J Psychiatry 1994;151(10): 1453–62.

[46] Andreasen NC, Grove WM. Thought, language, and communication in schizophrenia: diagnosis and prognosis. Schizophr Bull 1986;12(3):348–59.

[47] Kay SR, Opler LA, Lindenmayer JP. Reliability and validity of the positive and negative syndrome scale for schizophrenics. Psychiatry Res 1988;23(1):99–110.

[48] Kay SR, Fiszbein A, Opler LA. The Positive and Negative Syndrome Scale (PANSS) for schizophrenia. Schizophr Bull 1987;13(2):261–76.

[49] Bell M, Milstein R, Beam-Goulet J, et al. The Positive and Negative Syndrome Scale and the Brief Psychiatric Rating Scale. Reliability, comparability, and predictive validity. 1992;180(11):723–8.

[50] Kay SR. Positive-negative symptom assessment in schizophrenia: psychometric issues and scale comparison. Psychiatr Q 1990;61(3):163–78.

[51] Lindenmayer JP, Czobor P, Volavka J, et al. Effects of atypical antipsychotics on the syndromal profile in treatment-resistant schizophrenia. J Clin Psychiatry 2004;65(4):551–6.

[52] Kay SR, Opler LA, Lindenmayer JP. The Positive and Negative Syndrome Scale (PANSS): rationale and standardisation. Br J Psychiatry Suppl 1989;Nov(7):59–67.

[53] Singh MM, Kay SR. Is the positive-negative distinction in schizophrenia valid? Br J Psychiatry 1987;150:879–80.

[54] Opler LA, Kay SR, Lindenmayer J, et al. SCI-PANSS. Toronto: Multi-Health Systems Inc; 1992.

[55] Fields JH, Grochowski S, Lindenmayer JP, et al. Assessing positive and negative symptoms in children and adolescents. Am J Psychiatry 1994;151(2):249–53.

[56] Fenton WS, McGlashan TH. Testing systems for assessment of negative symptoms in schizophrenia. Arch Gen Psychiatry 1992;49(3):179–84.

[57] Alphs LD, Summerfelt A, Lann H, et al. The negative symptom assessment: a new instrument to assess negative symptoms of schizophrenia. Psychopharmacol Bull 1989;25(2): 159–63.

[58] American Psychiatric Association. Diagnostic and statistical manual of mental disorders 4th edition (DSM–IV). Washington, DC: American Psychiatric Associaton; 1994.

[59] Stahl SM, Alphs L. Negative symptom assessment: a clinical tool for negative symptoms of schizophrenia. San Diego (CA): Neuroscience Education Institute Press; 2006.

[60] Stauffer VL. An excitement subscale of the Positive and Negative Syndrome Scale. Schizophr Res 2004;68(2–3):331–7.

[61] Guy W. Clinical global impression. ECDEU assessment manual for psychopharmacology, revised. Rockville (MD): National Institute of Mental Health; 1976.

[62] Spearing MK, Post RM, Leverich GS, et al. Modification of the Clinical Global Impression scale for use in bipolar illness (BP): the CGI-BP. Psychiatry Res 1997;73:159–71.

[63] Leon AC, Shear K, Klerman GL, et al. A comparison of symptom determinants of patient and clinical global ratings in patients with panic disorder and depression. J Clin Psychopharmacol 1993;13:327–31.

[64] Dahlke F, Lohaus A, Gutzmann H. Reliability and clinical concepts underlying global judgments in dementia: implications for clinical research. Psychopharmacol Bull 1992;28(4): 425–32.

[65] Double DB. The factor structure of manic rating scales. J Affect Disord 1990;18:113–9.
[66] Weitkunat R, Letzel H, Kanowski S, et al. Clinical and psychometric evaluation of the efficacy of nootropic drugs: characteristics of several procedures. Zeitschrift für Gerontopsychologie undpsychiatrie 1993;61:51–60.
[67] Beneke M, Rasmus W. "Clinical Global Impressions" (ECDEU): some critical comments. Pharmacopsychiatry 1992;25(4):171–6.
[68] Haro JM, Kamath SA, Ochoa S, et al. on behalf of the SOHO Study Group. The global impression-schizophrenia scale: a simple instrument to measure the diversity of symptoms present in schizophrenia. Acta Psychiatr Scand 2003;107(Suppl 416):16–23.
[69] Collaborative Working Group on Clinical Trial Evaluations. Collaborative Working Group on Clinical Trial Evaluations. Atypical antipsychotics for treatment of depression in schizophrenia and affective disorders. J Clin Psychiatry 1998;59(Suppl 12):41–5.
[70] Addington D, Addington J, Atkinson M. A psychometric comparison of the Calgary Depression Scale for Schizophrenia and the Hamilton Depression Rating Scale. Schizophr Res 1996;19:205–12.
[71] Collins AA, Remington G, Coulter K, et al. Depression in schizophrenia: a comparison of three measures. Schizophr Res 1996;20:205–9.
[72] Yazaji El, Battas O, Agoub M, et al. Validity of the depressive dimension extracted from principal component analysis of the PANSS in drug-free patients with schizophrenia. Schizophr Res 2002;56:121–7.
[73] Endicott J, Tracy K, Burt D, et al. A novel approach to assess inter-rater reliability in the use of the Overt Aggression Scale-Modified. Psychiatry Res 2002;112(2):153–9.
[74] Reine G, Bernard D, Lancon C. Depression scales in schizophrenia: a critical review. Encephale 1998;24:530–40.
[75] Lancon C, Auquier P, Reine G, et al. Evaluation of depression in schizophrenia: psychometric properties of a French version of the Calgary Depression Scale. Psychiatry Res 1999;89:123–32.
[76] Müller MJ, Marx-Dannigkeit P, Schlosser R, et al. The Calgary Depression Rating Scale for Schizophrenia: development and interrater reliability of a German version (CDSS-G). J Psychiatr Res 1999;33:433–43.
[77] Reine G, Bernard D, Auquier P, et al. Psychometric properties of French version of the Calgary Depression Scale for Schizophrenia (CDSS). Encephale 2000;26:52–61.
[78] Sarro S, Duenas RM, Ramirez N, et al. Cross-cultural adaptation and validation of the Spanish version of the Calgary Depression Scale for Schizophrenia. Schizophr Res 2004;68:349–55.
[79] Bernard D, Lancon C, Auquier P, et al. The Calgary Depression Scale for Schizophrenia: a study of the validity of a French-language version in a population of schizophrenic patients. Acta Psychiatr Scand 1998;97:36–41.
[80] Coccaro EF, Harvey PD, Kupsaw-Lawrence E, et al. Development of neuropharmacologically based behavioral assessments of impulsive aggressive behavior. J Neuropsychiatry Clin Neurosci 1991;3(2):S44–51.
[81] Addington D, Addington J, Maticka-Tyndale E. Specificity of the Calgary Depression Scale for Schizophrenia. Schizophr Res 1994;11:239–44.
[82] Kontaxakis VP, Havaki-Kontaxaki BJ, Stamouli SS, et al. Comparison of four scales measuring depression in schizophrenic inpatients. Eur Psychiatry 2000;15:274–7.
[83] Lancon C, Auquier P, Reine G, et al. Study of the concurrent validity of the Calgary Depression Scale for Schizophrenics (CDSS). J Affect Disord 2000;58:107–15.
[84] Müller MJ, Kienzle B, Dahmen N. Depression, emotional blunting, and akinesia in schizophrenia: overlap and differentiation. Eur J Health Econ 2002;3:S99–103.
[85] Müller MJ. Overlap between emotional blunting, depression, and extrapyramidal symptoms in schizophrenia. Schizophr Res 2002;57:307–9.
[86] Kontaxakis VP, Havaki-Kontaxaki BJ, Margariti MM, et al. The Greek version of the calgary depression scale for schizophrenia. Psychiatry Res 2000;94(2):163–71.

[87] Lancon C, Auquier P, Reine G, et al. Relationships between depression and psychotic symptoms of schizophrenia during an acute episode and stable period. Schizophr Res 2001;47:135–40.

[88] Addington D, Addington J, Maticka-Tyndale E. Assessing depression in schizophrenia: the Calgary Depression Scale. Br J Psychiatry 1993;163(Suppl 22):39–44.

[89] Addington D, Addington J, Maticka-Tyndale E, et al. Reliability and validity of a depression rating scale for schizophrenics. Schizophr Res 1992;6:201–8.

[90] Addington D, Addington J, Schissel B. A depression rating scale for schizophrenics. Schizophr Res 1990;3:247–51.

[91] Lindenmayer JP, Czobor P, Alphs L, , et al. InterSePT Study Group. The InterSePT scale for suicidal thinking reliability and validity. Schizophr Res 2003;63(1–2):161–70.

[92] Taiminen T, Huttunen J, Heila H, et al. The Overt Aggression Scale for the objective rating of verbal and physical aggression. Am J Psychiatry 1986;143(1):35–9.

[93] Beck RW, Morris J, Lester D. Suicide notes and risk of future suicide. JAMA 1974;228(4): 495–6.

[94] Beck RW, Morris JB, Beck AT. Cross-validation of the Suicidal Intent Scale. Psychol Rep 1974;34(2):445–6.

[95] Hansen L, Kingdon D. Rating suicidality in schizophrenia: items on global scales (HoNOS and CPRS) correlate with a validated suicidality rating scale (InterSePT). Arch Suicide Res 2006;10(3):249–52.

[96] Holzman PS, Shenton ME, Solovay MR. Quality of thought disorder in differential diagnosis. Schizophr Bull 1986;12(3):360–71.

[97] Subotnik KL, Bartzokis G, Green MF, et al. Neuroanatomical correlates of formal thought disorder in schizophrenia. Cognit Neuropsychiatry 2003;8(2):81–8.

[98] Bond GR, Drake RE, Mueser KT, et al. An update on supported employment in schizophrenia. Psychiatr Serv 1997;48:335–46.

[99] Becker DR, Drake RE, Bond GR, et al. Job terminations among persons with severe mental illness participating in supported employment. Community Ment Health J 1998;34: 71–82.

[100] Mueser KT, Salyers MP, Mueser PR. A prospective analysis of work in schizophrenia. Schizophr Bull 2001;27(2):281–96.

[101] Sharma T, Antonova G. Cognitive function in schizophrenia. Deficits, functional consequences, and future treatment. Psychiatr Clin North Am 2003;26:25–40.

[102] Velligan DI, Mahurin RK, Diamond PL, et al. The functional significance of symptomatology and cognitive function in schizophrenia. Schizophr Res 1997;25:21–31.

[103] Velligan DI, Bow-Thomas CC, Huntzinger CD, et al. A randomized controlled trial of the use of compensatory strategies to enhance adaptive functioning in outpatients with schizophrenia. Am J Psychiatry 2000;157:1317–23.

[104] Dickerson FB, Ringel NB, Parente F. Subjective quality of life in out-patients with schizophrenia: clinical and utilization correlates. Acta Psychiatr Scand 1998;98: 124–7.

[105] Jaeger J, Berns SM, Szobor P. The multidimensional scale of independent functioning: a new instrument for measuring functional disability in psychiatric populations. Schizophr Bull 2003;29:153–68.

[106] Harvey PD, Howanitz E, Parrella M, et al. Symptoms, cognitive functioning, and adaptive skills in geriatric patients with lifelong schizophrenia: a comparison across treatment sites. Am J Psychiatry 1998;155:1080–6.

[107] Horan WP, Subotnik KL, Snyder KS, et al. Do recent-onset schizophrenia patients experience a "social network crisis"? Psychiatry 2006;69:115–29.

[108] Murray CJL, Lopez AD. Global mortality, disability, and the contributions of risk factors: global burden of disease study. Lancet 1997;349:1436–42.

[109] Murray CJL, Lopez AD. Alternative projections of mortality and disability by cause 1990–2020: global burden of disease study. Lancet 1997;349:1498–504.

[110] Bowie CR, Reichenberg A, Patterson TL, et al. Determinants of real world functional performance in schizophrenia: correlations with cognition, functional capacity, and symptoms. Am J Psychiatry 2006;163:418–25.
[111] Koren D, Seidman LJ, Poyurovsky M. The neuropsychological basis of insight in first-episode schizophrenia: a pilot metacognitive study. Schizophr Res 2004;70(2-3): 195–2021.
[112] Koren D, Poyurovsky M, Seidman LJ. The neuropsychological basis of competence to consent in first-episode schizophrenia: a pilot metacognitive study. Biol Psychiatry 2005;576: 609–16.
[113] Amador XF, Strauss DH, Yale SA, et al. Assessment of insight in psychosis. Am J Psychiatry 1993;150:873–9.
[114] McKibbin C, Patterson TL, Jeste DV. Assessing disability in older patients with schizophrenia: results from the WHODAS-II. J Nerv Ment Dis 2004;192:405–13.
[115] Keefe RSE, Poe M, Walker TM, et al. The Schizophrenia Cognition Rating Scale SCoRS: interview based assessment and its relationship to cognition, real world functioning and functional capacity. Am J Psychiatry 2006;163:426–32.
[116] Bowie CR, Twamley EW, Anderson H, et al. Self-assessment of functional status in schizophrenia. J Psychiatr Res 2006 Sep 30; [Epub ahead of print].
[117] Patterson TL, Semple SJ, Shaw WS, et al. Researching the caregiver: family members who care for older psychotic patients. Psychiatr Ann 1996;26:772–84.
[118] Harvey PD, Davidson M, Mueser KT, et al. Social-Adaptive Functioning Evaluation (SAFE): a rating scale for geriatric psychiatric patients. Schizophr Bull 1997;23:131–45.
[119] Bowie CR, Fallon C, Harvey PD. Convergence of clinical staff ratings and research ratings to assess patients with schizophrenia in nursing homes. Psychiatr Serv 2006;57: 838–43.
[120] Kirkpatrick B, Fenton WS, Carpenter WT Jr, et al. The NIMH-MATRICS consensus statement on negative symptoms. Schizophr Bull 2006;32(2):214–9.
[121] Kirkpatrick B, Kopelowicz A, Buchanan RW, et al. Assessing the efficacy of treatments for the deficit syndrome of schizophrenia. Neuropsychopharmacology 2000;22(3):303–10.
[122] Kraepelin E. Dementia praecox and paraphrenia. Melbourne (FL): Krieger Publishing Co; 1971 [originally published in 1919].
[123] Moller HJ, van Praag HM, Aufdembrinke B, et al. Negative symptoms in schizophrenia: considerations for clinical trials. Working group on negative symptoms in schizophrenia. Psychopharmacology (Berl) 1994;115(1–2):221–8.
[124] Kirkpatrick B, Buchanan RW, McKenney PD, et al. The schedule for the deficit syndrome: an instrument for research in schizophrenia. Psychiatry Res 1989;30(2):119–23.
[125] Carpenter WT Jr, Heinrichs DW, Wagman AM. Deficit and nondeficit forms of schizophrenia: the concept. Am J Psychiatry 1988;145(5):578–83.
[126] Dickerson F, Kirkpatrick B, Boronow J, et al. Deficit schizophrenia: association with serum antibodies to cytomegalovirus. Schizophr Bull 2006;32(2):396–400.
[127] Kirkpatrick B, Buchanan RW, Ross DE, et al. A separate disease within the syndrome of schizophrenia. Arch Gen Psychiatry 2001;58(2):165–71.
[128] Messias E, Kirkpatrick B, Bromet E, et al. Summer birth and deficit schizophrenia: a pooled analysis from 6 countries. Arch Gen Psychiatry 2004;61(10):985–9.
[129] Buchanan RW, Breier A, Kirkpatrick B, et al. Positive and negative symptom response to clozapine in schizophrenic patients with and without the deficit syndrome. Am J Psychiatry 1998;155(6):751–60.
[130] Kopelowicz A, Liberman RP, Mintz J, et al. Comparison of efficacy of social skills training for deficit and nondeficit negative symptoms in schizophrenia. Am J Psychiatry 1997;154(3):424–5.
[131] Kopelowicz A, Zarate R, Tripodis K, et al. Differential efficacy of olanzapine for deficit and nondeficit negative symptoms in schizophrenia. Am J Psychiatry 2000;157(6): 987–93.

Psychiatr Clin N Am 30 (2007) 365–399

PSYCHIATRIC CLINICS
OF NORTH AMERICA

ELSEVIER
SAUNDERS

Functional Genomics and Schizophrenia: Endophenotypes and Mutant Models

John L. Waddington, PhD, DSc[a,b,*],
Aiden P. Corvin, MRCPsych, PhD[c],
Gary Donohoe, DClinPsych[c], Colm M.P. O'Tuathaigh, PhD[a],
Kevin J. Mitchell, PhD[d], Michael Gill, MRCPsych, MD[c]

[a]Molecular & Cellular Therapeutics, Royal College of Surgeons in Ireland, Dublin 2, Ireland
[b]Cavan-Monaghan Mental Health Service, St. Davnet's Hospital, Monaghan, Ireland
[c]Department of Psychiatry, Trinity Centre for Health Sciences, Trinity College, St. James's Hospital, Dublin 8, Ireland
[d]Smurfit Institute of Genetics, Trinity College, Dublin 2, Ireland

Schizophrenia is a complex genetic disorder, the expression of which likely involves the interplay of multiple susceptibility genes, epigenetic factors, and environmental influences [1–6]. Recent progress in identifying and investigating the function of schizophrenia candidate genes is beginning to provide insights into cellular systems potentially involved in the disorder. This article reviews traditional and evolving methods of gene discovery, with a focus on the functional investigation of these genes. These procedures involve an impressive array of methodologies under the rubric functional genomics and range from molecular and cellular to clinical research, complemented by studies probing the functionality of these genes in mutant mice with targeted gene deletion. Integrating these data will inform the understanding of the molecular mechanisms involved in schizophrenia, will shape how the disorder might be defined in the future, and may answer wider questions about mental illness and human cognition.

This article summarizes the rationale, methods, and results of gene discovery programs in schizophrenia research and describes functional methods of investigating potential candidate genes. It focuses next on the most prominent current candidate genes and describes (1) the evidence for their association with schizophrenia and research into the function of each gene; (2) investigation

This work was supported by grants 02-IN1-B227 (JLW), 01-F1-B006 (KJM) and 02-IN1-B113 (MG) from Science Foundation Ireland. KJM is an EMBO Young Investigator.

*Corresponding author. Molecular & Cellular Therapeutics, Royal College of Surgeons in Ireland, Dublin 2, Ireland. E-mail address: jwadding@rcsi.ie (J.L. Waddington).

0193-953X/07/$ – see front matter
doi:10.1016/j.psc.2007.04.011
© 2007 Elsevier Inc. All rights reserved.
psych.theclinics.com

of the clinical phenotypes and endophenotypes associated with each gene, at the levels of psychopathologic, neurocognitive, electrophysiologic, neuroimaging, and neuropathologic findings; and (3) research into the ethologic, cognitive, social, and psychopharmacologic phenotype of mutants with targeted deletion of each gene at issue. It examines gene–gene and gene–environment interactions. Finally, it looks at future directions for research.

GENE DISCOVERY

The heritability of schizophrenia is substantial, but the etiology of the disorder is poorly understood [7]. With the emergence of molecular genetic and genomic methodologies, identifying the genes involved became a research priority, primarily as a prerequisite for understanding both cellular pathogenesis and gene–environment interaction. Positional cloning methods (linkage studies, cytogenetics, and association analyses) offered powerful tools for gene identification. Rather than depending on existing hypotheses (eg, targeting genes involved in dopamine metabolism), a hypothesis-free approach could be applied based on the coinheritance of genetic markers and disease within affected families (ie, genetic linkage analysis) or within populations (ie, genetic association analysis). These approaches aim to identify chromosomal loci or genes containing risk variants, which then can be investigated using fine-mapping and association analysis in families or case-control samples for positional cloning of the gene. A similar strategy can be used to follow up on chromosomal rearrangements identified through cytogenetic studies. These top-down approaches to gene discovery are indicated in Fig. 1.

More than 30 genome-wide linkage studies now have been reported, and significant linkage signals have emerged from several individual studies and from two meta-analyses of multiple studies [8,9]. This finding is surprising given that genes subsequently identified at several of these loci have modest effect sizes, may involve multiple risk variants at each gene (ie, allelic heterogeneity), and may contribute to susceptibility in certain populations but not in others. Indeed, at each of these loci the effect size subsequently reported for the associated variants was insufficient to account for the linkage signal in the families, suggesting that multiple risk variants or more than one susceptibility gene may be involved at each locus. By corollary, this finding also suggests that more modest genetic effects may evade detection using linkage paradigms in the family samples available.

Chromosomal abnormalities such as insertions, deletions, or translocations can disrupt gene function resulting in clinical disorders. Identifying such abnormalities is an opportunistic method for establishing loci that contribute to the risk of illness, but chromosomal abnormalities can occur in the general population with no adverse phenotypic consequence. In trying to infer causation, geneticists seek to identify abnormality either cosegregating with the disorder in affected families or coexisting with the disorder in independent cases or in chromosomal regions of interest identified by other methods such as linkage analyses [10]. For example, evidence for cosegregation of a (1;11)(q42;q14.3)

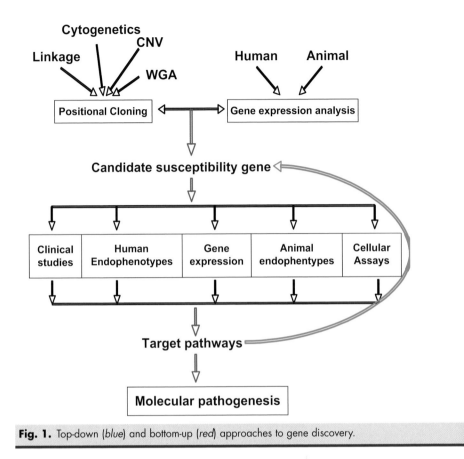

Fig. 1. Top-down (*blue*) and bottom-up (*red*) approaches to gene discovery.

chromosomal translocation cosegregating with clinical phenotypes in a large Scottish pedigree led to fine mapping of this region and identification of Disrupted in Schizophrenia-1 (*DISC-1*) as a candidate gene for schizophrenia at this locus [11], as discussed in detail later.

Small interstitial deletions of chromosome 22q11 are among the more common known chromosomal abnormalities, affecting 1 in 4000 live births. These abnormalities can result in the velo-cardio-facial syndrome (VCFS; Online Mendelian Inheritance in Man [OMIM] 192430), which is associated with at least a 20-fold increase in risk for psychosis and also presents with craniofacial dysmorphology, renal problems, and congenital heart disease [12,13]. The contribution of VCFS to susceptibility to schizophrenia is probably small, because the disorder is uncommon, and cytogenetic studies in schizophrenia samples rarely identify VCFS cases. This region also has been identified by schizophrenia linkage studies, suggesting that changes in gene dosage involving some of the 47 identified genes at this locus may contribute to risk of schizophrenia, and the disorder may be a useful model for investigating psychosis. The VCFS region contains three genes for which an association with schizophrenia has been reported: the catechol-O-methyltransferase (*COMT*), proline dehydrogenase (*PRODH*), and zinc finger DHHC domain-containing protein 8 (*ZDHHC8*) genes. Initial evidence for association with markers at *PRODH* in adult- and childhood-onset schizophrenia samples has not generally been supported in follow-up studies [14]. *ZDHHC8* emerged as a promising candidate gene based on association data and evidence that the associated single-nucleotide polymorphism (SNP) regulated the level of a functional transcript, thereby potentially affecting gene function; however, this association has not been supported by subsequent studies, including in a sample of more than 2000 individuals [15,16]. *COMT* is discussed in greater detail later.

Chromosomal abnormalities also have been reported in other psychosis populations, for example in individuals who have learning disability, but with less evidence to support causality. There are two case reports of deletions at 21q22 in individuals who had schizophrenia/learning disability and a third investigation identified four cases in a sample of 124 individuals who had schizophrenia, although this finding has yet to be replicated [17]. This region is not strongly supported as a susceptibility locus by linkage data but, interestingly, contains a promising schizophrenia candidate gene, oligodendrocyte lineage transcription factor 2 (*OLIG2*), which is discussed in more detail later.

The chromosomal abnormalities described thus far typically are large and are visible microscopically but represent a subset of total genomic copy number variation (CNV). Although submicroscopic CNV in DNA segments is found in all humans, it is only with the recent development of representational oligonucleotide microarray analysis and other technologies that they can be investigated at high resolution across the genome. Copy number variants involve more of the genome than previously suspected and represent a significant source of genetic variation between individuals [18,19]. Although their potential roles in complex disorders are underexplored, promising results from a recent study suggest they will be investigated further in schizophrenia [20]. These authors identified CNVs at four loci in persons who had schizophrenia and bipolar disorder that were not found in controls; three of the novel candidate genes identified (*GLUR7*, *CACNG2*, and *AKAP5*) were involved in glutamate signaling, and CNVs also were found at these loci in a second sample. CNVs also contribute a sizeable portion of the variance in gene expression across the genome [21].

Genetic association methods involve comparing the frequency of marker alleles in affected individuals with their frequency in unaffected individuals in a population rather than within families. Association methods are potentially more powerful than linkage studies for identifying common variants conferring moderate risk of a disorder [22]. Because there are millions of known variants in the genome, however, the probability of an investigated marker being involved in risk is very low. Recent advances in high-throughput genotyping and array-based expression platforms make it possible to assay most common genetic variations (SNP and CNV studies) across the whole genome in association studies (see the top-down approach illustrated in Fig. 1). This assay can be achieved by testing only a subset of the total variants, because common genetic variants share population ancestry and continue to be coinherited in populations over time, a phenomenon termed "linkage disequilibrium." This approach of genome-wide association analysis, comparing the frequencies of SNPs among affected individuals and controls across hundreds of thousands of markers, has successfully identified susceptibility genes for nonpsychiatric complex genetic disorders [23,24].

Functional investigation of genes in preclinical paradigms also can indicate new hypothesis-driven avenues for clinical research (see the bottom-up approach illustrated in Fig. 1). Thus, the increasing understanding of the pathogenic processes underlying the development of schizophrenia means that new genes identified as involved in these processes in animals may be good candidates for genetic studies in humans. In particular, such processes include neuronal migration, axon guidance, and synaptogenesis, together with control of synaptic activity and/or plasticity. Functional studies in normal and mutant mice that identify such genes, especially those with anatomic, physiologic, and behavioral phenotypes related to those of schizophrenia, thus are a powerful means for discovering candidate genes for the risk of schizophrenia. They also can be used to elucidate biochemical pathways that may yield further candidates, especially for studies assessing gene–gene interactions (epistasis). The distinction between top-down and bottom-up approaches will become increasingly artificial as bottom-up methods are used to interrogate and inform analysis of the vast datasets generated by top-down studies (see the section, "Future Directions").

GENE FUNCTION
Endophenotypic Approaches
One element in understanding how susceptibility genes may increase the risk for disease has been the endophenotypes approach. Endophenotypes, or intermediate phenotypes, have been described as "measurable components unseen by the unaided eye along the pathway between disease and distal genotype" [25]. The rationale for this approach is that if an endophenotype associated with a disorder is specific and represents a straightforward phenomenon, the number of genes required to produce variation in such traits may be fewer than those involved in producing a clinical disorder; this situation would facilitate identification of the genes involved. When specific susceptibility genes for a disorder already have been identified, endophenotypes may point toward the neural pathways by which individual genes contribute liability, using phenotypes that are dimensional rather than categorical.

Clinical endophenotypes continue to be studied to investigate what aspects of psychopathology might be associated with individual genetic variants. Investigating symptom dimensions, rather than categorical diagnoses, may be a powerful method of delineating the genetic architecture of, for example, mood-psychosis spectrum disorders [26]. This dimensional approach has led to analysis of genetic variants on the basis of both symptom clusters [27] and individual symptoms

[28,29] and may help define the relationship between clinical presentation and underlying genetic structure.

More incisively, neurocognitive deficits have been identified as potential endophenotypes in schizophrenia research. These deficits are present from an early stage of the disorder and often predate the emergence of clinical symptoms [30,31]. They are relatively stable over time and relate closely to functional outcome [32]. Furthermore, genetic epidemiologic research using family and twin studies indicates that these deficits have a substantial genetic component [33–36]. One issue in using cognitive deficits as endophenotypes is their independence from clinical state: performance on attentional measures, for example, has been shown to correlate with negative symptoms [37]. The amount of variance shared by these variables seems to be small, however, and in factor analysis cognitive function often emerges as a factor separate from clinical symptoms [38,39].

For cognitive endophenotypes, selecting suitable measures is complicated by the number of deficits involved, by different theories about their neurocognitive basis, and by differences in assessment. Higher stages of information processing have been targeted variously in terms of both general and specific aspects of cognitive functioning. A number of criteria already have been suggested for ensuring the suitability of endophenotypes [25,40], including evidence that the deficit is heritable and is associated with the illness. For neuropsychologic investigations, genetic epidemiologic studies, including family and twin studies, support a genetic contribution to deficits in working memory, attentional control, and episodic memory in affected families [33,34]. The heritability of general cognitive decline also has been demonstrated [41,42].

Similar rationales apply to the study of electrophysiologic correlates as endophenotypes. For example, deficits in early stages of information processing have been assessed using neurophysiologic indices such as mismatch negativity [43]. Furthermore, a number of components of later-stage processing show evidence of heritability, including the so-called "P50 component" associated with sensory gating deficits [40], the "P300 component" associated with attentional control, and, more recently, the "P1 component" of early visual processing [44]. Extensively documented neuroimaging findings, both structural [45,46] and functional [47], also are available for study as endophenotypes. Finally, although usually involving smaller numbers of subjects, neuropathologic findings offer the opportunity for direct examination of these processes at the molecular and cellular levels [2].

Mutant Models

Molecular biotechnology, through recombinant DNA techniques, allows the construction of mutant mice having deletion (knockout) or insertion (transgenesis) of individual genes that encode specific biologic entities. These are powerful approaches for elucidating specific mechanisms of neuronal function and disease. At a general level, the phenotype of a given central nervous system mutation may reveal mechanisms underlying normal structure and function and may increase the knowledge of mechanisms relevant to neuropsychiatric disorders. More specifically, the ability to delete genes shown to be associated with risk for schizophrenia is a powerful approach to identifying the functional role(s) of such genes, and the ability to insert genes associated with the disease, if and when identified, would offer new opportunities to investigate etiologic, pathophysiologic, and therapeutic processes [48–51].

Mutant models of susceptibility gene function (usually homozygous knock-outs) are not models of schizophrenia per se. Rather, given the probable polygenic basis of this disorder, they provide information about (1) the phenotypic role of each individual gene in the regulation of structure and function, assessed most commonly at the level of behavior; (2) whether the phenotype involves aspects of structure and function implicated in schizophrenia and can indicate relationships between anatomy, physiology, and behavior; (3) interactions between various risk genes; and (4) gene–environment interactions in the context of external biologic and psychosocial factors associated with risk for schizophrenia [6,48–51].

Such studies can provide converging support for the involvement of genes identified in linkage or association studies and a biologic framework to explore pathogenic mechanisms. They also provide the means to identify genes acting in the same cellular processes, which in turn may be good candidates to test in association studies or to examine for epistatic interactions. Extending this logic, the nonbiased identification of genes affecting neural development or synaptic connectivity in mutant mice is also likely to yield promising candidates for genetic studies in humans (the bottom-up approach). Dissecting these mechanisms will require filling in the blanks from genes to behavior through anatomy and physiology, together with more sophisticated genetic manipulations such as tissue-specific and temporally controlled knockouts (see the section, "Future Directions").

The phenotypic data considered in the present article have been collected primarily from mice with targeted mutation by gene knockout. Some have questioned the value of this approach because of the lack of clarity concerning the functional significance of the susceptibility allele in many cases [48]. In general terms, enthusiasm for the knockout approach must be tempered by the reported absence of material phenotypic effects in numerous central nervous system knockout mice and/or problems in replicating research findings across laboratories [50,52–54]. It now is evident that numerous factors, both genetic and epigenetic, contribute to the expression of mutant phenotype; these factors include genetic background, compensatory and redundancy processes, pleiotropy, and several environmental variables [50,51,54].

Although the impact of these factors complicates the interpretation of mutant phenotypes, these factors themselves have information value. Variable penetrance of susceptibility genes, both within and across populations, may be modeled and understood better by studying the mechanisms of action of modifier genes and epistatic interactions with the target gene in knockout mice. Furthermore, given that several of the best-supported schizophrenia susceptibility genes are implicated in diverse neurodevelopmental processes, it is likely that the relevant mutation is present throughout ontogeny, and compensatory and redundancy processes analogous to those in the knockout mouse may be present in humans also.

The development of valid endophenotypes, as outlined in the preceding section, has the potential to facilitate the modeling of psychopathologic and neurocognitive deficits that are demonstrable across species and are capable of being quantified reliably in existing mutant models. The pitfalls of attempting to assess some of the uniquely human features of psychosis are well documented in the literature, however; behavioral models based on cognitive (eg, sensorimotor gating) or social (eg, altered response to social novelty) endophenotypes may be more advantageous for modeling psychosis in animals.

At first glance the genes considered in this article seem to fall into two groups: those that have clear roles in neural development and those with more obvious roles in adult neuronal function. Among the best-replicated genes from human genetic studies, *DISC1* and *NRG1* each have prominent functions in aspects of cell migration in the cerebral cortex, together with additional roles in neural development; others, for example *DTNBP1*, *PLXNA2*, *AKT1*, and calcineurin, may have similar roles. Conversely, many other genes identified as risk factors for schizophrenia are implicated in the function of neural circuits rather than in their development; these genes include *RGS4*, *COMT*, *DAO*, *DAOA*, *PDE4B*, and *PRODH*. The distinction between these functions probably is artificial, however, with many such genes acting at both stages.

DYSBINDIN
Relationship to Schizophrenia

Evidence for the involvement of the dystrobrevin binding protein 1 (*DTNBP1*; dysbindin) gene came from a dense fine-mapping study of the chromosome 6p susceptibility locus in affected Irish families. The *DTNBP1* association now has been reported by many studies [55], but no functional variant has been identified, and studies have differed in the alleles/haplotypes reported. The expectation that single-risk variants and functional mutations would be identified at susceptibility genes underestimated the complexity of the gene. For a Mendelian disorder such as cystic fibrosis, more than 140 mutations of the *CFTR* gene are described in OMIM (602421). Multiple variants in a given gene (allelic heterogeneity) may contribute to a susceptibility to schizophrenia; that might explain the excess of rare variants that have been reported at *DTNBP1* and other candidate genes. Additionally, different genes may independently influence disease in different populations (locus heterogeneity). The same issues of gene complexity, heterogeneity, and lack of clear functional mutations apply equally to the other schizophrenia candidate genes detailed later.

In the case of *DTNBP1*, the association findings are supported by expression and functional studies. Reduced prefrontal and hippocampal expression of the gene and levels of the protein dysbindin have been reported in schizophrenia [56–58]. An allelic expression study reported association between different risk haplotypes of the gene and the cortical expression of dysbindin, demonstrating that different associations could contribute to a common mechanism, albeit without identifying the mechanism involved [56]. This mechanism may involve an action of the protein to affect and potentially to regulate neuronal glutamate release through its role as a component of the BLOC-1 protein complex. Several studies have identified genetic associations with other components of BLOC-1 and of epistasis between *DTNBP1* and *MUTED* in schizophrenia risk.

Although the cellular functions of dysbindin are not well understood, it has been shown to bind to snapin, a synaptic protein [59], and to a number of microtubule-interacting proteins [60]. Several of these *DTNBP1*-interacting proteins also interact with *DISC1*, suggesting a link between these two pathways and the possible involvement of *DTNBP1* in cell migration or other aspects of neural development.

Endophenotypes

As noted previously, investigating symptom dimensions or clusters rather than categorical diagnoses may be a useful method for specifying the clinical phenotype associated with individual risk variants. Two published studies suggest that variation in *DTNBP1* is associated with negative symptoms in schizophrenia [27,29]. Few studies investigating *DTNBP1* in affective disorders have been published, and the results, often based on modest sample sizes, have been mixed [61–63]. From these data, it has been suggested that *DTNBP1* may be part of a prototypical schizophrenia gene set on the mood-psychosis spectrum [64]. This view of *DTNBP1* is supported by recent evidence for its association with both child-onset psychosis and poor premorbid adjustment [65,66].

Further evidence that *DTNBP1* may be associated with a clinical presentation involving more enduring and disabling features of psychosis derives from a series of studies of its influence on cognitive function. *DTNBP1* risk variants have been associated with poorer performance in higher cognitive domains in controls [67,68] and with both general and domain-specific deficits in schizophrenia [65,69]. Using a composite measure derived from selected subtests of the Wechsler Adult Intelligence Scale, investigators found that carriers of a risk haplotype previously reported in their sample performed more poorly on this measure of general cognitive ability [65]. This association was independent of disease status (schizophrenia versus controls). In the present authors' study, patient carriers of the *DTNBP1* risk haplotype identified previously both in their sample and in a sample from the United Kingdom [70] performed more poorly on the Cambridge Neuropsychological Test Automated Battery (CANTAB) spatial working memory task. Working memory and general cognitive ability are highly correlated, so these results on apparently different indices may simply be two aspects of the same cognitive deficit. The association in controls between *DTNBP1* and P300 waveforms, an index of higher-level cognitive functions [68], may be described similarly.

Such methodologic differences in approaching cognitive assessment, however, preclude a definitive understanding of whether the role of *DTNBP1* in cognition is general or specific. Some commentators argue that the complex system of inter-action between genes contributing to brain function make a specific role unlikely [71], particularly for the genes involved in glutamate function (see the discussion of *DAOA*). Consistent with the role for glutamate signaling in regions throughout the brain, a recent study from the authors' group found that carriers of the *DTNBP1* risk variant, in addition to showing poorer spatial working memory, showed significant deficits in an electrophysiologic index of early visual process-ing (G. Donohoe, D.W. Morris, P. De Sanctis, E. Magno, J.L. Montesi, H.P. Garavan, I.H. Robertson, D.C. Javitt, M. Gill, A.P. Corvin, and J.J. Foxe, unpublished data). Because dysbindin is expressed throughout the brain, includ-ing in occipital cortex, it may be that poor sensory-level processing of information is responsible for the deficits at higher stages of cognitive function that already have been reported.

Mutant Models

A spontaneous mutant, subsequently named "sandy" (*sdy*) arose in the DBA/2J colony at Jackson Laboratories in the early 1980s. It later was demonstrated that Hermansky-Pudlak syndrome, a congenital disorder characterized by ocu-locutaneous albinism, prolonged bleeding, and albinism was attributable to a nonsense mutation in the dysbindin gene, and that the *sdy* mouse constituted a murine model of Hermansky-Pudlak syndrome [72]. It is caused by an in-frame deletion of two exons of the mouse *DTNBP1* gene, and *sdy* mice express no dysbindin protein. Preliminary behavioral data in *sdy* mutants (on a mixed genetic background) indicated no difference in prepulse inhibition (PPI) between homozygous mutants and wild-type controls [72]. The investigators also noted no further differences at a behavioral level, although they did not elaborate on the range of assessments used.

A recent report examining motor and exploratory function in the *sdy* mutant mice indicated decreased levels of spontaneous activity in the open field and a significant reduction in time spent in the center of the arena [73]; these data might suggest a role for this gene in the regulation of exploratory behavior in a novel environment. Changes in temporal and spatial patterns of hippocam-pal CA1 activation in homozygous *sdy* mutants, perhaps indicative of reduced inhibition in the hippocampus, were noted also [74]. Further investigation is required to ascertain the extent to which schizophrenia-related phenotypes, par-ticularly at the level of cognition as suggested by clinical data, are observed in mice mutant for the *DTNBP1* gene.

DISC1

Relationship to Schizophrenia

In 1970, a translocation was reported in an individual who had adolescent con-duct disorder and in other members of the extended family; follow-up of this family identified many additional members as having major psychiatric disorders and a (1;11)(q42;q14.3) translocation [75]. Detailed clinical investigation of the family and a linkage analysis generated a logarithm of odds score of 3.6 with schizophrenia as the phenotype, increasing to 7.1 when relatives who had bipolar disorder and recurrent major depression also were included [76]. This degree of linkage was strong evidence that the translocation was responsible for the mental illness, at least in this unusual family. Further suggestive linkage evidence was reported for both schizophrenia [77,78] and bipolar disorder [79,80].

The breakpoint on chromosome 1 disrupted two overlapping and opposite sense genes, *DISC1* and *DISC2*. *DISC1* is expressed as a protein, and the gene is disrupted within intron 8, removing exons 9 to 13 to chromosome 11. *DISC2* has no identified open reading frames and could be an RNA transcript. Identifying the gene allows association studies to be focused on DNA variants in and around the genes and the breakpoint. Such studies in Finnish [81,82], North American [83], and Scottish [84] populations have provided additional support. These findings suggest that, apart from the major disruption caused by the translocation, other DNA variation in the area seems to confer susceptibility to major mental illness in the general population.

The *DISC1* gene has at least 13 exons and spans more than 300 kilobases (kb) of genomic DNA, with the gene sequence and structure conserved across species. *DISC1* messenger RNA transcripts occur in the brain, heart, placenta, testis, and kidney [85]. In humans different mRNA transcripts have been reported [86], and a variety of protein signals have been detected using antibodies. The signal at 100 to 105 kd seems to reflect the entire translated product of 854 amino acids. Larger signals have been detected in developing brains, suggesting posttranslational modifications or protein complexes, including *DISC1* [87]. In human brain, *DISC1* is expressed in the cerebral cortex and hippocampus [11]; subcellular distribution may be altered in the brains of persons who have schizophrenia [88]. In cell lines derived from the translocation, there is a 50% reduction of the normal levels of *DISC1* [89]. In the mouse, *DISC1* is expressed from embryonic day 10 through to adult life [90,91], indicating a role in brain development. *DISC1* has multiple subcellular distributions, including the centrosome and microtubular fractions, postsynaptic densities, actin cytoskeletal fractions, mitochondria, and the nucleus [87].

To understand the role of *DISC1* in the brain, it is useful to identify the other proteins to which it binds. *DISC1* interacts with many other proteins, including the microtubule-associated proteins NUDEL, NUDE, dynactin, kendrin, MIPT3, and MAP1A; the nuclear proteins LIS1 and ATF4; the actin-associated proteins spectrin, FEZ1, and actinin1; the postsynaptic density–associated proteins citron and HAPOP; and others such as the phosphodiesterase PDE4B. These interactions suggest that *DISC1* has several functions, including neuronal migration, cytoskeletal function, and neuronal signaling.

Consistent with the haploinsufficiency model, cell and animal models that reduce the expression of endogenous *DISC1* by RNA interference indicate a role for *DISC1* in neuronal cell migration and neurite extension [92]. These authors showed that *DISC1* is a component of the microtubule-associated dynein motor complex and is required to keep the complex at the centromere [92]. The centrosome has a key role in neuronal migration, and the mutated *DISC1*, as seen in the translocation, functions as a dominant-negative mutation, disturbing the normal subcellular localization of the wild-type *DISC1* through self-association with wild-type *DISC1*. In differentiating neuronal cells, both suppression of *DISC1*, using RNA interference, and expression of mutated *DISC1* led to inhibition of neurite outgrowth. In the developing mouse embryo, the introduction of mutated *DISC1* resulted in delayed neuronal migration of some cells and the abnormal orientation of some pyramidal neurones. These subtle quantitative changes are reflective of the changes seen in neuropathologic studies in schizophrenia, demonstrating the basic cellular biology potentially underlying at least some forms of this disorder. How these changes might relate to clinical, neuropsychologic, and other manifestations of schizophrenia remains to be elucidated.

What is particularly striking about the *DISC1* story is the possibility that its role in centrosomes, neurite outgrowth, and neuronal migration might be only one of the functions of *DISC1* [93]. A binding partner of *DISC1* is the phosphodiesterase PDE4B, one of a family of proteins similar to the *Drosophila* learning and memory gene *dunce*. PDE4B is involved in the inactivation of cAMP, a signaling molecule involved in memory [94]. Thus, it has been suggested that *DISC1* and PDE4B regulate cellular responses to cAMP [95], indicating a cellular mechanism that might underlie some of the cognitive deficits seen in schizophrenia and other severe psychiatric disorders and that could account for some of the endophenotypic findings reviewed later.

Endophenotypes

Although *DISC1* has been associated with both schizophrenia and bipolar disorder [96], there has been little investigation of its clinical correlates in terms of individual symptoms or symptom clusters. Using a broad diagnosis of affected status to relatives (schizophrenia, schizoaffective disorder, schizotypal disorder, bipolar disorder, and recurrent major depression), investigators have reported that the HEP3 haplotype was significantly associated in women who had delusions, hallucinations, and negative symptoms but not in women who had manic or depressive symptoms; no such association was found in men [81].

Recent investigations have focused on the association between a *DISC1* haplotype, which includes the SER704CYS polymorphism, and positive symptom items from severe compromised immunodeficiency, selected because positive symptom severity has been associated with hippocampal dysfunction [28]. Significant differences in the severity of positive symptom were associated with being a carrier of both the overall haplotype and individual variants, including the SER704CYS polymorphism. Although it is of interest, particularly because the same SER allele is associated with both positive symptoms and impaired memory function, this finding is reported in the absence of an association with the broader schizophrenia phenotype and will require confirmation in other samples.

Evidence for associations between *DISC1* and cognitive deficits has been reviewed recently [96]. Association between performance on neurocognitive measures and variants at the *DISC1* locus has been reported in independent samples [33,76,81,97–104]. For studies reporting association with markers within *DISC1*, interpretation of the data is complicated by the diversity in both genetic markers and cognitive measures. Nonetheless, aspects of memory function seem to be a common denominator among positive associations with cognition. This finding is consistent with the suggestion that *DISC1* is important in the development of hippocampal neurons [105] and is most strongly expressed in the hippocampal formation in mammals [106].

The SER704CYS polymorphism has been investigated using neuropsychologic measures of memory and structural/functional imaging of associated brain regions [99]; SER carriers were observed to show reduced hippocampal volume and less efficient hippocampal activation, as well as more subtle decrements in verbal episodic memory. Following evidence for linkage of cognitive deficits to the *DISC1* region of 1q42 in their sample [104], a Finnish group reported similar associations between *DISC1* and memory function using haplotypes spanning *DISC1* and *TRAX* (HEP1, HEP2, HEP3). A HEP3 haplotype was reported to be associated with poorer performance on the Wechsler Memory Scale visual span task, both for the attentional (visual span forward) and working memory (visual span backward components of the task [82].

Based on a separate twin study, an association between HEP2 and HEP3 and spatial working memory has been reported [100], using a task distinct from that employed previously [82], together with an association between verbal episodic memory and each of the HEP haplotypes considered. Furthermore, evidence suggests some association between reduced hippocampal volume and HEB1 [100]. Association between *DISC1* variation (rs2255340 in intron 8) and verbal working memory also has been reported in an African American sample but not in a white sample [98].

Mutant Models

An intriguing finding reported recently has shown that mice belonging to the commonly employed 129S6 Sv/Ev strain carry a 25-bp deletion in exon 6 of the *DISC1* gene relative to six other inbred mouse strains (BALB/cJ, CBA/J, C3H/HeJ, C57BL/6J, DBA/2J, and AKR/J) [107]. Spatial working memory was assessed using the delayed non-match to place task in C57BL/6J mice carrying the modified 129 Sv/Ev *DISC1* allele. The parameters of the spatial working memory task employed were chosen to recruit maximally the prefrontally mediated cognitive function involving the use of retention intervals in the working memory range and short intertrial intervals. Learning performance in the task was found to be intact in *DISC1* mutant mice.

In contrast, both heterozygous and homozygous *DISC1* mutants demonstrated significant disruption in performance during the working memory component of the task. These data are consistent with studies in humans (see the previous section, "Endophenotypes") that have suggested an association between *DISC1* variants and working memory function. In contrast, no significant deficit in PPI (a measure of preattentional processing that is disrupted in schizophrenia) was observed in *DISC1*-mutant mice, and basal locomotor activity levels were unaffected.

Other groups recently have generated mice mutant for the *DISC1* gene, although these data have yet to be elaborated in full publications. Several inducible dominant negative transgenic strains that express different truncated *DISC1* proteins suggest that disruption of *DISC1* function during development produces impairments in latent inhibition (a measure of selective attention), social approach behaviors, and spatial working memory [108]. The generation of a transgenic mouse model involving inducible forebrain-selective expression of the truncated *DISC1* protein indicated deficits in PPI and spatial working performance in the water maze, together with hyperactivity in a novel environment [109]. The same investigators subsequently reported increased intermale aggression in the same *DISC1* mutant [110].

A different *DISC1* transgenic line, expressing the truncated form of the *DISC1* protein under the CaMKII promoter, exhibited sex-specific disruption of PPI only in males, intact motor function and impaired olfactory function [111]. The same authors also described enlarged lateral ventricles (measured using MRI) in this *DISC1* mutant. Lateral ventricular enlargement is a feature observed in alternative genetic models of psychosis (ie, the *chakragati* mouse [112]) and has been demonstrated repeatedly in patients who have schizophrenia [6]. The existing data from the various available *DISC1*-mutant lines implicate the gene in working memory function; this finding is consistent with the previous suggestion that aspects of memory function may represent the common denominator underlying the role of *DISC1* in cognition.

NEUREGULIN 1

Relationship to Schizophrenia

In a study of 33 Icelandic families, the deCODE group reported suggestive evidence of linkage to a chromosome 8p locus that previously had been implicated in schizophrenia susceptibility by several studies and in a linkage meta-analysis [9]. Following up this finding in a larger case-control sample, the authors identified several risk haplotypes that mapped to a region containing the neuregulin 1 (*NRG1*) gene [113]. The core risk haplotype (HAPBICE) at the 5′ end of the gene was replicated in the Scottish population, and a truncated form of the haplotype (HAPIRE) was seen in an Irish sample [114,115]. Subsequent studies have produced negative and positive reports; for example, markers in a separate haplotype block were reported as associated in the Chinese population. A recent meta-analysis of the 13 reported *NRG1* studies confirmed evidence of association but indicated evidence for genetic heterogeneity, with different but adjacent haplotype blocks being associated in white and Asian populations [116]. Functional risk variants have not been identified at the gene.

The Neuregulins are a family of growth and differentiation factors that interact with the ErbB tyrosine kinase transmembrane receptors inducing growth and differentiation of epithelial, neuronal, glial, and other cell types. Neuregulin 1 is a large, complex gene that spans more than 1.1 megabase (Mb) and contains at least 25 alternatively spliced exons that can produce multiple promoters upstream of the protein-coding sequences [117]. Neuregulin 1 signaling by means of ErbB receptors has been implicated in neuronal differentiation and myelination and in the development and functioning of glutamatergic N-methyl-D-aspartate (NMDA) receptor systems. A C-terminal fragment of the gene also can translocate into the nucleus and interact with transcription factors to enhance expression of genes including *PSD-95*, which has many functions including facilitation of erbB4 activation.

Animal and human postmortem studies suggest that *NRG1* stimulation suppresses NMDA receptor activation in the prefrontal cortex and that this suppression may be more pronounced in schizophrenia [118]. These findings are compatible with the view that *NRG1* signaling is involved in NMDA hypofunction in schizophrenia but come with the caveat that *NRG1* contributes to multiple aspects of brain function, many of which are poorly understood. *NRG1* also is involved in early processes in neurodevelopment that may be relevant to its role in schizophrenia. For example, it is required to attract γ–aminobutyric acid–producing (GABAergic) interneurons toward the cortex, through its ErbB4 receptor [119] and also has secondary effects on thalamocortical connectivity [120,121]; additionally, it has well-characterized functions in later aspects of synapse development [122].

Endophenotypes

Despite being one of the candidate genes associated most frequently with schizophrenia in independent samples, the cognitive and clinical correlates of Neuregulin have received little attention to date. No functional mutation has been identified that is associated causally with schizophrenia. This lack, together with the complexity of the gene, makes it difficult to identify suitable risk variants for functional analysis in terms of endophenotypes.

There now is initial evidence for an association between a Neuregulin variant (SNP8NRG243177, part of the original DeCODE haplotype) and cognitive performance in a population at high risk of schizophrenia [123]. Carriers of the risk genotype (T/T) scored lower on premorbid IQ, as measured by the National Adult Reading Test. Similarly, in a functional (fMRI) study of prefrontal activation using the Hayling sentence completion task, subjects who had the risk genotype showed decreased activation of the medial prefrontal and right temporo-occipital cortex relative to carriers of the nonrisk genotype.

Although these findings remain to be replicated in other samples, it is interesting to compare them with results for *DTNBP1*. For both these genes putatively involved in NMDA signaling, there is evidence of association between identified risk variants and deficits in both general and executive cognitive functions. One interpretation of these data is that, given the ubiquitous distribution of glutamate-regulated neurons throughout brain, genes that affect glutamate function are likely to have wide-ranging effects on cognition.

Mutant Models

To date, a number of groups have developed several variants of *NRG1* knockouts, each targeting a particular domain and/or selective for *NRG1* types I through III. Generally, targeted knockout of *NRG1* or its ErbB receptor results in midembryonic lethality, with homozygotes dying during early embryologic development because of cardiac failure; however, heterozygous mice are viable and fertile [113,124]. Phenotypic studies in mice containing deletion of the transmembrane (TM) domain of the *NRG1* gene have implicated this gene in the regulation of several aspects of behavior related to schizophrenia. Heterozygous TM-domain *NRG1* knockouts display sex-specific abnormalities in the process by which individual elements of behavior in the mouse repertoire change and interchange over an extended time-frame of interaction with the environment, from initial exploration, through habituation, to quiescence (ie, the ethogram) [125].

Other studies have reported disruption to a number of schizophrenia-related phenotypes in heterozygous TM-domain *NRG1* mutants: reduction in NMDA receptor expression, impaired PPI, spontaneous hyperactivity, and reversal by clozapine of such hyperactivity [113,126]. Data from the authors' own studies [127] suggest that spatial learning and working memory processes are intact in TM-domain *NRG1* mutants, with any changes in these measures being mediated by higher basal activity levels. In contrast, these *NRG1* mutants show abnormal patterns of social behavior relative to controls. Specifically, when assessed for social affiliative behavior and behavioral response to social novelty, TM-domain *NRG1* mutants evidence the same number of social approach behaviors as wild types; however, response to social novelty is diminished in *NRG1* mutants.

Recent evidence from the authors' own studies also suggests altered behavioral responsivity to subchronic phencyclidine (an NMDA antagonist that possesses psychotomimetic properties) in TM-domain *NRG1* mutants at the level of social interaction behaviors and locomotor activity (C.M.P. O'Tuathaigh, G.J. O'Sullivan, J.J. Clifford, O. Tighe, R. Harvey, D.T. Croke, J.L. Waddington, unpublished data, 2007). Similarly, others have shown the modulatory effects of delta-9-tetrahydrocannabinol (the active constituent of cannabis) on PPI and locomotor behavior to be modified in TM-domain *NRG1* mutants [128]. These findings are intriguing because they provide insight into a putative gene–environment interaction, suggesting that the effect of mutation of the *NRG1* gene may be modified in vivo by environmental manipulations relevant to psychosis. For example, the *COMT* gene can differentially influence risk for schizophrenia in individuals who are exposed to cannabis during adolescence [129]. It has been postulated that stresses such as drug use at developmentally specific periods can propel the developmentally compromised individual across the "psychosis threshold," resulting in full-blown expression of the disease.

In contrast, no evidence for a hyperactive phenotype was observed in mutants heterozygous for an immunoglobulin domain–specific mutation of the *NRG1* gene (*Ig-NRG1*); however, these mutants exhibited disruption of latent inhibition, perhaps indicative of a deficit in selective attention [130]. Together with the evidence from TM-domain *NRG1* mutants, these data indicate a role for the *NRG1* gene in social functioning and selective elements of cognition (preattentional processing and selective attention) relevant to schizophrenia.

The extent to which knockout or partial loss of function of *NRG1* models functional alterations associated with the genetic contribution of *NRG1* to psychosis is unclear, however. Although there is indirect evidence that *NRG1* signaling may be enhanced in patients who have schizophrenia [118], this enhancement may reflect a compensatory response to diminished *NRG1* function.

DAOA
Relationship to Schizophrenia
Following up a chromosome 13q32-34 susceptibility locus in French-Canadian and Russian schizophrenia samples, an association with markers in a region containing two overlapping genes, *DAOA* (previously *G72*) and *G30*, was reported [131]. Functional experiments indicated that only the *DAOA* gene is actively translated and that the resultant protein activates the enzyme D-amino acid oxidase (*DAO*; OMIM 124050). Based on evidence that oxidation of D-serine by DAO attenuates NMDA receptor function through the glycine modulation site, these authors speculated that variation at the *DAOA/G30* (and *DAO*; see later discussion) loci influences the efficiency of glutamate gating of the NMDA ion channel and in this manner contributes to susceptibility to schizophrenia.

A series of independent studies support the involvement of *DAOA/G30* in susceptibility to schizophrenia [132–139], although negative studies also have been reported. Interpretation of these data is complicated by differences between studies in the populations ascertained, markers tested, and risk variants/haplotypes identified [140]. A detailed meta-analysis, involving 1292 persons who had schizophrenia and 1392 controls, supported association at four *DAOA* markers, including a putative functional polymorphism (rs2391191) that is predicted to cause an arginine-to-lysine substitution at codon 30 of the gene [141]. This strong genetic support is not yet sustained by functional studies because of difficulties in isolating and investigating the predicted DAOA protein.

Endophenotypes
As with *DTNBP1* and *NRG1*, a putative influence of *DAOA* on the efficiency of glutamate gating of the NMDA channel may make cognitive phenotypes particularly useful for understanding the role of this gene in brain function. The recruitment of NMDA receptors during high presynaptic glutamatergic activity results in a permanent increase in synaptic efficacy known as "long-term potentiation," particularly in hippocampal regions. Long-term potentiation has been suggested as the likely biologic basis of associative learning assessed in cognitive memory tasks [142,143]. NMDA receptors also have been hypothesized

to have a role in prefrontally mediated aspects of cognition (attentional control and working memory), either directly or possibly by means of a reciprocal influence on dopaminergic functioning [144].

A *DAOA* marker, although not associated with increased schizophrenia risk, is associated with poorer performance on neuropsychologic measures of working memory and attention [36]. Using the N-back task to index working memory and the continuous performance task to index attention, these authors reported that the risk genotype in one of the SNPs (T/T genotype at SNP10) associated with schizophrenia in the original association study [131] was associated with poorer performance on both measures. Furthermore, in addition to showing a trend-level association with verbal episodic memory deficits, their fMRI study in normal controls revealed a significant association between the same marker and levels of hippocampal activation during an episodic memory paradigm. Again, carriers of the risk genotype showed lower hippocampal activation during the memory tasks than carriers of the nonrisk genotype. The authors recently sought to confirm this cognitive finding, based on a risk variant associated with schizophrenia in their sample [133] and found evidence that this variant (ARG30LYS, the arginine-to-lysine substitution at codon 30 described previously) was associated with poorer immediate and delayed verbal episodic memory performance [145]. In addition to being consistent with an earlier report [36], this association is in a mis-sense and possibly functional polymorphism, although the impact of this variant will be known only when its associated protein is identified and characterized.

Several studies also have reported association between *DAOA* and bipolar disorder [140]. These reports have led to speculation that the gene may have a more general role and may contribute to susceptibility across psychotic disorders or have a wider role in susceptibility to a psychiatric disorder [146].

Mutant Models

The human *DAOA/G30* gene locus is not conserved in mice, excluding the possibility of conventional knockout or transgenic technologies. Identification of expressed transcripts has proved problematic. Alternative genetic techniques may be used to introduce the human gene locus into the mouse genome, but such a model has not yet been described in the literature.

DAO

Relationship to Schizophrenia

D-amino acid oxidase (*DAO*) is a peroxisomal enzyme involved in oxidizing D-serine, an activator of the NMDA receptor. Using yeast-2-hybrid methods, a protein interaction between the schizophrenia susceptibility gene *G72* (subsequently *DAOA*; see previous discussion) and *DAO* was identified, with in vitro evidence that *G72* was an activator of *DAO* [131]. The authors also presented evidence of association between *DAO* and schizophrenia in a French-Canadian population and evidence of statistical interaction suggesting epistasis between *DAOA* and *DAO* in contributing to risk for schizophrenia.

At least five independent studies support the involvement of *DAO* in susceptibility to schizophrenia, with some consistency in the associations [133,135,147–149]. In particular, two studies of white populations have now replicated association with the T allele of the marker rs3918346 reported originally [133,149]. Involvement of this gene is supported indirectly by functional studies, in which reduced serum levels of D-serine and a decreased ratio of D-serine/*DAO* expression have been identified in persons who have schizophrenia [147,148]. Endophenotypic studies are sparse, however.

Mutant Models

A mouse strain lacking *DAO* activity because of a point mutation in the *DAO* gene has been described [150,151]. *DAO*-deficient mice exhibit elevated levels of D-amino acids in serum and brain [152,153]. *DAO* mutants exhibit increased occupancy of the NMDA receptor–associated glycine site, with a resultant increase in NMDA receptor function. This increase is accompanied by reduced behavioral responsivity to acute administration of the NMDA antagonist phencyclidine [154]. Furthermore, the number of stereotyped behaviors and ataxic movements induced by acute administration of the NMDA antagonist MK-801 was reduced in *DAO* mutants [155]. *DAO* mutants also demonstrated hypoactivity in a novel environment, with intact PPI [154]. Superior performance in a test of spatial working memory was observed in *DAO* mutants, together with enhanced long-term potentiation in the hippocampus [156].

RGS4

Relationship to Schizophrenia

The regulator of G-protein signaling-4 (*RGS4*) gene is involved in the regulation and timing of duration of G-protein–mediated receptor signaling. This action may be important in the adrenergic modulation of prefrontal NMDA receptor function [157]. *RGS4* maps to chromosome 1q23.3 and was investigated for linkage and association in United States and Indian schizophrenia family and case-control samples [158]. This gene, which was selected for investigation based on position and also because of the expression of *RGS4* transcript, was reduced in the cortex of postmortem brain samples from patients who had schizophrenia, a finding that subsequently has been replicated independently [159,160].

To address inconsistency across multiple subsequent association studies, a genotype-based meta-analysis of family-based and case-control samples from published and unpublished sources (13,807 subjects) found no single-marker associations [161]; however, there was evidence for overtransmission of two common haplotypes in the family samples and evidence of single-marker association in the case-control samples, suggesting a complex pattern of association at the gene.

Endophenotypes

Among sparse endophenotypic data, variation at an *RGS4* SNP (rs951436) has recently been reported [162] to affect frontoparietal and frontotemporal function during a working memory task and on the volume of these regions. Further studies are required to confirm these findings.

Mutant Models

An *RGS4* knockout (Cre-deleted *RGS4$_{lacZ/lacZ}$* on a mixed 129/B6D2/C57Bl/6 background) has been reported [163]. Homozygous *RGS4* mutants evidenced no differences in spontaneous activity in the open field; working memory, as assessed in the spontaneous alternation test, was intact; PPI was unaffected, as was acoustic startle reactivity. The failure to observe any material phenotypic effect may be attributable to a number of factors, including mixed genetic background, compensation, or redundancy. Alternatively, *RGS4* may not contribute materially to the risk for schizophrenia [161]. Given the involvement of *RGS4* in cellular processes thought to be relevant to schizophrenia and the reduction in *RGS4* mRNA observed in patients who have schizophrenia, further phenotypic studies in *RGS4* mutants are required to clarify the functional role of this gene vis-à-vis a schizophrenia-like phenotype.

COMT

Relationship to Schizophrenia

The gene encoding the enzyme catechol-O-methyltransferase (*COMT*) has been scrutinized intensively as a positional and functional candidate gene for schizophrenia. *COMT* maps to a chromosomal 22q11 susceptibility locus identified from several linkage studies and by the strong association between the chromosomal microdeletion syndrome involving this locus (VCFS; as discussed previously) and schizophrenia [12,13]. *COMT* has a key role in dopamine catabolism, and a functional polymorphism that substitutes a valine for methionine reduces the thermal stability and activity of the enzyme. Hypothetically, having more copies of the methionine allele would result in higher dopamine levels and thus might be expected to increase the risk for schizophrenia; however, a counterintuitive association with the opposite valine allele has been reported in several schizophrenia samples. These findings, including association with several haplotypes at the *COMT* locus, have not been replicated consistently by suitably powered studies and are not supported by a recent meta-analysis [64,164].

Endophenotypes

Although evidence from association studies implicating *COMT* is weak, neuropsychologic, electrophysiologic, and neuroimaging studies suggest that variation at *COMT* may have an important modulatory role both in normal prefrontal cortical function and in the dysfunction thereof in schizophrenia, as recently reviewed *in extensio* elsewhere [2,165,166].

Mutant Models

Although a comprehensive study of putative schizophrenia-related phenotypes has not been performed in *COMT* knockouts, studies have found spontaneous activity in a novel environment to be unaffected in both heterozygous and homozygous mutants on a mixed 129J/C57BL/6 [167,168]. In the light-dark apparatus, a measure of anxiety, only female homozygous mutants displayed an anxiolytic profile, whereas increased aggression toward an unfamiliar C57Bl/6 mouse was observed only in male heterozygous mutants. This observation provides evidence for sexually dimorphic phenotypic expression of the *COMT* mutation [167]. Locomotor and stereotyped behaviors were attenuated in male homozygous *COMT* mutants following administration of the psychotomimetic drugs amphetamine and cocaine [169]. Preliminary evidence from the authors' own group (D.S. Babovic, C.M.P. O'Tuathaigh, G.J. O'Sullivan, J.J. Clifford, O. Tighe, D.T. Croke, M. Karayiorgou, J.A. Gogos, D. Cotter, and J.L. Waddington, unpublished data, 2007) indicates sex-specific disruption of social interaction in homozygous *COMT* mutants. Sex-specific effects are of particular relevance in relation to genes associated with risk for psychiatric disorders such as schizophrenia that are characterized by sexual dimorphism [51].

PPI was found to be intact in both heterozygous and homozygous *COMT* mutants [167]. Further studies are required to establish whether *COMT* knockout produces effects across murine analogues of tasks that access diverse cognitive processes in humans. Pharmacologically induced *COMT* inhibition in rats has been demonstrated to enhance attentional performance; this improvement was associated with increased dopamine (DA) efflux in the medial prefrontal cortex (mPFC), consistent with better performance on tests of PFC-mediated cognition in human carriers of the low-activity Met–Met allele [170–172]. Further studies in *COMT* mutants are indicated.

AKT1

The AKT signaling pathway was targeted for candidate gene analysis based on evidence for decreases in phosphorylation of components of the pathway and in levels of the AKT1 protein in schizophrenia [173]. These authors reported evidence for association with a single SNP and several haplotypes at the V-AKT Murine Tymoma Viral Oncogene Homolog 1 (*AKT1*) locus, one of which was significant when corrected for the number of tests performed. *AKT1* is a protein kinase that may be involved in many processes that modulate the growth, proliferation, differentiation, and survival of cells. Two subsequent studies from Asian populations found no evidence and weak evidence for association, respectively. More recently, Schwab and colleagues [167] confirmed the original finding and reported association with additional haplotypes in a European family sample. These association data are supported by functional studies, but further systematic investigation of this locus in suitably powered samples is warranted.

Mutant Models

Using exploratory transcriptional profiling, alterations in prefrontal cortical expression of genes involved in neuronal development, synaptic function, myelination, and cytoskeleton structure have been reported in *AKT1*-deficient mice [174]. These mutants also demonstrated abnormal working memory retention under neurochemical challenge of diverse neurotransmitter systems. *AKT1* is known to be a signaling intermediary downstream of the D2 DA receptor, an established target for antipsychotic drugs.

OTHER CANDIDATE GENES

Convergent functional genomics, using bottom-up as well as top-down approaches, is now leading to the identification of a number of other putative schizophrenia candidate genes. Two genes involved in the regulation of oligodendrocyte function, oligodendrocyte lineage transcription factor 2 (*OLIG2*) and 2'3'-cyclic nucleotide 3'-phosphodiesterase (*CNP*), have been implicated in schizophrenia [175,176]. Each of these findings requires further genetic investigation in independent samples. Many other positive and negative candidate gene studies in schizophrenia have been reported. Among these, the metabotropic glutamate receptor 3 gene (*GRM3*) has been investigated in at least five studies; however, in each instance the association identified is weak, and there is no consistency as to the associations identified.

Semaphorin6A (*SEMA6A*) is a member of a family of genes involved in cell migration, axon guidance, and synaptogenesis. Mutant mice with deletion of this gene have a spectrum of subtle defects in cell migration and axon guidance in the brain, including the thalamocortical system [177], hippocampus [178], cerebellum [179], and various other structures. Thus, there is some overlap between these defects and those reported in neuropathologic and neuroimaging studies of putative network disconnectivity in schizophrenia [2,6,47,180,181]. This gene falls into a well-replicated linkage peak for schizophrenia on 5q21 [182], as do all the other members of this family (*SEMA6B*, *-C*, and *-D*) together with several of the *PlexinA* (*PLXNA1-4*) family of genes that encode interacting proteins [178,183].

The authors' recent functional studies indicate that *SEMA6A* mutants show behavioral defects associated with schizophrenia, including hyperactivity that is reversed by clozapine and impaired working memory, together with a general alteration in cortical electroencephalographic patterns, particularly an increase in alpha power that also is reversed by clozapine. At the same time, an unbiased whole-genome association study identified *PLXNA2*, the receptor for *SEMA6A*, as a risk factor for schizophrenia [184]. These initial observations suggest that the Semaphorin and Plexin gene families may be viable general candidates for involvement in schizophrenia, endophenotypes, or involved in related disorders. For example, *PLXNA2* also has been associated with anxiety in a separate study [185], whereas variants in *PLXNB3* are associated with differences in spatial memory [186].

Another example of the bottom-up approach is provided by investigations in mice mutant for the calcineurin gene, which encodes a serine-threonine phosphatase. The calcineurin pathway is involved in many different processes, both in neural development and in adult neural function [187]. Mutants with forebrain-specific deletion of calcineurin show a number of behavioral phenotypes related to schizophrenia, including impaired working memory, re-duced social interaction, and increased responsiveness to a glutamatergic antag-onist, suggesting the possible involvement of this pathway in schizophrenia [188]. Using detailed knowledge of the biochemical signaling pathway of calci-neurin, association analyses have revealed positive associations with schizo-phrenia for the gene encoding the gamma regulatory subunit of calcineurin, *PPP3CC* [189]. This association has been replicated, and another association has been found with one of the downstream targets of calcineurin, the early growth response gene *EGR3* [190]. *EGR3*, which encodes a transcription factor, also is downstream of *NRG1* signaling [191].

GENE–GENE INTERACTIONS

Identifying that specific genes contribute to disease risk is important, but under-standing the relationships between risk-inducing (or protective) genes is prob-ably more so. The effects of some genes may depend on their interactions with others (ie, epistasis; gene–gene interactions), and statistical evidence of interaction may guide researchers to investigate specific molecular pathways contributing to complex disorders. For example, although *COMT* variation may not contribute directly to the risk of schizophrenia, a study in United States and European samples suggests epistasis with a number of other candi-date genes, most significantly with *RGS4* [192]; in this study, the contribution of markers at *RGS4* to schizophrenia risk was dependent on *COMT* genotype.

Most such studies in schizophrenia to date have been prompted by existing biologic evidence of a relationship between the genes being investigated. For example, in a study of *DAOA* and *DAO*, an epistatic interaction between markers at *DAOA* and *DAO* was greater than the single-locus effects at either gene [131]. Only one of three reported replication studies found evidence for epistasis between these genes, and this observation involved different markers [133]. Assessing whether this finding is confirmatory is difficult, because differ-ent variants may contribute to risk in different populations. Among alternatives to analyzing pairs of SNP–SNP interactions, gene-based tests that simulta-neously consider all SNPs in a pair of genes may be more powerful.

Neuregulin-1 isoforms are ligands for the erbB3 and erbB4 tyrosine kinase receptors. In particular, erbB4 can regulate neuronal migration, GABAergic in-terneurone function, and NMDA receptor signaling [118]. That *erbB4* mutants behave similarly to *NRG1* mutants [113] suggests a potential role for this gene and its interaction with *NRG1* in schizophrenia risk. In a large schizophrenia case-control sample from the United Kingdom, individuals heterozygous for *IVS12-15* C-T genotypes exhibited higher risk of disease as the number of cop-ies of the *NRG_{ICE}* haplotype increased; a similar trend was seen in an indepen-dent sample [193]. The same group performed a more intensive investigation of oligodendrocyte/myelination related (*OMR*) genes and identified significant ev-idence for interaction between *erbB4* and *OLIG2* and between *OLIG2* and *CNP* [175]. These findings clearly indicate a need for more formal investigation of epistasis between *OMR* genes.

If alterations in the levels of dysbindin are disrupting the assembly and function of *BLOC-1* and possibly affecting intracellular lysosomal trafficking and glutamate function in patients who have schizophrenia, then other genes encoding BLOC-1 proteins may be susceptibility genes for the disorder. This hypothesis has been investigated by at least two studies, one of which performed gene-based tests of epistasis among all the genes coding for BLOC-1 components and found significant evidence for epistasis between dysbindin and the gene *MUTED* [194]. The *MUTED* SNP that contributed most strongly to the allele-based signal (rs10458217) was independently associated with schizophrenia in a case-control sample from the United States and also interacted with *DTNBP1* in that sample. Several groups are now investigating genes involved in other components of the presynaptic vesicular transport system for evidence of additive and epistatic effects on risk for schizophrenia.

These preliminary findings emphasize the importance of considering each potential risk-inducing gene not in isolation but rather as an entity having putative interactions with other genes at a functional level that ultimately determine the risk for schizophrenia and phenotypic profile [195].

GENE–ENVIRONMENT INTERACTIONS

Although the previous analysis indicates the need for investigating interactions between genes, it is essential to recognize that the effects of some genes also may depend on their interaction with environmental factors (gene–environment interactions). Although evidence for a genetic contribution to the risk for schizophrenia is overwhelming, it must be juxtaposed with primarily epidemiologic studies that indicate a role for environmental factors, both biologic [196] and psychosocial [197,198], and, by implication, for gene–environment interactions.

Only recently have traditional, indirect arguments for such interactions been sustained by the first systematic studies to combine contemporary molecular genetics with prospectively collected data on environmental variables. A landmark investigation showed that, in a prospectively identified birth cohort, *COMT* genotype influences the association between adolescent exposure to cannabis and subsequent risk for schizophreniform disorder in adulthood [129]. Further studies of this type, together with the ability to address in detail the mechanistic interplay between genetic and environmental variables in mutant models, may be powerfully heuristic in elucidating the functional genomics of schizophrenia.

FUTURE DIRECTIONS

The first wave of large-scale whole-genome association studies of schizophrenia will soon be in press, to be followed over the next several years by multiple additional reports. These studies will assay a majority of the genomic variation in the samples investigated but in turn will be superceded by sequencing platforms providing complete sequence information. Carefully investigating and comparing these datasets will be important in identifying novel candidate genes. With such a wealth of data, however, it also will be important to distinguish signal from noise in period when the methodology for analyzing these data is still evolving. Ultimately, statistical evidence for the association between a gene and schizophrenia is a step in a process that ends with functional understanding of the mechanisms involved. A key question, not yet resolved, will be what criteria should be used in deciding which genes should be brought forward to this next step of functional genomic studies. Additionally, investigators already are beginning to understand the importance of interactions between genes. Epistasis analysis at the level of the genome has been proposed but would be computationally intensive [199]. Nevertheless, one study suggests that mining whole-genome association data for all pairwise interactions is feasible and for certain allele frequencies and effect sizes could identify genes that would not be detected by single-gene association values [199]. Reviewing the breadth and depth of methodologies involved in investigating epistasis is beyond the scope of this article; the interested reader is referred to an authoritative text [200].

To dissect the links from schizophrenia risk genes to abnormal behavior, it will be necessary to understand (1) the functions of the proteins concerned; (2) the cells in which they are expressed; (3) the time during which they function; (4) the circuits in which they function; (5) how mutations lead to circuit dysfunction; and (6) how circuit dysfunction leads to altered behavior and psychopathology. To explore this sequence in model organisms, from gene and protein through cellular morphology and physiology to behavior, will require the generation of more sophisticated genetic lesions than typically have been made to date.

Null mutations in mice are a powerful route for discovering protein function and can provide evidence to support involvement in psychiatric disease; however, they are less incisive for dissecting pathogenic mechanisms. Still more informative will be temporally controlled and tissue-specific gene deletions [188,201–203]. For example, these deletions could be used, respectively, to assess whether the function of a protein is required in development or in an ongoing fashion in adults, and to link (dys)function in specific circuits to (dys)function in specific behaviors. Analysis of double and triple mutants also may reveal epistatic interactions that could be relevant to human population studies, although the link between biologic epistasis and statistical epistasis probably is not direct [195,200].

Such studies will benefit hugely from greater integration across different levels of analysis. This integration will be important at two levels: first within species, moving from developmental and anatomic studies to physiologic, pharmacologic, and behavioral analyses; and second, between species, translating from anatomic defects in mutant mice to neuropathologic and MRI studies in humans, or from cellular physiology and behavior in mutant mice to electroencephalographic and fMRI studies in humans. Recent advances in MRI techniques such as diffusion tensor imaging should make it possible to assess circuitry directly rather than inferring differences in connectivity from functional studies.

The schizophrenia susceptibility genes identified to date probably represent a small fraction of the genetic architecture of psychotic illness. Progressive elaboration of endophenotypic assessments and analyses will allow functional relationships, from cellular to psychopathologic, to be explored in even greater breadth and depth.

References

[1] Freedman R. Schizophrenia. N Engl J Med 2003;349(18):1738–49.

[2] Harrison PJ, Weinberger DR. Schizophrenia genes, gene expression, and neuropathology: on the matter of their convergence. Mol Psychiatry 2005;10(1):40–68.

[3] Karayiorgou M, Gogos JA. Schizophrenia genetics: uncovering positional candidate genes. Eur J Hum Genet 2006;14(5):512–9.

[4] Owen MJ, Craddock N, O'Donovan MC. Schizophrenia: genes at last? Trends Genet 2005;21(9):518–25.

[5] Thaker GK, Carpenter WT Jr. Advances in schizophrenia. Nat Med 2001;7(6):667–71.

[6] Waddington JL. Neuroimaging and other neurobiological indices in schizophrenia: relationship to measurement of functional outcome. Br J Psychiatry; in press.

[7] Cardno AG, Gottesman II. Twin studies of schizophrenia: from bow-and-arrow concordances to Star Wars Mx and functional genomics. Am J Med Genet 2000;97:12–7.

[8] Badner JA, Gershon ES. Meta-analysis of whole-genome linkage scans of bipolar disorder and schizophrenia. Mol Psychiatry 2002;7(4):405–11.

[9] Lewis CM, Levinson DF, Wise LH, et al. Genome scan meta-analysis of schizophrenia and bipolar disorder, part II: schizophrenia. Am J Hum Genet 2003;73(1):34–48.

[10] MacIntyre DJ, Blackwood DH, Porteous DJ, et al. Chromosomal abnormalities and mental illness. Mol Psychiatry 2003;8(3):275–87.

[11] Millar JK, James R, Brandon NJ, et al. DISC1 and DISC2: discovering and dissecting molecular mechanisms underlying psychiatric illness. Ann Med 2004;36(5):367–78.

[12] Murphy KC. Schizophrenia and velo-cardio-facial syndrome. Lancet 2002;359(9304): 426–30.

[13] Murphy KC, Jones LA, Owen MJ. High rates of schizophrenia in adults with velo-cardio-facial syndrome. Arch Gen Psychiatry 1999;56(10):940–5.

[14] Liu H, Heath SC, Sobin C, et al. Genetic variation at the 22q11 PRODH2/DGCR6 locus presents an unusual pattern of susceptibility to schizophrenia. Proc Natl Acad Sci USA 2002;99:3717–22.

[15] Glaser B, Moskvina V, Kirov G, et al. Analysis of ProDH, COMT and ZDHHC8 risk variants does not support individual or interactive effects on schizophrenia susceptibility. Schizophr Res 2006;87(1–3):21–7.

[16] Mukai J, Liu H, Burt RA, et al. Evidence that the gene encoding ZDHHC8 contributes to the risk of schizophrenia. Nat Genet 2004;36(7):725–31.

[17] Murtagh A, McTigue O, Hegarty AM, et al. Interstitial deletion of chromosome 21 and schizophrenia. Schizophr Res 2005;78(2-3):353–6.

[18] Redon R, Ishikawa S, Fitch KR, et al. Global variation in copy number in the human genome. Nature 2006;444(7118):444–54.

[19] Sebat J, Lakshmi B, Troge J, et al. Large-scale copy number polymorphism in the human genome. Science 2004;305(5683):525–8.

[20] Wilson GM, Flibotte S, Chopra V, et al. DNA copy-number analysis in bipolar disorder and schizophrenia reveals aberrations in genes involved in glutamate signaling. Hum Mol Genet 2006;15(5):743–9.

[21] Stranger BE, Forrest MS, Dunning M, et al. Relative impact of nucleotide and copy number variation on gene expression phenotypes. Science 2007;315(5813):848–53.

[22] Risch N, Merikangas K. The future of genetic studies of complex human diseases. Science 1996;273:1516–7.

[23] Duerr RH, Taylor KD, Brant SR, et al. A genome-wide association study identifies IL23R as an inflammatory bowel disease gene. Science 2006;314(5804):1461–3.

[24] Klein RJ, Zeiss C, Chew EY, et al. Complement factor H polymorphism in age-related macular degeneration. Science 2005;308:385–9.

[25] Gottesman II, Gould TD. The endophenotype concept in psychiatry: etymology and strategic intentions. Am J Psychiatry 2003;160:636–45.

[26] Cardno AG, Sham PC, Murray RM, et al. Twin study of symptom dimensions in psychoses. Br J Psychiatry 2001;179:39–45.

[27] Fanous AH, van den Oord EJ, Riley BP, et al. Relationship between a high-risk haplotype in the DTNBP1 (dysbindin) gene and clinical features of schizophrenia. Am J Psychiatry 2005;162(10):1824–32.

[28] Derosse P, Hodgkinson CA, Lencz T, et al. Disrupted in schizophrenia 1 genotype and positive symptoms in schizophrenia. Biol Psychiatry 2007;61(10):1208–10.

[29] Derosse P, Funke B, Burdick KE, et al. Dysbindin genotype and negative symptoms in schizophrenia. Am J Psychiatry 2006;163(3):532–4.

[30] Erlenmeyer-Kimling L, Rock D, Roberts SA, et al. Attention, memory, and motor skills as childhood predictors of schizophrenia-related psychoses: the New York High-Risk Project. Am J Psychiatry 2000;157:1416–22.

[31] Niendam TA, Bearden CE, Rosso IM, et al. A prospective study of childhood neurocognitive functioning in schizophrenic patients and their siblings. Am J Psychiatry 2003;160:2060–2.

[32] Green MF, Kern RS, Heaton RK. Longitudinal studies of cognition and functional outcome in schizophrenia: implications for MATRICS. Schizophr Res 2004;72:41–51.

[33] Cannon TD, Huttunen MO, Lonnqvist J, et al. The inheritance of neuropsychological dysfunction in twins discordant for schizophrenia. Am J Hum Genet 2000;67(2):369–82.

[34] Goldberg TE, Ragland JD, Torrey EF, et al. Neuropsychological assessment of monozygotic twins discordant for schizophrenia. Arch Gen Psychiatry 1990;47:1066–72.

[35] Goldberg TE, Torrey EF, Gold JM, et al. Genetic risk of neuropsychological impairment in schizophrenia: a study of monozygotic twins discordant and concordant for the disorder. Schizophr Res 1995;17:77–84.

[36] Sullivan PF, Kendler KS, Neale MC. Schizophrenia as a complex trait: evidence from a meta-analysis of twin studies. Arch Gen Psychiatry 2003;60(112):1187–92.

[37] Nieuwenstein MR, Aleman A, de Haan EH. Relationship between symptom dimensions and neurocognitive functioning in schizophrenia: a meta-analysis of WCST and CPT studies. J Psychiatr Res 2001;35:119–25.

[38] Donohoe G, Robertson IH. Can specific deficits in executive functioning explain the negative symptoms of schizophrenia? A review. Neurocase 2003;9(2):97–108.

[39] Good KP, Rabinowitz J, Whitehorn D, et al. The relationship of neuropsychological test performance with the PANSS in antipsychotic naive, first-episode psychosis patients. Schizophr Res 2004;68:11–9.

[40] Freedman R, Adler LE, Leonard S. Alternative phenotypes for the complex genetics of schizophrenia. Biol Psychiatry 1999;45:551–8.

[41] Egan MF, Goldberg TE, Kolachana BS, et al. Effect of COMT Val108/158 Met genotype on frontal lobe function and risk for schizophrenia. Proc Natl Acad Sci U S A 2001;98:6917–22.

[42] Hughes C, Kumari V, Das M, et al. Cognitive functioning in siblings discordant for schizophrenia. Acta Psychiatr Scand 2005;111(3):185–92.

[43] Javitt DC, Strous RD, Grochowski S, et al. Impaired precision, but normal retention, of auditory sensory ("echoic") memory information in schizophrenia. J Abnorm Psychol 1997;106:315–24.

[44] Yeap S, Kelly SP, Sehatpour P, et al. Early visual sensory deficits as endophenotypes for schizophrenia: high-density electrical mapping in clinically unaffected first-degree relatives. Arch Gen Psychiatry 2006;63(11):1180–8.

[45] Honea R, Crow TJ, Passingham D, et al. Regional deficits in brain volume in schizophrenia: a meta-analysis of voxel-based morphometry studies. Am J Psychiatry 2005;162(12): 2233–45.

[46] Vita A, De Peri L, Silenzi C, et al. Brain morphology in first-episode schizophrenia: a meta-analysis of quantitative magnetic resonance imaging studies. Schizophr Res 2006;82(1): 75–88.

[47] Tost H, Ende G, Ruf M, et al. Functional imaging research in schizophrenia. Int Rev Neurobiol 2005;67:95–118.

[48] Arguello PA, Gogos JA. Modeling madness in mice: one piece at a time. Neuron 2006;52: 179–96.

[49] Chen J, Lipska BK, Weinberger DR. Genetic mouse models of schizophrenia: from hypothesis-based to susceptibility gene-based models. Biol Psychiatry 2006;59:1180–8.

[50] O'Sullivan GJ, O'Tuathaigh CM, Clifford JJ, et al. Potential and limitations of genetic manipulation in animals. Drug Disc Today: Tech 2006;3(2):173–80.

[51] O'Tuathaigh CMP, Babovic D, O'Meara G, et al. Susceptibility genes for schizophrenia: phenotypic characterisation of mutant models. Neurosci Biobehav Rev 2007;31: 60–78.

[52] Barthold SW. Genetically altered mice: phenotypes, no phenotypes, and faux phenotypes. Genetica 2004;122:75–88.

[53] Crusio WE. Flanking gene and genetic background problems in genetically manipulated mice. Biol Psychiatry 2004;56:381–5.

[54] Waddington JL, O'Tuathaigh C, O'Sullivan G, et al. Phenotypic studies on dopamine receptor subtype and associated signal transduction mutants: insights and challenges from 10 years at the psychopharmacology-molecular biology interface. Psychopharmacology 2005;181:611–38.

[55] Williams NM, O'Donovan MC, Owen MJ. Is the dysbindin gene (DTNBP1) a susceptibility gene for schizophrenia? Schizophr Bull 2005;31:800–5.

[56] Bray NJ, Preece A, Williams NM, et al. Haplotypes at the dystrobrevin binding protein 1 (DTNBP1) gene locus mediate risk for schizophrenia through reduced DTNBP1 expression. Hum Mol Genet 2005;14:1947–54.

[57] Talbot K, Eidem WL, Tinsley CL, et al. Dysbindin-1 is reduced in intrinsic, glutamatergic terminals of the hippocampal formation in schizophrenia. J Clin Invest 2004;113: 1353–63.

[58] Weickert CS, Straub RE, McClintock BW, et al. Human dysbindin (DTNBP1) gene expression in normal brain and in schizophrenic prefrontal cortex and midbrain. Arch Gen Psychiatry 2004;61:544–55.

[59] Talbot K, Cho DS, Ong WY, et al. Dysbindin-1 is a synaptic and microtubular protein that binds brain snapin. Hum Mol Genet 2006;15:3041–54.

[60] Camargo LM, Collura V, Rain JC, et al. Disrupted in Schizophrenia 1 interactome: evidence for the close connectivity of risk genes and a potential synaptic basis for schizophrenia. Mol Psychiatry 2007;12:74–86.

[61] Breen G, Prata D, Osborne S, et al. Association of the dysbindin gene with bipolar affective disorder. Am J Psychiatry 2006;163(9):1636–8.

[62] Pae CU, Serretti A, Mandelli L, et al. Effect of 5-haplotype of dysbindin gene (DTNBP1) polymorphisms for the susceptibility to bipolar I disorder. Am J Med Genet B Neuropsychiatr Genet; in press.

[63] Raybould R, Green EK, MacGregor S, et al. Bipolar disorder and polymorphisms in the dysbindin gene (DTNBP1). Biol Psychiatry 2005;57:696–701.

[64] Craddock N, O'Donovan MC, Owen MJ. Genes for schizophrenia and bipolar disorder? Implications for psychiatric nosology. Schizophr Bull 2006;32(1):9–16.

[65] Burdick KE, Goldberg TE, Funke B, et al. DTNBP1 genotype influences cognitive decline in schizophrenia. Schizophr Res 2007;89(1-3):169–72.

[66] Gornick MC, Addington AM, Sporn A, et al. Dysbindin (DTNBP1, 6p22. 3) is associated with childhood-onset psychosis and endophenotypes measured by the Premorbid Adjustment Scale (PAS). J Autism Dev Disord 2005;35:831–8.

[67] Burdick KE, Lencz T, Funke B, et al. Genetic variation in DTNBP1 influences general cognitive ability. Hum Mol Genet 2006;15:1563–8.

[68] Fallgatter AJ, Herrmann MJ, Hohoff C, et al. DTNBP1 (dysbindin) gene variants modulate prefrontal brain function in healthy individuals. Neuropsychopharmacology 2006;31: 2002–10.

[69] Donohoe G, Morris DW, Clarke S, et al. Variance in neurocognitive performance is associated with dysbindin-1 in schizophrenia: a preliminary study. Neuropsychologia 2007;45:454–8.

[70] Williams NM, Preece A, Morris DW, et al. Identification in 2 independent samples of a novel schizophrenia risk haplotype of the dystrobrevin binding protein gene (DTNBP1). Arch Gen Psychiatry 2004;61:336–44.

[71] Plomin R, Spinath FM. Genetics and general cognitive ability (g). Trends Cogn 2002;6(4): 169–76.

[72] Li W, Zhang Q, Oiso N, et al. Hermansky-Pudlak syndrome type 7 (HPS-7) results from mutant dysbindin, a member of the biogenesis of lysosome-related organelles complex 1 (BLOC-1). Nat Genet 2003;35:84–9.

[73] Hattori S, Chiba S, Takeda M, et al. Dysbindin knockout mouse reveals abnormal behaviour in a novel environment. Program No. 188.2. 2006 Neuroscience Meeting Planner. Atlanta, GA: Society for Neuroscience; 2006. Available at: http://www.sfn.org/am2006. Accessed April 1, 2007.

[74] Arnold SE, Carlson GC, Talbot K, et al. Failure of inhibition in the hippocampus of the dysbindin mutant "Sandy" mouse. Program No. 936.13. 2005 Neuroscience Meeting Planner. Washington, DC: Society for Neuroscience; 2005. Available at: http://www.sfn.org/am2005. Accessed April 1, 2007.

[75] St Clair D, Blackwood D, Muir W, et al. Association within a family of a balanced autosomal translocation with major mental illness. Lancet 1990;336(8706):13–6.

[76] Blackwood DH, Fordyce A, Walker MT, et al. Schizophrenia and affective disorders–cosegregation with a translocation at chromosome 1q42 that directly disrupts brain-expressed genes: clinical and P300 findings in a family. Am J Hum Genet 2001;69(2): 428–33.

[77] Ekelund J, Hovatta I, Parker A, et al. Chromosome 1 loci in Finnish schizophrenia families. Hum Mol Genet 2001;10(15):1611–7.

[78] Hovatta I, Varilo T, Suvisaari J, et al. A genomewide screen for schizophrenia genes in an isolated Finnish subpopulation, suggesting multiple susceptibility loci. Am J Hum Genet 1999;65(4):1114–24.

[79] Detera-Wadleigh SD, Badner JA, Berrettini WH, et al. A high-density genome scan detects evidence for a bipolar-disorder susceptibility locus on 13q32 and other potential loci on 1q32 and 18p11.2. Proc Natl Acad Sci USA 1999;96(10):5604–9.

[80] Gejman PV, Martinez M, Cao Q, et al. Linkage analysis of fifty-seven microsatellite loci to bipolar disorder. Neuropsychopharmacology 1993;9(1):31–40.

[81] Hennah W, Varilo T, Kestila M, et al. Haplotype transmission analysis provides evidence of association for DISC1 to schizophrenia and suggests sex-dependent effects. Hum Mol Genet 2003;12(23):3151–9.

[82] Hennah W, Tuulio-Henriksson A, Paunio T, et al. A haplotype within the DISC1 gene is associated with visual memory functions in families with a high density of schizophrenia. Mol Psychiatry 2005;10:1097–103.

[83] Hodgkinson CA, Goldman D, Jaeger J, et al. Disrupted in schizophrenia 1 (DISC1): association with schizophrenia, schizoaffective disorder, and bipolar disorder. Am J Hum Genet 2004;75(5):862–72.

[84] Thomson PA, Harris SE, Starr JM, et al. Association between genotype at an exonic SNP in DISC1 and normal cognitive aging. Neurosci Lett 2005;389(1):41–5.

[85] Ma L, Liu Y, Ky B, et al. Cloning and characterization of Disc1, the mouse ortholog of DISC1 (Disrupted-in-Schizophrenia 1). Genomics 2002;80(6):662–72.

[86] Taylor MS, Devon RS, Millar JK, et al. Evolutionary constraints on the Disrupted in Schizophrenia locus. Genomics 2003;81(1):67–77.

[87] Ishizuka K, Paek M, Kamiya A, et al. A review of Disrupted-In-Schizophrenia-1 (DISC1): neurodevelopment, cognition, and mental conditions. Biol Psychiatry 2006;59(12): 1189–97.

[88] Sawamura N, Sawamura-Yamamoto T, Ozeki Y, et al. A form of DISC1 enriched in nucleus: altered subcellular distribution in orbitofrontal cortex in psychosis and substance/alcohol abuse. Proc Natl Acad Sci USA 2005;102(4):1187–92.

[89] Millar JK, James R, Christie S, et al. Disrupted in schizophrenia 1 (DISC1): subcellular targeting and induction of ring mitochondria. Mol Cell Neurosci 2005;30(4):477–84.

[90] Schurov IL, Handford EJ, Brandon NJ, et al. Expression of disrupted in schizophrenia 1 (DISC1) protein in the adult and developing mouse brain indicates its role in neurodevelopment. Mol Psychiatry 2004;9(12):1100–10.

[91] Sawamura N, Sawa A. Disrupted-in-schizophrenia-1 (DISC1): a key susceptibility factor for major mental illnesses. Ann N Y Acad Sci 2006;1086:126–33.

[92] Kamiya A, Kubo K, Tomoda T, et al. A schizophrenia-associated mutation of DISC1 perturbs cerebral cortex development. Nat Cell Biol 2005;7(12):1167–78.

[93] Porteous DJ, Millar JK. Disrupted in schizophrenia 1: building brains and memories. Trends Mol Med 2006;12(6):255–61.

[94] Alberini CM, Ghirardi M, Huang YY, et al. A molecular switch for the consolidation of long-term memory: cAMP-inducible gene expression. Ann N Y Acad Sci 1995;758: 261–86.

[95] Millar JK, Pickard BS, Mackie S, et al. DISC1 and PDE4B are interacting genetic factors in schizophrenia that regulate cAMP signaling. Science 2005;310(5751):1187–91.

[96] Porteous DJ, Thomson P, Brandon NJ, et al. The genetics and biology of DISC1—an emerging role in psychosis and cognition. Biol Psychiatry 2006;60(2):123–31.

[97] Altshuler LL, Ventura J, van Gorp WG, et al. Neurocognitive function in clinically stable men with bipolar I disorder or schizophrenia and normal control subjects. Biol Psychiatry 2004;56:560–9.

[98] Burdick KE, Hodgkinson CA, Szeszko PR, et al. DISC1 and neurocognitive function in schizophrenia. Neuroreport 2005;16:1399–402.

[99] Callicott JH, Straub RE, Pezawas L, et al. Variation in DISC1 affects hippocampal structure and function and increases risk for schizophrenia. Proc Natl Acad Sci USA 2005;102(24): 8627–32.

[100] Cannon TD, Hennah W, van Erp TG, et al. Association of DISC1/TRAX haplotypes with schizophrenia, reduced prefrontal gray matter, and impaired short- and long-term memory. Arch Gen Psychiatry 2005;62:1205–13.

[101] Elvevag B, Goldberg TE. Cognitive impairment in schizophrenia is the core of the disorder. Crit Rev Neurobiol 2000;14(1):1–21.

[102] Ferrier IN, Thompson JM. Cognitive impairment in bipolar affective disorder: implications for the bipolar diathesis. Br J Psychiatry 2002;180:293–5.

[103] Gold JM. Cognitive deficits as treatment targets in schizophrenia. Schizophr Res 2004;72(1):21–8.

[104] Paunio T, Tuulio-Henriksson A, Hiekkalinna T, et al. Search for cognitive trait components of schizophrenia reveals a locus for verbal learning and memory on 4q and for visual working memory on 2q. Hum Mol Genet 2004;13:1693–702.

[105] Austin CP, Ky B, Ma L, et al. Expression of Disrupted-In-Schizophrenia-1, a schizophrenia-associated gene, is prominent in the mouse hippocampus throughout brain development. Neuroscience 2004;124(1):3–10.

[106] Miyoshi K, Honda A, Baba K, et al. Disrupted-In-Schizophrenia 1, a candidate gene for schizophrenia, participates in neurite outgrowth. Mol Psychiatry 2003;8(7): 685–94.

[107] Koike H, Arguello PA, Kvajo M, et al. Disc1 is mutated in the 129S6/SvEv strain and modulates working memory in mice. Proc Natl Acad Sci USA 2006;103(10):3693–7.

[108] Li W, Tinsley M, Ehninger D, et al. Disrupting DISC1 function during development results in schizophrenia-like behaviors in mutant mice. Program No. 1021.3. 2005 Neuroscience Meeting Planner. Washington, DC: Society for Neuroscience; 2006. Available at: http://www.sfn.org/am2006. Accessed April 1, 2007.

[109] Xu Y, Kasda E, Hikida T, et al. Inducible mutant DISC1 mouse model: insights into the pathogenesis of schizophrenia. Program No. 1021.4. 2005 Neuroscience Meeting Planner. Washington, DC: Society for Neuroscience; 2005. Available at: http://www.sfn.org/am2005. Accessed April 1, 2007.

[110] Xu Y, Lancaster K, Sawa A, et al. Inducible expression of mutant disrupted in schizophrenia 1 (DISC1) in mouse forebrain: a time course of behavioral effects related to schizophrenia. Program No.488.4. 2006 Neuroscience Meeting Planner. Atlanta (GA): Society for Neuroscience; 2006. Available at: http://www.sfn.org/am2006. Accessed April 1, 2007.

[111] Hikida T, Morita M, Pletnikov M.V, et al. In vivo MRI and behavioral analyses of transgenic mice expressing the C- terminal truncated mutant DISC1 under the CaMKII promoter. Program No. 674.8. 2005 Neuroscience Meeting Planner. Washington, DC: Society for Neuroscience; 2005. Available at: http://www.sfn.org/am2005. Accessed April 1, 2007.

[112] Torres G, Meeder BA, Hallas BH, et al. Ventricular size mapping in a transgenic model of schizophrenia. Brain Res Dev Brain Res 2005;154:35–44.

[113] Stefansson H, Sigurdsson E, Steinthorsdottir V, et al. Neuregulin 1 and susceptibility to schizophrenia. Am J Hum Genet 2002;71(4):877–92.

[114] Corvin A, Morris DW, McGhee KA, et al. Confirmation and refinement of an 'at risk' haplotype for SZ suggests the EST cluster, Hs.97362, as a potential susceptibility gene in addition to Neuregulin 1. Mol Psychiatry 2004;9(2):208–13.

[115] Stefansson H, Sarginson J, Kong A, et al. Association of neuregulin 1 with schizophrenia confirmed in a Scottish population. Am J Hum Genet 2003;72:83–7.

[116] Li D, Collier DA, He L. Meta-analysis shows strong positive association of the neuregulin 1 (NRG1) gene with schizophrenia. Hum Mol Genet 2006;15(12): 1995–2002.

[117] Steinthorsdottir V, Stefansson H, Ghosh S, et al. Multiple novel transcription initiation sites for NRG1. Gene 2004;342(1):97–105.

[118] Hahn CG, Wang HY, Cho DS, et al. Altered neuregulin 1-erbB4 signaling contributes to NMDA receptor hypofunction in schizophrenia. Nat Med 2006;12(7):824–8.

[119] Flames N, Long JE, Garratt AN, et al. Short- and long-range attraction of cortical GABAergic interneurons by neuregulin-1. Neuron 2004;44:251–61.

[120] Lopez-Bendito G, Cautinat A, Sanchez JA, et al. Tangential neuronal migration controls axon guidance: a role for neuregulin-1 in thalamocortical axon navigation. Cell 2006;125:127–42.

[121] Marin O, Valdeolmillos M, Moya F, et al. Neurons in motion: same principles for different shapes? Trends Neurosci 2006;29(12):655–61.

[122] Harrison PJ, Law AJ. Neuregulin 1 and schizophrenia: genetics, gene expression, and neurobiology. Biol Psychiatry 2006;60:132–40.

[123] Hall J, Whalley HC, Job DE, et al. A neuregulin 1 variant associated with abnormal cortical function and psychotic symptoms. Nat Neurosci 2006;9:1477–8.

[124] Gerlai R, Pisacane P, Erickson S. Heregulin, but not ErbB2 or ErbB3, heterozygous mutant mice exhibit hyperactivity in multiple behavioural tasks. Behav Brain Res 2000;109: 219–27.

[125] O'Tuathaigh CM, O'Sullivan GJ, Kinsella A, et al. Sexually dimorphic changes in the exploratory and habituation profiles of heterozygous neuregulin-1 knockout mice. Neuroreport 2006;17:79–83.

[126] Karl T, Duffy L, Scimone A, et al. Altered motor activity, exploration and anxiety in heterozygous neuregulin 1 mutant mice: implications for understanding schizophrenia. Genes Brain Behav, in press.

[127] O'Tuathaigh CMP, Babovic D, O'Sullivan G, et al. Phenotypic characterisation of spatial cognition and social behaviour in mice with 'knockout' of the schizophrenia risk gene neuregulin 1. Neuroscience; in press.

[128] Boucher AA, Arnold JC, Duffy L, et al. Heterozygous neuregulin 1 mice are more sensitive to the behavioural effects of Delta(9)-tetrahydrocannabinol. Psychopharmacology; 2007;192(3):325–36.

[129] Caspi A, Moffitt TE, Cannon M, et al. Moderation of the effect of adolescent-onset cannabis use on adult psychosis by a functional polymorphism in the catechol-O-methyltransferase gene: longitudinal evidence of a gene x environment interaction. Biol Psychiatry 2005;57:1117–27.

[130] Rimer M, Barrett DW, Maldonado MA, et al. Neuregulin-1 immunoglobulin-like domain mutant mice: clozapine sensitivity and impaired latent inhibition. Neuroreport 2005;16:271–5.

[131] Chumakov I, Blumenfeld M, Guerassimenko O, et al. Genetic and physiological data implicating the new human gene G72 and the gene for D-amino acid oxidase in schizophrenia. Proc Natl Acad Sci USA 2002;99(21):13675–80.

[132] Addington AM, Gornick M, Sporn AL, et al. Polymorphisms in the 13q33.2 gene G72/G30 are associated with childhood-onset schizophrenia and psychosis not otherwise specified. Biol Psychiatry 2004;55(10):976–80.

[133] Corvin A, McGhee KA, Murphy K, et al. Evidence for association and epistasis at the DAOA/G30 and D-amino acid oxidase loci in an Irish schizophrenia sample. Am J Med Genet; in press.

[134] Hall D, Gogos JA, Karayiorgou M. The contribution of three strong candidate schizophrenia susceptibility genes in demographically distinct populations. Genes Brain Behav 2004;3(4):240–8.

[135] Korostishevsky M, Kaganovich M, Cholostoy A, et al. Is the G72/G30 locus associated with schizophrenia? Single nucleotide polymorphisms, haplotypes and gene expression analyses. Biol Psychiatry 2004;56(3):169–76.

[136] Korostishevsky M, Kremer I, Kaganovich M, et al. Transmission disequilibrium and haplotype analyses of the G72/G30 locus: suggestive linkage to schizophrenia in Palestinian Arabs living in the north of Israel. Am J Med Genet B Neuropsychiatr Genet 2006;141(1):91–5.

[137] Schumacher J, Abon Jamra R, Freudenberg J, et al. Examination of G72 and D-amino acid oxidase as genetic risk factors for schizophrenia and bipolar affective disorder. Mol Psychiatry 2004;9:203–7.

[138] Wang X, He G, Gu N, et al. Association of G72/G30 with schizophrenia in the Chinese population. Biochem Biophys Res Commun 2004;319(4):1281–6.

[139] Zou F, Li C, Duan S, et al. A family-based study of the association between the G72/G30 genes and schizophrenia in the Chinese population. Schizophr Res 2005;73(2–3):257–61.

[140] Detera-Wadleigh SD, McMahon FJ. G72/G30 in schizophrenia and bipolar disorder: review and meta-analysis. Biol Psychiatry 2006;60(2):106–14.

[141] Li D, He L. G72/G30 genes and schizophrenia: a systematic meta-analysis of association studies. Genetics 2007;175(2):917–22.

[142] Poo MM. Neurotrophins as synaptic modulators. Nat Rev Neurosci 2001;2:24–32.

[143] Tyler WJ, Alonso M, Bramham CR, et al. From acquisition to consolidation: on the role of brain-derived neurotrophic factor signaling in hippocampal-dependent learning. Learn Mem 2002;9(5):224–37.

[144] Goff DC, Coyle JT. The emerging role of glutamate in the pathophysiology and treatment of schizophrenia. Am J Psychiatry 2001;158(9):1367–77.

[145] Donohoe G, Morris DW, Robertson IH, et al. DAOA ARG30LYS and verbal memory function in Schizophrenia. Mol Psychiatry; in press.

[146] Williams NM, Green EK, Macgregor S, et al. Variation at the DAOA/G30 locus influences susceptibility to major mood episodes but not psychosis in schizophrenia and bipolar disorder. Arch Gen Psychiatry 2006;63(4):366–73.

[147] Hashimoto K, Fukushima T, Shimizu E, et al. Decreased serum levels of D-serine in patients with schizophrenia: evidence in support of the N-methyl-D-aspartate receptor hypofunction hypothesis of schizophrenia. Arch Gen Psychiatry 2003;60(6):572–6.

[148] Toro CT, Kasher PR, Deakin JFW. Altered D-serine metabolism in schizophrenia? A post-mortem study using the Stanley Consortium brains. Schizophr Res 2004;67: 125S–6S.

[149] Wood LS, Pickering EH, Decairo BM. Significant support for DAO as a schizophrenia susceptibility locus: examination of five genes putatively associated with schizophrenia. Biol Psychiatry, 2007;61(10):1195–9.

[150] Hamase K, Takagi S, Morikawa A, et al. Presence and origin of large amounts of D-proline in the urine of mice lacking D-amino oxidase activity. Anal Bioanal Chem 2006;386(3): 705–11.

[151] Konno R, Yasumura Y. Mouse mutant deficient in D-amino acid oxidase activity. Genetics 1983;103(2):277–85.

[152] Hashimoto A, Nishikawa T, Konno R, et al. Free D-serine, D-aspartate and D-alanine in central nervous system and serum in mutant mice lacking D-amino acid oxidase. Neurosci Lett 1993;152:33–6.

[153] Morikawa A, Hamase K, Inoue T, et al. Determination of free d-aspartic acid, d-serine and d-alanine in the brain of mutant mice lacking d-amino acid oxidase activity. J Chromatogr B Biomed Sci Appl 2001;757:119–25.

[154] Almond SL, Fradley RL, Armstrong EJ, et al. Behavioral and biochemical characterization of a mutant mouse strain lacking D-amino acid oxidase activity and its implications for schizophrenia. Mol Cell Neurosci 2006;32(4):324–34.

[155] Hashimoto A, Yoshikawa M, Niwa A, et al. Mice lacking D-amino acid oxidase activity display marked attenuation of stereotypy and ataxia induced by MK-801. Brain Res 2005;1033(2):210–5.

[156] Maekawa M, Watanabe M, Yamaguchi S, et al. Spatial learning and long-term potentiation of mutant mice lacking d-amino-acid oxidase. Neurosci Res 2005;53: 34–8.

[157] Liu W, Yuen EY, Allen PB, et al. Adrenergic modulation of NMDA receptors in prefrontal cortex is differentially modulated by RGS proteins and spinophilin. Proc Natl Acad Sci USA 2006;103(48):18338–43.

[158] Chowdari KV, Mirnics K, Semwal P, et al. Association and linkage analyses of RGS4 polymorphisms in schizophrenia. Hum Mol Genet 2002;11(12):1373–80.

[159] Bowden NA, Scott RJ, Tooney PA. Altered expression of regulator of G-protein signaling 4 (RGS4) mRNA in the superior temporal gyrus in schizophrenia. Schizophr Res 2007;89(1-3):165–8.

[160] Mirnics K, Middleton FA, Stanwood GD, et al. Disease-specific changes in regulator of G-protein signaling 4 (RGS4) expression in schizophrenia. Mol Psychiatry 2001;6(3): 293–301.

[161] Talkowski ME, Seltman H, Bassett AS, et al. Evaluation of a susceptibility gene for schizophrenia: genotype based meta-analysis of RGS4 polymorphisms from thirteen independent samples. Biol Psychiatry 2006;60(2):152–62.

[162] Buckholtz JW, Meyer-Lindenberg A, Honea RA, et al. Allelic variation in RGS4 impacts functional and structural connectivity in the human brain. J Neurosci 2007;27(7): 1584–93.

[163] Grillet N, Pattyn A, Contet C, et al. Generation and characterization of Rgs4 mutant mice. Mol Cell Biol 2005;25:4221–8.

[164] Munafo MR, Bowes L, Clark TG, et al. Lack of association of the COMT (Val158/108 Met) gene and schizophrenia: a meta-analysis of case-control studies. Mol Psychiatry 2005;10(8):765–70.

[165] Meyer-Lindenberg A, Weinberger DR. Intermediate phenotypes and genetic mechanisms of psychiatric disorders. Nat Rev Neurosci 2006;7(10):818–27.

[166] Tunbridge EM, Harrison PJ, Weinberger DR. Catechol-o-methyltransferase, cognition, and psychosis: Val158Met and beyond. Biol Psychiatry 2006;60(2):141–51.

[167] Schwab SG, Hoefgen B, Hanses C, et al. Further evidence for association of variants in the AKT1 gene with schizophrenia in a sample of European sib-pair families. Biol Psychiatry 2005;58(6):446–50.

[168] Huotari M, Santha M, Lucas LR, et al. Effect of dopamine uptake inhibition on brain catecholamine levels and locomotion in catechol-o-methyltransferase-disrupted mice. J Pharmacol Exp Ther 2002;303:1309–16.

[169] Huotari M, Garcia-Horsman JA, Karayiorgou M, et al. D-amphetamine responses in catechol-O-methyltransferase (COMT) disrupted mice. Psychopharmacology 2004;172:1–10.

[170] Mattay VS, Goldberg TE, Fera F, et al. Catechol-O-methyltransferase Val158-Met genotype and individual variation in the brain response to amphetamine. Proc Natl Acad Sci USA 2003;100:6186–91.

[171] Nolan KA, Bilder RM, Lachman HM, et al. Catechol-O-methyltransferase Val158Met polymorphism in schizophrenia: differential effects of Val and Met alleles on cognitive stability and flexibility. Am J Psychiatry 2004;161:359–61.

[172] Tunbridge EM, Bannerman DM, Sharp T, et al. Catechol-O-methyltransferase inhibition improves set-shifting performance and elevates stimulated dopamine release in the rat prefrontal cortex. J Neurosci 2004;24(23):5331–5.

[173] Emamian ES, Hall D, Birnbaum MR, et al. Convergent evidence for impaired AKT1-GSK3 signaling in schizophrenia. Nat Genet 2005;36:131–7.

[174] Lai WS, Xu B, Westphal KG, et al. Akt1 deficiency affects neuronal morphology and predisposes to abnormalities in prefrontal cortex functioning. Proc Natl Acad Sci U S A 2006;103(45):16906–11.

[175] Georgieva L, Moskvina V, Peirce T, et al. Convergent evidence that oligodendrocyte lineage transcription factor 2 (OLIG2) and interacting genes influence susceptibility to schizophrenia. Proc Natl Acad Sci U S A 2006;103(33):12469–74.

[176] Peirce TR, Bray NJ, Williams NM, et al. Convergent evidence for 2',3'-cyclic nucleotide 3'-phosphodiesterase as a possible susceptibility gene for schizophrenia. Arch Gen Psychiatry 2006;63(1):18–24.

[177] Leighton PA, Mitchell KJ, Goodrich LV, et al. Defining brain wiring patterns and mechanisms through gene trapping in mice. Nature 2001;410:174–9.

[178] Suto F, Tsuboi M, Kamiya H, et al. Interactions between Plexin-A2, Plexin-A4, and semaphorin 6A control lamina-restricted projection of hippocampal mossy fibers. Neuron 2007;53:535–47.

[179] Kerjan G, Dolan J, Haumaitre C, et al. The transmembrane semaphorin Sema6A controls cerebellar granule cell migration. Nat Neurosci 2005;8:1516–24.

[180] Kanaan RA, Kim JS, Kaufmann WE, et al. Diffusion tensor imaging in schizophrenia. Biol Psychiatry 2005;58(12):921–9.

[181] Stephan KE, Baldeeb T, Friston KJ. Synaptic plasticity and dysconnection in schizophrenia. Biol Psychiatry 2006;59(10):929–39.

[182] Straub RE, MacLean CJ, O'Neill FA, et al. Support for a possible schizophrenia vulnerability locus in region 5q22–31 in Irish families. Mol Psychiatry 1997;2(2):148–55.

[183] Toyufuku T, Zhang H, Kumanogoh A, et al. Dual roles of Sema6D in cardiac morphogenesis through region-specific association of its receptor, Plexin-A1, with off-track and vascular endothelial growth factor receptor type 2. Genes Dev 2004;18(4):435–47.

[184] Mah S, Nelson MR, Delisi LE, et al. Identification of the semaphorin receptor PLXNA2 as a candidate for susceptibility to schizophrenia. Mol Psychiatry 2006; 11:471–8.

[185] Wray NR, James MR, Mah SP, et al. Anxiety and comorbid measures associated with PLXNA2. Arch Gen Psychiatry 2007;64(3):318–26.

[186] Rujescu D, Meisenzahl EM, Krejcova S, et al. Plexin B3 is genetically associated with verbal performance and white matter volume in human brain. Mol Psychiatry 2007;12: 190–4.

[187] Winder DG, Sweatt JD. Roles of serine/threonine phosphatases in hippocampal synaptic plasticity. Nat Rev Neurosci 2001;2(9):670.

[188] Miyakawa T, Leiter LM, Gerber DJ, et al. Conditional calcineurin knockout mice exhibit multiple abnormal behaviors related to schizophrenia. Proc Natl Acad Sci USA 2003;100(15):8987–92.

[189] Gerber DJ, Hall D, Miyakawa T, et al. Evidence for association of schizophrenia with genetic variation in the 8p21.3 gene, PPP3CC, encoding the calcineurin gamma subunit. Proc Natl Acad Sci USA 2003;100(15):8993–8.

[190] Yamada K, Gerber DJ, Iwayama Y, et al. Genetic analysis of the calcineurin pathway identifies members of the EGR gene family, specifically EGR3, as potential susceptibility candidates in schizophrenia. Proc Natl Acad Sci USA 2007;104:2815–20.

[191] Hippenmeyer S, Shneider NA, Birchmeier C, et al. A role for neuregulin 1 signaling in muscle spindle differentiation. Neuron 2002;36(6):1035–49.

[192] Nicodemus KK, Kolachana BS, Vakkalanka R, et al. Evidence for statistical epistasis between catechol-O-methyltransferase (COMT) and polymorphisms in RGS4, G72 (DAOA), GRM3, and DISC1: influence on risk of schizophrenia. Hum Genet 2007; 120(6):889–906.

[193] Norton N, Moskvina V, Morris DW, et al. Evidence that interaction between neuregulin 1 and its receptor erbB4 increases susceptibility to schizophrenia. Am J Med Genet B Neuropsychiatr Genet 2006;141(1):96–101.

[194] Morris DW, Murphy K, Kenny N, et al. Dysbindin (DTNBP1) and the BLOC-1 protein complex: main and epistatic interactions are potential contributors to schizophrenia susceptibility. Biol Psychiatry; in press.

[195] Mitchell KJ. The genetic of brain wiring; from molecules to mind. PLoS Biol; 2007;5(4):e113.

[196] Brown AS. Prenatal infection as a risk factor for schizophrenia. Schizophr Bull 2006;32(2):200–2.

[197] Spauwen J, Krabbendam L, Lieb R, et al. Impact of psychological trauma on the development of psychotic symptoms: relationship with psychosis proneness. Br J Psychiatry 2006;188:527–33.

[198] Van Os J, Krabbendam L, Myin-Germeys I, et al. The schizophrenia envirome. Curr Opin Psychiatry 2005;18(2):141–5.

[199] Evans DM, Marchini J, Morris AP, et al. Two-stage two-locus models in genome-wide association. PLoS Genet 2006;2(9):e157.

[200] Moore JH. The ubiquitous nature of epistasis in determining susceptibility to common human diseases. Hum Hered 2003;56:73–82.

[201] Gaveriaux-Ruff C, Kieffer BL. Conditional gene targeting in the mouse nervous system: Insights into brain function and diseases. Pharmacol Ther 2007;113(3):619–34.

[202] Hong HK, Chong JL, Song W, et al. Inducible and reversible Clock gene expression in brain using the tTa system for the study of circadian behaviour. PLoS Genet 2007;3(2):e33.

[203] Lewandoski M. Conditional control of gene expression in the mouse. Nat Rev Genet 2001;2(10):743–55.

Psychiatr Clin N Am 30 (2007) 401–416

PSYCHIATRIC CLINICS
OF NORTH AMERICA

Real-World Antipsychotic Treatment Practices

Troy A. Moore, PharmD, MS[a], Nancy H. Covell, PhD[b,c], Susan M. Essock, PhD[d,e], Alexander L. Miller, MD[a,*]

[a]Division of Schizophrenia and Related Disorders, Department of Psychiatry, The University of Texas Health Science Center at San Antonio, Related Disorders–MSC 7792, 7703 Floyd Curl Drive, San Antonio, TX 78229-3900, USA
[b]Division of Health Services Research, Department of Psychiatry, Mount Sinai School of Medicine, One Gustave L. Levy Place, New York, NY 10029-6574, USA
[c]Research Division, Department of Mental Health and Addiction Services, 410 Capitol Ave., MS 14RSD, Hartford, CT 06134, USA
[d]Department of Psychiatry, College of Physicians and Surgeons, Columbia University, Room 2702, Box 100, 1051 Riverside Drive, New York, NY 10032, USA
[e]Department of Mental Health Services and Policy Research, New York State Psychiatric Institute, Room 2702, Box 100, 1051 Riverside Drive, New York, NY 10032, USA

This article examines real-world antipsychotic use in the treatment of schizophrenia by comparing real-world prescribing with medication algorithms and guidelines, by evaluating the evidence underlying recommendations and guidelines, and by examining the roles of side effects and medication adherence in real-world prescribing decisions. The authors first examine patterns of use of antipsychotic agents and of frequently coprescribed psychotropic agents and compare actual use with recommendations found in widely cited medication algorithms and guidelines. They then evaluate the strength of the evidence underlying common recommendations. Next they review recent evidence pertaining to side effects from the Clinical Antipsychotic Trials of Intervention Effectiveness (CATIE) trial [1] that may help inform the selection of antipsychotic for individual patients. Finally, they address the possible impact of adherence to medication on prescribing decisions and review evidence concerning treatments to improve medication adherence.

GUIDELINES AND ALGORITHMS FOR ANTIPSYCHOTIC MEDICATION

One way to evaluate real-world prescribing of antipsychotic medications is to compare actual practice with the recommendations of guidelines and

This work was supported by grants R01 MH59312 (SME), R03 MH 071663 (NHC), and R24 MH072830 (ALM) from the National Institutes of Mental Health.

*Corresponding author. E-mail address: millera@uthscsa.edu (A.L. Miller).

0193-953X/07/$ – see front matter
doi:10.1016/j.psc.2007.04.008

© 2007 Elsevier Inc. All rights reserved.
psych.theclinics.com

algorithms for medication treatment of schizophrenia, which reflect a combination of evidence and expert consensus. Some of the widely cited treatment guidelines for schizophrenia include the American Psychiatric Association (APA) Schizophrenia Treatment Guideline [2,3], the Expert Consensus Guideline on Treatment of Schizophrenia [4], the Texas Medication Algorithm Project (TMAP) Schizophrenia Algorithm [5], the Schizophrenia Patient Outcomes Research Team (PORT) recommendations [6], and the International Psychopharmacology Algorithm Project Schizophrenia Algorithm [7].

Guideline and algorithm recommendations for the use of antipsychotic agents at various points of treatment for schizophrenia are shown in Table 1. Although these algorithms and guidelines differ in some details, the following three recommendations stand out as common to many or all: (1) preferential use of second-generation antipsychotics (SGAs) for first-episode schizophrenia, (2) use of clozapine after one or two failed trials of other antipsychotics, and (3) no or last-resort use of combination antipsychotic medications. Given the considerable consensus around each of these recommendations, one might expect that real-world practices using antipsychotic agents would mirror these recommendations closely. In the following sections the authors review the real-world prescribing practices in each area and the evidence underlying each of these recommendations. When recommendation and practice differ, they explore possible reasons for the discrepancies.

Table 1
Guideline and algorithm recommendations for treatment with antipsychotic agents

	Expert Opinion Guidelines 1999	Texas Medication Algorithm Project 2003	APA[a] 2004	Patient Outcomes Research Team 2004	International Psychopharmacology Algorithm Project 2005
First episode	SGA	SGA	SGA	SGA, FGA	SGA
Second choice	SGA	SGA	SGA, FGA, Clozapine	SGA, FGA	SGA
Third choice	Clozapine	Clozapine, SGA, FGA	Clozapine	Clozapine	Clozapine
Fourth choice	Clozapine augmentation	Clozapine augmentation	Clozapine augmentation	—	Clozapine augmentation, SGA
Fifth choice	—	SGA, FGA	—	—	—
Sixth choice	—	Combinations	—	—	—

Abbreviations: FGA, first-generation antipsychotic; SGA, second-generation antipsychotic.
[a] American Psychiatric Association Practice Guideline for the Treatment of Patients with Schizophrenia.

RECOMMENDATION 1: SECOND-GENERATION ANTIPSYCHOTICS ARE PREFERRED FOR TREATMENT OF PATIENTS PRESENTING WITH FIRST-EPISODE SCHIZOPHRENIA

Algorithms and Guidelines

With the exception of the PORT recommendations, each of these expert panels concluded that a second-generation antipsychotic agent should be used to treat a person's first episode of schizophrenia [2–5,7]. PORT lists both first-generation antipsychotics (FGAs) and SGAs as options [6].

Real-World Practice

Statistics on prescribing antipsychotic agents for schizophrenia in North America do not differentiate between first- and multi-episode cases, but 2001 Medicaid data from California for antipsychotic prescriptions indicated SGAs were used in 69% of schizophrenia-spectrum disorders [8]. Data from IMS Health show the use of SGAs in the United States in 2002 was over 70% [9]. It seems likely, based on clinician reports, that the use of SGAs in first-episode patients is even higher, supporting the conclusion that most first-episode patients are treated with SGAs.

Evidence

Studies of the use of SGAs in first-episode schizophrenia have examined clozapine [10,11], risperidone [12–15], olanzapine [14–17], and quetiapine [15]. These studies indicate that these agents are effective but also find that first-episode patients are particularly prone to weight gain. In the Comparison of Atypicals in First Episode (CAFÉ) study, all groups had substantial weight gains, but patients taking olanzapine had almost twice the increases as patients taking quetiapine or risperidone [15]. The Preventing Morbidity trial comparing risperidone and olanzapine showed no difference in cumulative response rates after 16 weeks of treatment and significantly more weight gain in patients taking olanzapine [14]. Ziprasidone and aripiprazole have lower tendencies to cause weight gain, but studies of these agents in first-episode schizophrenia are lacking [18].

In examining the evidence comparing SGAs and FGAs for first-episode schizophrenia, no differences in symptom response rates were found in studies comparing risperidone with haloperidol [12,13], olanzapine with haloperidol [16,17], and clozapine with chlorpromazine [10]. More subjects were adherent to olanzapine than to haloperidol during the 12-week acute phase of a 104-week study (67% versus 54%, respectively) [16]. The 2-year data from the study found patients taking olanzapine had a longer time to discontinuation of medication than patients taking haloperidol (322 days versus 230 days) and had greater rates of remission (57% versus 44%) [17]. The median time to relapse was substantially better with risperidone than with haloperidol (466 days versus 205 days) [13]. At 52 weeks, 85% of patients taking clozapine remained in the study, versus 77.5% in the chlorpromazine group [10].

The risk of tardive dyskinesia (TD) with antipsychotic agents increases with age [19]. A study examining TD in patients who had first-episode schizophrenia treated with low-dose haloperidol found a 12.3% incidence of TD [20]. In a review of 11 studies analyzing the risk of TD, the weighted mean annual incidence risk of TD was 2.1% with SGAs, versus 5.4% in patients receiving haloperidol [19].

Thus, although guideline recommendations favor the use of SGAs for first-episode schizophrenia, the evidence from randomized, controlled trials does not indicate efficacy advantages for SGAs in short-term studies. The advantage of risperidone over haloperidol in time to relapse during maintenance treatment is an important finding that needs replication in comparisons with other SGAs and other FGAs. The same is true of the finding that patients discontinue haloperidol sooner than olanzapine. Although agents clearly differ in side effects, it is not so clear which side effects should take precedence when selecting an antipsychotic agent for this population of patients. A number of key gaps in the evidence remain:

1. Is the course of illness different with SGAs versus FGAs over the long term (eg, 5 years or longer)?
2. Do the relative risks of TD in this population differ with SGAs versus FGAs, and do the SGAs differ from one another in the risk of TD?
3. Are side-effects profiles the only basis for choosing among antipsychotics for first episode schizophrenia?

In summary, expert recommendations and real-world prescribing practices for antipsychotic agents are quite congruent in the preferential use of SGAs for first-episode schizophrenia. The evidence supporting this practice is not definitive, however, and further studies are needed.

RECOMMENDATION 2: CLOZAPINE SHOULD BE USED FOR TREATMENT-RESISTANT SCHIZOPHRENIA

Algorithms and Guidelines

The various algorithms and guidelines differ somewhat in the number of failed trials suggested before a trial of clozapine is undertaken, but the range is not great. The APA guideline indicates clozapine as an option after failure of only one SGA or FGA. The others suggest that two failed trials are sufficient to warrant a clozapine trial, although the TMAP does present the option of a third trial before clozapine. None of the algorithms or guidelines specifies the duration of nonresponse that should warrant a clozapine trial.

Real-World Practice

Data obtained in 1999 from Novartis estimated that treatment with clozapine had been used in 160,000 patients who had schizophrenia-spectrum disorder in the United States [21]. If one assumes that 20% to 30% of the 2.6 million patients who had schizophrenia in the United States at that time were treatment resistant (25% = 650,000), only 25% of the patients who had treatment-resistant schizophrenia had been treated with clozapine [21].

Evidence

It is estimated that 20% to 30% of patients who have schizophrenia are treatment resistant, and only a modest fraction of these patients are being treated with clozapine [21]. Clozapine has been shown to be more effective than FGAs in treating patients who have not responded to trials with FGAs [22–27]. Clozapine also has been shown to be more effective than other SGAs in treating patients who have had an inadequate response to FGAs [28–30]. Recent data from the CATIE trial show that patients for whom an initial SGA was ineffective have a longer median time to discontinuation of clozapine than with quetiapine, risperidone, or olanzapine (10.5 months versus 2.7–3.3 months) [31].

Many factors may play a role in the diminished used of clozapine; among them are the required laboratory monitoring, increased frequency of physician and clinic visits, and medication side effects (agranulocytosis, weight gain, hyperlipidemia, and increased risk of diabetes). In many clinical settings clinicians refer treatment-resistant patients to a separate team for clozapine management. Although this practice may improve efficiency, it also means that, to receive clozapine, patients often must change prescribers and sometimes even the treatment location. The need to make such changes probably acts as an additional disincentive for patients to try clozapine. An unintended consequence of the use of specialized clozapine clinics also may be that many psychiatry trainees have little, if any, practice in initiating treatment with clozapine, and this lack of familiarity may contribute to their later hesitancy to initiate use of this medication.

In summary, the guidelines and algorithms and the evidence support the use of clozapine after one or two failed trials of an antipsychotic agent. Conversely, data from real-world prescribing practices indicate that the rate of clozapine use is much lower than the incidence of treatment-resistant schizophrenia.

RECOMMENDATION 3: ANTIPSYCHOTIC POLYPHARMACY SHOULD BE A LAST OPTION

Algorithms and Guidelines

Prescribing more than one antipsychotic medication (hereafter, "polypharmacy") other than in combination with clozapine is omitted from consideration in all but one guideline, TMAP, in which polypharmacy is listed as a last resort [5].

Real-World Practice

Increasingly, patients who have schizophrenia are being treated with antipsychotic polypharmacy [32–40], with recent studies reporting an FGA plus SGAs as the most common combinations [41–43]. Reports of the prevalence of antipsychotic polypharmacy among people who have schizophrenia-spectrum disorders vary, with most reporting rates of 10% to 30% [42–53]. Additionally, studies examining prescribing practices through time have shown a trend toward the increasing use of antipsychotic polypharmacy [42,54–56]. For example, a recent report examining antipsychotic polypharmacy in more than 30,000 Medicaid recipients who had schizophrenia found an increase from 32% in 1998 to 41% in 2000 [42].

Evidence

A recent review examining 52 published studies of antipsychotic polypharmacy from 1976 to 2002 concluded that definitive evidence to support this practice was lacking [57]. In one small (n = 40) randomized, double-blind, controlled trial comparing risperidone augmentation with placebo for individuals who continued to experience significant psychotic symptoms despite adequate treatment with clozapine, risperidone augmentation was associated with significant improvements in psychiatric symptoms and was as well tolerated as placebo [58]. Several small, uncontrolled studies also have reported improvement in psychotic symptoms when clozapine has been augmented with risperidone, olanzapine, pimozide, or loxapine [59–64]. Several additional studies report symptomatic improvements after combining FGAs and SGAs [65–67]. On the other hand, one pre-/post study suggests that switching from combined antipsychotic therapy to a single antipsychotic agent does not necessarily destabilize individuals and may even lead to improvement [68].

In the small literature of rigorous studies assessing antipsychotic polypharmacy, most studies have examined clozapine augmented with another agent [57]. Although two studies reported superior results when clozapine was combined with sulpiride [69] or with risperidone [58], two others did not find any benefit of augmenting clozapine with risperidone [70,71]. To date, in the only controlled study evaluating the efficacy and safety of antipsychotic combinations that did not include clozapine, the authors found no significant differences between polypharmacy combining two FGAs and monotherapy with a third FGA [72]. Rigorous trials examining the combination of an FGA and a SGA are completely lacking, even though these combinations are most common forms of antipsychotic polypharmacy.

Although there is no definitive evidence to support the practice of prescribing more than one antipsychotic medication, some studies have documented an increase in adverse events with this practice. For example, an elevated risk for treatment-emergent diabetes mellitus was associated with the use of two SGAs [73], and significantly greater increases in fasting glucose levels were seen in individuals taking clozapine and risperidone than in those taking placebo [71]. Moreover, higher rates of sedation [70], hyperprolactinemia [69], and other adverse effects (mostly movement disorders) [74] have been observed more often in individuals treated with antipsychotic polypharmacy than in those receiving monotherapy.

RECOMMENDATION 4: ADJUNCTIVE PSYCHOTROPIC MEDICATIONS, SUCH AS ANTIDEPRESSANTS AND MOOD STABILIZERS, SHOULD BE USED WHEN INDICATED

Algorithms and Guidelines

These algorithms and guidelines do not provide a great deal of direction on the use of adjunctive psychotropic agents other than antipsychotics to treat schizophrenia. Each, however, encourages treatment of comorbid conditions and/or symptoms as clinically indicated. The APA guideline goes into the greatest detail in reviewing the evidence on the use of antidepressants, mood stabilizers, beta-blockers, and other psychotropic medications.

Real-World Practice

The adjunctive medications most commonly used in schizophrenia are antidepressants, mood stabilizers, anxiolytics, and sedative hypnotics. Baseline data on patients entering the CATIE study found that patients taking antipsychotic agents frequently used adjunctive medication: 38% of the patients were taking antidepressants, 22% were taking anxiolytics, 19% were taking sedative hypnotics, 4% were taking lithium, and 15% were taking other mood stabilizers [75]. Patients participating in the CATIE study had a number of adjunctive medications added to their antipsychotic regimen during the initial treatment period (mean duration of 6 months), including anticonvulsants (3.5%), antidepressants (12%), anxiolytics (12%), and sedative hypnotics (7%) [1].

A retrospective cohort study that lasted 1 year (1995) evaluating patients who had schizophrenia showed that nearly 90% of the patients received a concomitant medication during the year [76]. A variety of studies have shown that a number of patients who have schizophrenia are treated with adjunctive medications such as antidepressants, anxiolytics, and mood stabilizers [75–78]. The use of these agents seems to be increasing since the introduction of the SGAs [77,78].

Evidence

Most of these adjunctive medications have not been studied specifically in schizophrenia. The evidence for the efficacy of antidepressants for comorbid depressive symptoms is not as robust as one might expect [79–83].

Because the use of concomitant psychotropic medications is so common in persons who have schizophrenia, there have been recent efforts to assess the effects of reducing concomitant psychotropic medication burden. In 37 patients who had schizophrenia, gradual tapering of concomitant psychotropic medications (antidepressants, mood stabilizers, and miscellaneous agents) from an average of one to zero over a 3- to 6-month period did not affect the Clinical Global Impression outcome in most patients, and the number of patients worsening during the taper was equivalent to the number improving [84].

The paucity of studies highlights the need for further examination of the efficacy of adjunctive medications in schizophrenia, as well as the need to consider discontinuing these agents once target symptoms or conditions have resolved.

RECOMMENDATION 5: MOST PATIENTS WHO HAVE SCHIZOPHRENIA WILL RESPOND TO, AND SHOULD BE TREATED WITH, DOSAGES OF ANTIPSYCHOTIC MEDICATIONS WITHIN A THERAPEUTIC RANGE

Algorithms and Guidelines

With the exception of the International Psychopharmacology Algorithm Project, the guidelines and algorithms reviewed here contain specific recommended ranges of dosages for antipsychotic agents. As discussed later, the dosing recommendations are not uniform across guidelines, reflecting the dynamic nature of knowledge about optimal dosing.

Real-World Practice

The PORT study showed that real-world treatments for schizophrenia often did not follow dosing recommendations, especially in outpatients [85]. Antipsychotic medications were prescribed for 89.2% of inpatients and for 92.3% of outpatients. Only 62% of inpatients and 29% of outpatients were receiving antipsychotic medications at dosages that were in the therapeutic range defined by an expert panel. A recent survey of physicians in the APA practice network, however, found that dosages of antipsychotics were within recommended ranges 83% of the time [86].

A study examining national Department of Veterans Affairs data in fiscal year 2000 found 27.8% (14,932 patients) of patients who had schizophrenia were dosed below PORT dosing recommendations, and 10.1% (5425 patients) were dosed above PORT dosing recommendations. Patients who were black, who had a greater than 50% service connection, who were prescribed SGAs, and who were treated in facilities with higher proportions of total cost spent on mental health or research and education were more likely to be dosed above PORT recommendations. Patients who were elderly (age 65 years or over), who were female, who had a less than 50% service connection, or who had co-morbid psychiatric disorders were more likely to be dosed below recommended PORT dosing ranges [87].

In a Medicaid beneficiary sample of patients who had schizophrenia and were at high-risk for hospitalization, 144 patients (40.7%) were receiving antipsychotic agents at dosages above 1000 chlorpromazine (CPZ) equivalents [88]. A trend toward increased side effects ($P = .07$) was seen in patients treated with higher dosages of antipsychotic agents.

Antipsychotic dosing outside the recommended dosage range occurs 17% to 36% of the time during inpatient treatment [85,86]. Although based on a small number of studies, this percentage range is what one might expect, given that treatment-resistant patients and outliers may need higher dosages to obtain a response. Out-of-range antipsychotic dosing in outpatient settings is harder to decipher because of the lack of easily obtainable pharmacy and diagnostic data in the United States.

Evidence

Because dosage ranges are determined on the basis of large-scale studies designed to enroll typical, physically healthy patients, it is inevitable that in real-world practice prescribers will encounter patients who require dosages above or below the recommended range. What is lacking, in terms of evidence, are studies that systematically examine the effects of changing the dosage of patients who are stable on dosages outside the recommended range so that the dosage is within the recommended range.

After the US Food and Drug Administration (FDA) has approved a drug, clinical practice and postmarketing studies may indicate the need to change the recommended dosage range of a medication. Risperidone is a good example. The dosage range in clinical trials ranged from 4 to 16 mg/d, and the FDA approved dosage within this range [89]. Postmarketing studies, however, found the maximal benefits of risperidone to be achieved with dosages between 4 and 8 mg/d. Higher doses were not associated with additional benefits but did result in increased extrapyramidal side effects. The experience was similar with haloperidol, an extensively studied FGA [90,91]. Postmarketing studies also can lead to the use antipsychotic dosages higher than those approved by the FDA. In the CATIE study, for instance, the dosing range of olanzapine was extended to 30 mg/d, although the FDA-approved maximum dose is 20 mg/d [1]. Additionally, positron emission tomography and single-photon emission CT allow in vivo measurement of the central effects of antipsychotic agents on neurotransmitter receptors to determine the optimal doses required to provide benefit while not inducing extrapyramidal side effects [92].

Dosing of antipsychotics outside the recommended dosage ranges should be performed judiciously. Practitioners need to monitor symptoms and effects of subsequent dose changes objectively to justify dosages of antipsychotic agents outside the recommended range. One also must be aware that outliers and treatment-resistant patients may benefit from higher or lower dosages.

RECOMMENDATION 6: SIDE EFFECTS SHOULD GUIDE MEDICATION SELECTION AND SHOULD BE MONITORED AFTER INITIATION OF ANTIPSYCHOTIC TREATMENT

Algorithms and Guidelines

The Expert Consensus Guidelines for the treatment of schizophrenia provide the best-detailed recommendations for selecting medications to avoid side effects [4]. Depending on patient presentation, the practitioner can use patient-specific information to guide the choice of an appropriate antipsychotic agent to avoid or help alleviate side effects.

Real-World Practice

Medication selection in psychiatry is individualized to the specific needs of each patient. The type of antipsychotic chosen depends on the patient's medication history, risk factors for side effects (TD, metabolic side effects, and others), and likelihood of adherence. The antipsychotic agent with the greatest likelihood of benefit and least likelihood of risk should be chosen. Unfortunately, these decisions are complex because of conflicting evidence about the degree and severity of the side effects caused by the antipsychotic medications.

The CATIE and Cost Utility of the Latest Antipsychotic Drugs in Schizophrenia Study (CUtLASS) studies provide data on the frequency of switching antipsychotic agents because of adverse medication effects. In phase I of the CATIE study, 15% of patients discontinued because of side effects [1]. In the CUtLASS study, 51% of those enrolling did so because of medication-induced adverse events [93]. These studies made every effort to enroll typical patients who had schizophrenia, and these numbers illustrate the range of frequencies of side effects as a basis for changing antipsychotics.

Evidence

The CATIE study is particularly helpful in evaluating the comparative likelihood of side effects when various antipsychotics are used. These data can help guide drug selection and information given to patients. Two major domains of side effects well addressed by CATIE data are extrapyramidal side effects and metabolic syndrome.

With regard to extrapyramidal side effects, there were no significant differences in the number of patients who had a Simpson-Angus Extrapyramidal Signs Scale mean score of 1 or higher among the medications, including perphenazine, in the dosage ranges used in the CATIE study [1]. The perphenazine group had the largest percentage of patients taking anticholinergic agents, and there was a significant difference across treatment groups in the percentage of patients having an anticholinergic agent added to their regimen. There also was a significant difference across the treatment groups in the percentage of patients discontinuing treatment because of extrapyramidal side effects, with the perphenazine group being highest but not by a large margin. There was no difference in Abnormal Involuntary Movement Scale (AIMS) global severity score of 2 or higher in the medication groups, but CATIE was too brief a study to allow conclusions about relative likelihood of new-onset TD [1].

There were significant differences across treatment groups in metabolic measures. Of the antipsychotic medications tested, the largest increases in weight and in glycosylated hemoglobin, total cholesterol, and triglycerides levels were seen with olanzapine [1]. Reductions in weight and in glycosylated hemoglobin, total cholesterol, and triglycerides levels were seen with ziprasidone [1]. Similar results were found in phase II of CATIE, with patients taking olanzapine having greater weight gain, total cholesterol level, and triglycerides level, and patients taking ziprasidone having a reduction in these parameters [94].

A follow-up analysis of CATIE data examining the effectiveness of switching antipsychotic medications found that patients randomly assigned to olanzapine or risperidone at baseline and then re-randomized to stay on the same medication had significantly longer times to discontinuation than patients randomly assigned to switch medications (>11.6 and 8.4 weeks, respectively, versus 7.7 and 4.7 weeks, respectively; $P = .007$) [95]. Therefore, for patients who have problems with side effect, an argument can be made for trying to ameliorate the side effects rather than changing antipsychotic agents, if adequate symptom relief has been achieved.

THE ROLE OF ADHERENCE IN REAL-WORLD PRESCRIBING

In real-world prescribing, the importance of evaluating adherence to antipsychotic medication cannot be overestimated. High rates of partial adherence and nonadherence to antipsychotic medications are well documented, with mean rates across studies of 40% to 50% [96]. Nonadherence to antipsychotic medications may be second only to poor adherence to weight loss treatments [97]. Consequences of nonadherence or partial adherence with antipsychotic medication include increased rates of relapse and hospitalization and increased costs [98].

Providers in real-world settings probably factor into their prescribing decisions their sense of whether individuals will take medications as prescribed, and the published literature can inform this assessment. In a review of 39 studies published from 1980 through 2002 examining predictors of adherence to antipsychotic medications, poor insight, negative attitude or subjective response to medication, prior nonadherence, shorter illness duration, poor therapeutic alliance, and poor environment following discharge from hospital were all associated with lower adherence to antipsychotic medication [96]. Use of injectable antipsychotic medications and the presence of and/or severity of side effects were not consistently related to medication adherence, although the authors note that systematic assessments of side effects, particularly subjective side effects, were rarely obtained [96].

Even with awareness of predictors of nonadherence, given the magnitude of the problem overall, providers in real-world settings probably will find themselves intervening with about half of the individuals in their caseload in the hopes of improving adherence. A review of 21 studies published between 1980 and 2001 examining treatments to improve adherence to antipsychotic medications concluded that interventions using a combination of educational, behavioral, and affective (including appeals to feeling and emotion or social relationships and supports) strategies were more effective in increasing adherence to medication than those offering a purely educational approach [99]. Further, when adherence improved, individuals also experienced secondary gains including reduced relapse and hospitalization, decreased psychopathology, improvements in social functioning, and increased insight [99], suggesting that the time invested in such strategies may provide long-lasting benefits for multiple stakeholders.

Before leaving the discussion of adherence, it is important to mention a growing concern regarding how adherence is measured and categorized. In a recent review examining 161 articles published between 1970 and February 2006 reporting studies examining adherence to oral antipsychotic medications, the method most commonly used to assess adherence was self-report; in only 23% of the studies were direct or objective measures (eg, pill counts, blood or urine analyses, electronic monitoring, or electronic refill records) used to assess adherence [100]. Additionally, because definitions of adherence varied broadly across studies, an individual could be categorized as adherent in one study and nonadherent in another [100]. Given these inconsistencies, and given that those who decline to take all medication probably differ from those who are partially adherent, Velligan and colleagues [100] suggest distinguishing these groups in both research and targeted interventions. Further, the authors suggest that future studies should include at least two measures of adherence, with at least one direct or objective measure [100].

References

[1] Lieberman JA, Stroup TS, McEvoy JP, et al. Effectiveness of antipsychotic drugs in patients with chronic schizophrenia. N Engl J Med 2005;353(12):1209–23.

[2] Lehman AF, Lieberman JA, Dixon LB, et al. Work Group on Schizophrenia. American Psychiatric Association practice guideline for the treatment of patients with schizophrenia. 2nd edition. 2004. Available at: http://www.psych.org/psych_pract/treatg/pg/Schizophrenia2ePG_05-15-06.pdf. Accessed October 13, 2006.

[3] McIntyre JS, Charles SC, Anzia DJ, et al. American Psychiatric Association. Treating schizophrenia: a quick reference guide. Available at: http://www.psych.org/psych_pract/treatg/quick_ref_guide/Schizophrenia_QRG.pdf. Accessed October 13, 2006.

[4] McEvoy JP, Scheifler PL, Frances A. The Expert Consensus Guideline Series: treatment of schizophrenia 1999. J Clin Psychiatry 1999;60(Suppl 11):1–81.

[5] Miller AL, Hall CS, Buchanan RW, et al. The Texas Medication Algorithm Project antipsychotic algorithm for schizophrenia: 2003 update. J Clin Psychiatry 2004;65:500–8.

[6] Lehman AF, Kreyenbuhl J, Buchanan RW, et al. The Schizophrenia Patient Outcomes Research Team (PORT): updated treatment recommendations 2003. Schizophr Bull 2004;30(2):193–217.

[7] The International Psychopharmacology Algorithm Project. IPAP schizophrenia algorithm. Available at: www.ipap.org/schiz. Accessed October 13, 2006.

[8] Duggan M. Do new prescription drugs pay for themselves? The case of second-generation antipsychotics. J Health Econ 2005;24:1–31.

[9] IMS Health. Atypical antipsychotics: generating evidence to inform policy and practice. Available at: http://research.imshealth.com/research_schizophrenia.htm. Accessed December 18, 2006.

[10] Lieberman JA, Phillips M, Gu H, et al. Atypical and conventional antipsychotic drugs in treatment-naive first-episode schizophrenia: a 52-week randomized trial of clozapine vs chlorpromazine. Neuropsychopharmacology 2003;28(5):995–1003.

[11] Woerner MG, Robinson DG, Alvir JMJ, et al. Clozapine as a first treatment of schizophrenia. Am J Psychiatry 2003;160(8):1514–6.

[12] Emsley RA. Risperidone in the treatment of first-episode psychotic patients: a double-blind multicenter study. Risperidone Working Group. Schizophr Bull 1999;25(4):721–9.

[13] Schooler N, Rabinowitz J, Davidson M, et al. Risperidone and haloperidol in first-episode psychosis: a long-term randomised trial. Am J Psychiatry 2005;162:947–53.

[14] Robinson DG, Woerner MG, Napolitano B, et al. Randomized comparison of olanzapine versus risperidone for the treatment of first-episode schizophrenia: 4-month outcomes. Am J Psychiatry 2006;163:2096–102.

[15] McEvoy JP, Lieberman JA, Perkins D, et al. Efficacy and tolerability of olanzapine, quetiapine, and risperidone in the treatment of early psychosis: a randomized, double-blind, 52-week comparison. Am J Psychiatry, in press.

[16] Lieberman JA, Tollefson G, Tohen M, et al, HGDH Study Group. Comparative efficacy and safety of atypical and conventional antipsychotic drugs in first-episode psychosis: a randomized, double-blind trial of olanzapine versus haloperidol. Am J Psychiatry 2003; 160(8):1396–404.

[17] Green AI, Lieberman JA, Hamer RM, et al, HGDH Study Group. Olanzapine and haloperidol in first episode psychosis: two-year data. Schizophr Res 2006;86:234–43.

[18] Lublin H, Eberhard J, Levander S. Current therapy issues and unmet clinical needs in the treatment of schizophrenia: a review of the new generation antipsychotics. Int Clin Psychopharmacol 2005;20:183–98.

[19] Corell CU, Leucht S, Kane JM. Lower risk for tardive dyskinesia associated with second-generation antipsychotics: a systematic review of 1-year studies. Am J Psychiatry 2004;161(3):414–25.

[20] Oosthuizen PP, Emsley RA, Maritz JS, et al. Incidence of tardive dyskinesia in first-episode psychosis patients treated with low-dose haloperidol. J Clin Psychiatry 2003;64: 1075–80.

[21] Buckley P, Miller AL, Olsen J, et al. When symptoms persist: clozapine augmentation strategies. Schizophr Bull 2001;27:615–28.

[22] Claghorn J, Honigfeld G, Abuzzahab FS, et al. The risks and benefits of clozapine versus chlorpromazine. J Clin Psychopharmacol 1987;7:377–84.

[23] Kane JM, Honigfeld G, Singer J, et al. Clozapine for the treatment–resistant schizophrenic: a double-blind comparison with chlorpromazine. Arch Gen Psychiatry 1988;45:789–96.

[24] Pickar D, Owen RR, Litman RE, et al. Clinical and biological response to clozapine in patients with schizophrenia: crossover comparison with fluphenazine. Arch Gen Psychiatry 1992;49:345–53.

[25] Breier A, Buchanan RW, Kirkpatrick B, et al. Clozapine in schizophrenic outpatients: effects on positive and negative symptoms. Arch Gen Psychiatry 1994;151:20–6.

[26] Carpenter WT Jr, Conley RR, Buchanan RW, et al. Patient response and resource management: another view of clozapine treatment of schizophrenia. Am J Psychiatry 1995;152: 827–32.

[27] Essock SM, Hargreaves WA, Covell NH, et al. Clozapine's effectiveness for patients in state hospitals: results from a randomized trial. Psychopharmacol Bull 1996;32: 683–97.

[28] Volavka J, Czobor P, Sheitman B, et al. Clozapine, olanzapine, risperidone, and haloperidol in the treatment of patients with chronic schizophrenia and schizoaffective disorder. Am J Psychiatry 2002;159:255–62 [erratum: 159: 2132].

[29] Chakos M, Lieberman J, Hoffman E, et al. Effectiveness of second-generation antipsychotics in patients with treatment-resistant schizophrenia: a review and meta-analysis of randomized trials. Am J Psychiatry 2001;158:518–26.

[30] Conley RR, Kelly DL, Richardson CM, et al. The efficacy of high-dose olanzapine in treatment-resistant schizophrenia: a double-blind, crossover study. J Clin Psychopharmacol 2003;23(6):668–71.

[31] McEvoy JP, Lieberman JA, Stroup TS, et al. Effectivness of clozapine versus olanzapine, quetiapine, and risperidone in patients with chronic schizophrenia who did not respond to prior atypical antipsychotic treatment. Am J Psychiatry 2006;163:600–10.

[32] Ereshefsky L. Pharmacologic and pharmacokinetic considerations in choosing an antipsychotic. J Clin Psychiatry 1999;60(Suppl 10):20–30.

[33] Fourrier A, Gasquet I, Allicar MP, et al. Patterns of neuroleptic drug prescription: a national cross-sectional survey of a random sample of French psychiatrists. Br J Clin Pharmacol 2000;49(1):80–6.

[34] Ito C, Kubota Y, Sato M. A prospective survey on drug choice for prescriptions for admitted patients with schizophrenia. Psychiatry Clin Neurosci 1999;53(Suppl):S35–40.

[35] Keks NA, Altson K, Hope J, et al. Use of antipsychosis and adjunctive medications by an inner urban community psychiatric service. Aust N Z J Psychiatry 1999;33(6):896–901.

[36] Meltzer HY, Kostaoglu AE. Combining antipsychotics: is there evidence for efficacy? Psychiatric Times 2000;17(9):25–34.

[37] Rittmannsberger H, Meise U, Schauflinger K, et al. Polypharmacy in psychiatric treatment. Patterns of psychotropic drug use in Austrian psychiatric clinics. Eur Psychiatry 1999;14(1):33–40.

[38] Stahl SM. Antipsychotic polypharmacy, part 2: tips on use and misuse. J Clin Psychiatry 1999;60(8):506–7.

[39] Stahl SM. Antipsychotic polypharmacy, part 1: therapeutic option or dirty little secret? J Clin Psychiatry 1999;60(7):425–6.

[40] Tapp A, Wood AE, Secrest L, et al. Combination antipsychotic therapy in clinical practice. Psychiatr Serv 2003;54(1):55–9.

[41] Centorrino F, Fogarty KV, Sani G, et al. Use of combinations of antipsychotics: McLean Hospital inpatients, 2002. Hum Psychopharmacol 2005;20:482–92.

[42] Ganguly R, Kotzan JA, Miller LS, et al. Prevalence, trends, and factors associated with antipsychotic polypharmacy among Medicaid-eligible schizophrenia patients, 1998–2000. J Clin Psychiatry 2004;65:1377–88.

[43] Ito H, Koyama A, Higuchi T. Polypharmacy and excessive dosing: psychiatrists' perceptions of antipsychotic drug prescription. Br J Psychiatry 2005;187:243–7.

[44] Biancosino B, Barbui C, Marmai L, et al. Determinants of antipsychotic polypharmacy in psychiatric inpatients: a prospective study. Int Clin Psychopharmacol 2005;20:305–9.

[45] Brunot A, Lachaux B, Sontag H, et al [Pharmaco-epidemiological study on antipsychotic drug prescription in French Psychiatry: patient characteristics, antipsychotic treatment, and care management for schizophrenia]. Encephale 2002;28(2):129–38 [French].

[46] Centorrino F, Eakin M, Bahk WM, et al. Inpatient antipsychotic drug use in 1998, 1993, and 1989. Am J Psychiatry 2002;159:1932–5.

[47] Chee YK, Ungvari GS, Kin CH, et al. A survey of antipsychotic treatment for schizophrenia in Hong Kong. Chin Med J (Engl) 1997;110:792–6.

[48] Covell NH, Jackson CT, Evans AC, et al. Antipsychotic prescribing practices in Connecticut's public mental health system: rates of changing medications and prescribing styles. Schizophr Bull 2002;28:17–29.

[49] Frangou S, Lewis M. Atypical antipsychotics in ordinary clinical practice: a pharmaco-epidemiologic survey in a south London service. Eur Psychiatry 2000;15(3):220–6.

[50] Leslie DL, Rosenheck RA. Use of pharmacy data to assess quality of pharmacotherapy for schizophrenia in a national health care system: individual and facility predictors. Med Care 2001;39(9):923–33.

[51] Procyshyn RM, Kennedy NB, Tse G, et al. Antipsychotic polypharmacy: a survey of discharge prescriptions from a tertiary care psychiatric institution. Can J Psychiatry 2001;46(4):334–9.

[52] Wang PS, West JC, Tanielian T, et al. Recent patterns and predictors of antipsychotic medication regimens used to treat schizophrenia and other psychotic disorders. Schizophr Bull 2000;26(2):451–7.

[53] Weissman EM. Antipsychotic prescribing practices in the Veterans Healthcare Administration–New York metropolitan region. Schizophr Bull 2002;28(1):31–42.

[54] Clark RE, Bartels SJ, Mellman TA, et al. Recent trends in antipsychotic combination therapy of schizophrenia and schizoaffective disorder: implications for state mental health policy. Schizophr Bull 2002;28(1):75–84.

[55] Johnson DAW, Wright NF. Drug prescribing for schizophrenic outpatients on depot injections: repeat surveys over 18 years. Br J Psychiatry 1990;156:827–34.

[56] Taylor D, Holmes R, Hilton T, et al. Evaluating and improving the quality of risperidone prescribing. Psychiatr Bull R Coll Psychiatr 1997;22:680–3.

[57] Patrick V, Levin E, Schleifer S. Antipsychotic polypharmacy: is there evidence for its use? J Psychiatr Pract 2005;11:248–57.

[58] Josiassen RC, Joseph A, Kohegyi E, et al. Clozapine augmented with risperidone in the treatment of schizophrenia: a randomized, double-blind, placebo-controlled trial. Am J Psychiatry 2005;162:130–6.

[59] Friedman J, Ault K, Powchik P. Pimozide augmentation for the treatment of schizophrenic patients who are partial responders to clozapine. Biol Psychiatry 1997;42(6):522–3.

[60] Gupta S, Sonnenberg SJ, Frank B. Olanzapine augmentation of clozapine. Ann Clin Psychiatry 1998;10(3):113–5.

[61] Henderson DC, Goff DC. Risperidone as an adjunct to clozapine therapy in chronic schizophrenics. J Clin Psychiatry 1996;57(9):395–7.

[62] Morera AL, Barreiro P, Cano-Munoz JL. Risperidone and clozapine combination for the treatment of refractory schizophrenia. Acta Psychiatr Scand 1999;99(4):305–6 [discussion: 306–7].

[63] Mowerman S, Siris SG. Adjunctive loxapine in a clozapine-resistant cohort of schizophrenic patients. Ann Clin Psychiatry 1996;8(4):193–7.

[64] Raskin S, Katz G, Zislin Z, et al. Clozapine and risperidone: combination/augmentation treatment of refractory schizophrenia: a preliminary observation. Acta Psychiatr Scand 2000;101(4):334–6.

[65] Bacher NM, Kaup BA. Combining risperidone with standard neuroleptics for refractory schizophrenic patients. Am J Psychiatry 1996;153(1):137.

[66] Goss JB. Concomitant use of thioridazine with risperidone. Am J Health Syst Pharm 1995;52(9):1012.

[67] Waring EW, Devin PG, Dewan V. Treatment of schizophrenia with antipsychotics in combination. Can J Psychiatry 1999;44(2):189–90.

[68] Suzuki T, Uchida H, Tanaka KF, et al. Revising polypharmacy to a single antipsychotic regimen for patients with chronic schizophrenia. Int J Neuropsychopharmacol 2004;7: 133–42.

[69] Shiloh R, Zemishlany Z, Aizenberg D, et al. Sulpiride augmentation in people with schizophrenia partially responsive to clozapine. A double-blind, placebo-controlled study. Br J Psychiatry 1997;171:569–73.

[70] Anil Yagcioglu AE, Kivircik Akdede BB, Turgut TI, et al. A double-blind controlled study of adjunctive treatment with risperidone in schizophrenic patients partially responsive to clozapine: efficacy and safety. J Clin Psychiatry 2005;66(1):63–72.

[71] Honer WG, Thornton AE, Chen EY, et al. Clozapine alone versus clozapine and risperidone with refractory schizophrenia. N Engl J Med 2006;354(5):472–82.

[72] Knight RG, Harrison A. A double-blind comparison of thiothixene and trifluoperazine/chlorpromazine composite in the treatment of schizophrenia. N Z Med J 1979;89:302–4.

[73] Citrome L, Jaffe A, Levine J, et al. Relationship between antipsychotic medication treatment and new cases of diabetes among psychiatric inpatients. Psychiatr Serv 2004;55(9): 1006–13.

[74] Centorrino F, Goren JL, Hennen J, et al. Multiple versus single antipsychotic agents for hospitalized psychiatric patients: case-control study of risks versus benefits. Am J Psychiatry 2004;161:700–6.

[75] Chakos MH, Glick ID, Miller AL, et al. Baseline use of concomitant psychotropic medications to treat schizophrenia in the CATIE trial. Psychiatr Serv 2006;57(8):1094–101.

[76] Williams CL, Johnstone BM, Keterson JG, et al. Evaluation of antipsychotic and concomitant medication use patterns in patients with schizophrenia. Med Care 1999;37(4): AS81–6.

[77] McCue RE, Waheed R, Urcuyo L. Polypharmacy in patients with schizophrenia. J Clin Psychiatry 2003;64(9):984–9.

[78] Edlinger M, Hausmann A, Kemmler G, et al. Trends in the pharmacological treatment of patients with schizophrenia over a 12 year observation period. Schizophr Res 2005;77:25–34.

[79] Siris SG. Akinesia and postpsychotic depression: a difficult differential diagnosis. J Clin Psychiatry 1987;48:240–3.

[80] Siris SG, Bermanzohn PC, Mason SE, et al. Maintenance imipramine therapy for secondary depression in schizophrenia: a controlled trial. Arch Gen Psychiatry 1994;51: 109–15.

[81] Kirli S, Caliskan M. A comparative study of sertraline versus imipramine in postpsychotic depressive disorder of schizophrenia. Schizophr Res 1998;33:103–11.

[82] Addington D, Addington J, Patten S, et al. Double-blind, placebo-controlled comparison of the efficacy of sertraline as treatment for a major depressive episode in patients with remitted schizophrenia. J Clin Psychopharmacol 2002;22:20–5.

[83] Kasckow JW, Mohamed S, Thallasinos A, et al. Citalopram augmentation of antipsychotic treatment in older schizophrenia patients. Int J Geriatr Psychiatry 2001;16:1163–7.

[84] Glick ID, Pham D, Davis JM. Concomitant medications may not improve outcome of anti-psychotic monotherapy for stabilized patients with nonacute schizophrenia. J Clin Psychiatry 2006;67(8):1261–5.

[85] Buchanan RW, Kreyenbuhl J, Zito JM, et al. The schizophrenia PORT pharmacological treatment recommendations: conformance and implications for symptoms and functional outcome. Schizophr Bull 2002;28(1):63–73.

[86] West JC, Wilk JE, Olfson M, et al. Patterns and quality of treatment for patients with schizophrenia in routine psychiatric practice. Psychiatr Serv 2005;56(3):283–91.

[87] Leslie DL, Rosenheck RA. Adherence of schizophrenia pharmacotherapy to published treatment recommendations: patient, facility, and provider predictors. Schizophr Bull 2004;30(3):649–58.

[88] Dickey B, Normand SLT, Eisen S, et al. Associations between adherence to guidelines for antipsychotic dose and health status, side effects, and patient care experiences. Med Care 2006;44:827–34.

[89] Risperdal [package insert]. Available at: http://www.risperdal.com/active/janus/en_US/assets/common/company/pi/risperdal.pdf. Accessed December 18, 2006.

[90] McEvoy JP, Hogarty GE, Steingard S. Optimal dose of neuroleptic in acute schizophrenia. A controlled study of the neuroleptic threshold and higher haloperidol dose. Arch Gen Psychiatry 1991;48(8):739–45.

[91] Rifkin A, Doddi S, Karajgi B, et al. Dosage of haloperidol for schizophrenia. Arch Gen Psychiatry 1991;48(2):166–70.

[92] Tauscher J, Kapur S. Choosing the right dose of antipsychotics in schizophrenia: lessons from neuroimaging studies. CNS Drugs 2001;15(9):671–8.

[93] Jones PB, Barnes TRE, Davies L, et al. Randomized controlled trial of the effect on quality of life of second- vs first-generation antipsychotic drugs in schizophrenia. Cost utility of the latest antipsychotic drugs in schizophrenia study (CUtLASS 1). Arch Gen Psychiatry 2006;63(10):1079–87.

[94] Stroup TS, Lieberman JA, McEvoy JP, et al. Effectiveness of olanzapine, quetiapine, risperidone, and ziprasidone in patients with chronic schizophrenia following discontinuation of a previous atypical antipsychotic. Am J Psychiatry 2006;163(4):611–22.

[95] Essock SM, Covell NH, Davis SM, et al. Effectiveness of switching antipsychotic medications. Am J Psychiatry 2006;163:2090–5.

[96] Lacro JP, Dunn LB, Dolder CR, et al. Prevalence of and risk factors for medication nonadherence in patients with schizophrenia: a comprehensive review of recent literature. J Clin Psychiatry 2002;63:892–909.

[97] Kane JM. Review of treatments that can ameliorate nonadherence in patients with schizophrenia. J Clin Psychiatry 2006;67(Suppl 5):9–14.

[98] Leucht S, Heres S. Epidemiology, clinical consequences, and psychosocial treatment of nonadherence in schizophrenia. J Clin Psychiatry 2006;67(Suppl 5):3–8.

[99] Dolder CR, Lacro JP, Leckband S, et al. Interventions to improve antipsychotic medication adherence: review of recent literature. J Clin Psychopharmacol 2003;23:389–99.

[100] Velligan DI, Lam YWF, Glahn DC, et al. Defining and assessing adherence to oral antipsychotics: a review of the literature. Schizophr Bull 2006;32:724–42.

Pharmacogenetics and Schizophrenia

Adriana Foster, MD[a],*, Del D. Miller, PharmD, MD[b],
Peter F. Buckley, MD[a]

[a]Department of Psychiatry and Health Behavior, Medical College of Georgia, 1515
Pope Avenue, Augusta, GA 30912, USA
[b]University of Iowa, Carver College of Medicine, Psychiatry Research, #2-105 Medical
Education Building, 500 Newton Rd., Iowa City, IA 52242-1000, USA

S chizophrenia is a major focus of genetic research in psychiatry. There is strong support from meta-analyses of linkage studies for susceptibility genes on chromosomes 8p and 22q, whereas other regions like 2q, 5q, 3p, 11q, 6p, 1q, 20q are less supported [1]. Other molecular genetic studies in schizophrenia explored positional candidate genes, such as *neuregulin* on chromosome 8 and dystrobrevin-binding protein 1 *(dysbindin)* on chromosome 6. Catecholamine O-methyltransferase *(COMT)* and *proline dehydrogenase*, associated with deletions on chromosome 22 and disrupted in schizophrenia genes *DISC1* and *DISC2*, genes disrupted by a translocation on chromosome 1, also were studied for their association with schizophrenia. From the large amount of literature about functional candidate genes in schizophrenia, the genes coding for dopamine receptors DRD2 and DRD3 or serotonin receptor HT2A emerge as potential risk factors. *Dysbindin* and *neuregulin* are considered strong susceptibility genes for schizophrenia [2].

First-generation antipsychotics have well-known movement-related side effects, and second-generation drugs have equally concerning metabolic complications. In addition, patients often have incomplete clinical response or do not respond at all to antipsychotic drugs. Thus, clinicians treating patients who have schizophrenia are in dire need of new ways to optimize the outcome, minimize side effects, and individualize their patients' treatment. The emerging field of pharmacogenetics and/or pharmacogenomics aims to uncover and use genetic variations so clinicians can select the drugs that have the highest likelihood of benefit and least likelihood of adverse events in individual patients based on their genetic make-up [3]. Various factors such as age, sex, ethnicity, concomitant disease, liver and kidney function, diet, smoking, and drug–drug interactions can influence the response to drugs. In addition, inherited variations in the DNA sequence of the genes responsible for drug-metabolizing enzymes, drug receptors, transporters, and signal transducers are believed to have significant effects on the

*Corresponding author. E-mail address: afoster@mcg.edu (A. Foster).

0193-953X/07/$ – see front matter
doi:10.1016/j.psc.2007.04.004
© 2007 Elsevier Inc. All rights reserved.

efficacy and toxicity of drugs. Predicting polymorphisms in the drug-metaboliz-ing enzymes, drug receptors, and transporters could increase the clinician's ability to individualize antipsychotic treatment, reduce the time to drug response, avoid potential side effects, and lower the overall burden of mental health treatment [4–6]. Moreover, the use of genetic analyses to predict efficacy and safety in drug discovery and development is becoming a frequently used technology [7].

Far from being all-inclusive, this article summarizes the current findings about the pharmacogenetics of antipsychotic drug response, especially of second-gener-ation antipsychotics (SGAs), and the association of genetic factors with the devel-opment of adverse effects of antipsychotic drugs in schizophrenia.

Terms used in this article are defined in Box 1 [4,8].

PHARMACOGENETICS IN ANTIPSYCHOTIC TREATMENT

Because of the complexity of the human brain, it is not surprising that knowl-edge about the interaction between genetics and the treatment of psychiatric

---

Box. 1: Terms used in this article

Allele: one of several alternative forms of a gene at a given locus (a single-nucle-otide polymorphism [SNP] has 2 alleles)

Diplotype: a combination of two haplotypes

Exon: a segment of a gene that contains the genetic code for an amino acid

Haplotype: a combination of alleles at two or more closely linked gene loci on the same chromosome (for example, the human leukocyte antigen system) [9]

Heritability: ratio of additive genetic variance

Linkage disequilibrium: same block of DNA containing the SNP as well other polymorphisms in the same block, which are not independently inherited but which "travel together"

Nonsynonymous: functional polymorphism, that is, genetic variance that pro-duces changes in protein function

p: the short arm of chromosome

Pharmacogenetics: the role of genetic factors in predicting drug response and potential side effects

Pharmacogenomics: the relationship between whole-genome factors and drug response and potential side effects

Phenotypic variance: the result of the interaction of genetic and nongenetic factors in a population

Polymorphism: a genetic variation that occurs with a frequency of 1% or more in a population

Promoter: the region of a gene that controls the initiation of protein production

q: the long arm of chromosome

Single nucleotide polymorphism (SNP): the substitution of one nucleotide for another (eg, cytosine for timine) creating a mutation in DNA.

Synonymous: SNPs in coding regions that do not influence the structure of the protein illnesses is limited [6]. To date, little progress has been made in elucidating the precise mechanisms of action of new antipsychotics, which have a combined effect on positive, negative, and cognitive symptoms. Part of the reason for this failure is the limited number of appropriate animal models that can manifest these symptoms and be used for drug screening [10,11]. Thus, in the future, it will be of great importance to determine how antipsychotics improve and prevent positive, negative, and cognitive symptoms in patients who have schizophrenia.

CLINICAL RESPONSE TO ANTIPSYCHOTICS

There is a growing literature on the role that pharmacogenetics plays in response to antipsychotic medications in schizophrenia. The preponderance of data relating genetic variations to antipsychotic drug response in schizophrenia was obtained in treatment-refractory patients who had schizophrenia treated with clozapine. Dopamine–serotonin receptor antagonism is believed to be the fundamental basis of atypical antipsychotic action [12], and both monoamine systems have been studied extensively in relation to antipsychotic drug response.

Association Studies of the Treatment Response to Second-Generation Antipsychotics with Polymorphisms in the Dopamine Receptor DRD2 Genes

In second-generation antipsychotics other than clozapine, some work has been done, primarily focusing on acute response. *DRD2* blockade is a property of all known antipsychotic medications, and several polymorphisms have been described in this gene [13,14]. It has been suggested that a diplotype of the *DRD2* receptor, comprised of the *Ins-A2/Del-A1* alleles, may predict better response to risperidone and that the *Ser311Cys* polymorphism may play a role in determining risperidone efficacy for positive, negative, and cognitive symptoms and may affect the general treatment response of several atypical agents.

Functionally, the *DRD2 Taq1A* polymorphism has been associated with lower D2 binding, although its location downstream from *DRD2* itself makes its significance for gene expression unclear [15]. Two *DRD2*-promoter single-nucleotide polymorphisms (SNPs) have been identified: a cytosine insertion/deletion (Ins/Del) at position *-141 (-141C Ins/Del)*, and a guanine-to-adenine transition at position *-241 (A-241G)*. No significant association has been found between the *A-241G* polymorphism and in vitro expression [16] Functionally, the *-141C Ins/Del* has been demonstrated to alter gene expression in vitro [16], and an imaging study in healthy volunteers showed increased striatal receptor density in *Del* carriers [17]. Although one pharmacogenetics study of this polymorphism has indicated reduced chlorpromazine response in *Del* carriers [18], other studies have found inconsistent results [4]. Recently, the *-141C Ins/Del* and *Taq1A* polymorphisms of *DRD2* were tested in 77 risperidone- and 107 olanzapine-treated subjects who had schizophrenia [19]. Neither polymorphism was associated with treatment response to risperidone or olanzapine.

Yamanouchi and colleagues [20] examined these same polymorphisms in 73 Japanese patients who had schizophrenia and who were given risperidone for the treatment of an acute exacerbation of psychosis. A combination of the *-41C Ins/Del* and *Taq 1A* polymorphisms tended to correlate with better clinical performance: subjects who had the *Ins-A2/Del-A1* diplotype (n = 10) showed 40% greater improvement (*P* = .03) on Positive and Negative Syndrome Scale (PANSS) [21] total scores than the patients who had the *Ins-A2/ Ins-A2* diplotype (n = 25). In a recent study of 117 Chinese Han antipsychotic-naive patients who had schizophrenia and who were treated with risperidone or chlorpromazine for 10 weeks, Reynolds and colleagues [22] found that the *Taq1A* polymorphism was not significantly associated with changes in PANSS total scores.

Lencz and colleagues [23] examined the promoter region of the *DRD2* gene as a predictor of the time course of response to risperidone or olanzapine in first-episode schizophrenia. Using Kaplan-Meier curves, they found that carriers of the *-241G* allele showed significantly faster time until sustained response, and carriers of the *-141C Del* allele showed significantly longer time until sustained response. The diplotype of no *-241G* allele and a *-141C Del* allele was associated with a significantly lower response rate.

A functional polymorphism in which there is a substitution of cytosine for serine at position -311 (*Ser311Cys*) in the *DRD2* gene also has been identified. This polymorphism was found to be associated with risperidone treatment response in acutely ill patients who had schizophrenia [24]. Compared with patients who were homozygous for the *Ser* allele (n = 111), patients with a *Ser311Cys* genotype (n = 12) had better clinical response in all dimensions, including positive symptoms, negative symptoms, general psychopathology, cognitive symptoms, and social function. This study was the first to investigate an association between SGA effects and the *Ser311Cys* polymorphism in the *DRD2* gene. These findings support the involvement of the DRD2 receptor in the response to second-generation antipsychotics [25]. Thus, functional differences between *DRD2* variants may be related to genetically determined differences in response to antipsychotic treatment.

Association Studies of Response to Second-generation Antipsychotics with Polymorphisms in the Serotonin (5-hydroxytryptamine, 5HT) Genes

Initial findings by Arranz [26] showed association between the serotonin *5HT2A* allele *102C* and failure to respond to clozapine, but these findings were not replicated by subsequent studies [4]. A more recent study by Lane and colleagues [27] with risperidone showed an association in the opposite direction, between *5HT2A 102C* and response to risperidone in Chinese Han patients.

For the serotonin *5HT2A* receptor and antipsychotic response in schizophrenia, the *T102C* and the *-1438G/A* SNPs, which are in complete linkage disequilibrium, may influence treatment response to risperidone or olanzapine for schizophrenia's negative symptoms (eg, blunted affect and social withdrawal).

In addition, the *5HTR6 T267C* polymorphism has been linked to risperidone response for positive symptoms (delusions and hallucinations).

5HTR2A *Single-nucleotide polymorphisms*
Studies regarding associations between *5HTR2A* receptor polymorphisms and clinical response to clozapine have yielded conflicting results [4]. Lane and colleagues [27], after controlling for nongenetic confounders, evaluated the effect of the *5HT2A 102T/C* polymorphism on risperidone efficacy based on changes in the PANSS. *102T/C* is a synonymous SNP, and although it does not alter amino acid sequence, there is evidence that individuals who have the *C/C* genotype express lower *5HT2A* mRNA and protein than those who have a *T/T* genotype [28]. After 6 weeks of risperidone therapy individuals with the C/C genotype (n = 10) had lower scores in the PANSS total and in the PANSS-negative and the PANSS-general subscales, but not in the PANSS-positive subscale, than those who had the *T/C* genotype (n = 47) [27]. The *T/C* and *T/T* (n = 43) genotypes were comparable in each subscale score. These investigators concluded that the *5HTR2A 102T/C* polymorphism or, alternatively, another genetic variation that is in linkage disequilibrium with this SNP, may influence clinical response for negative symptoms but not for positive symptoms. This study was the first to reveal genetic effects on the antipsychotic efficacy of risperidone for negative symptoms.

Consistent with these findings, Ellingrod and colleagues [29] determined relationships between the *5HTR2A* -1438G/A polymorphism (which is in complete linkage disequilibrium with the *102T/C* polymorphism) and negative symptom response to olanzapine in 41 subjects who had schizophrenia. The *-1438G/A* polymorphism and percent change in negative symptoms showed a borderline trend (P = .054). The *A/A* genotype group had a 45% reduction in negative symptoms, compared with 19% in the other groups. The investigators suggested that the *A/A* genotype may be associated with negative symptom response to olanzapine, seen as a twofold greater percent reduction in negative symptoms. Earlier, Ellingrod and colleagues [30] investigated relationships between clinical response and other *5HTR2A* polymorphisms (*102T/C, 516C/T, Thr25Asn,* and *His452Tyr*) in these 41 subjects. No statistical relationships were found for these polymorphisms.

Yamanouchi and colleagues [20] examined candidate polymorphisms (including *5HTR2A -1438G/A, 102T/C, His452Tyr*) in the 73 Japanese patients mentioned previously, who were given risperidone treatment. After adjustment for the effects of patient-related variables, the *5HTR2A* diplotype did not significantly influence the clinical response. The investigators cautioned that the results could be limited because of the small sample size and heterogeneity of patients with respect to past antipsychotic use history.

In an effort to find out if the *5HT2A* SNPs could explain the differences in antipsychotic response, Davies and colleagues [31] explored in vitro the pharmacology of four nonsynonymous SNPs, which determine the *5HT2A* serotonin receptor variants, compared with the wild type. The in vitro affinity of aripiprazole, clozapine, olanzapine, quetiapine, risperidone, and ziprasidone to the wild type and *T25N*, *I197V*, *A447V*, and *H452Y* variants of the *5HT2A* receptor were measured. There were statistically significant but modest changes in antipsychotic affinity between the wild type and three of the variants of the *5HT2A* receptor. The largest effect noted was in the affinity of aripiprazole for the *1197V* variant of the receptor, which was more than twofold higher than the affinity for wild type. Because a mutation in *5HT2A* receptors could affect their functional activity without changing their affinity, Davies also estimated the apparent antagonist potency of the atypical antipsychotics clozapine, olanzapine, risperidone, quetiapine, and ziprasidone (because aripiprazole is a partial agonist) in wild type and variants of the *5HT2A* receptor. There was a 10-fold increase in clozapine's apparent potency to *I194V* receptor compared with wild type, a fourfold increase in quetiapine's apparent potency to *T25N* receptor compared with wild type, and a threefold increase in risperidone's apparent potency at *H452Y* receptor compared with wild type. The group also compared the potency of aripiprazole (among other agonists) in the previously mentioned receptor variants and in the wild type. Significantly, aripiprazole displayed a 30-fold decrease in agonist potency at the *T25N* *5HT2A* receptor compared with the wild type, but its potency did not differ more than twofold at any other receptor variant compared with the wild type. The authors postulate that the loss of potency in patients who have this receptor variant could be related to clinical side effects such as akathisia.

5HTR2C *Single-nucleotide polymorphisms*

The *5HT2C* receptor was implicated in behaviors such as hypophagia, anxiety, motor function, and dyskinesia. *Cys23Ser* is the most frequently studied of the 5-HT2C polymorphisms in psychopharmacology. Research has investigated response to antidepressants as well as to antipsychotics.

Ellingrod and colleagues [29] investigated the relationship between clinical response to olanzapine in schizophrenia and the *Cys23Ser* polymorphism for the *5HTR2C* receptor in 41 subjects. No statistical relationship was found for this nonsynonymous polymorphism. Promoter-region polymorphisms such as *-995G/A*, *-759C/T*, and *-697G/C* are all in linkage disequilibrium [32]. In the described previously study of 117 Chinese Han antipsychotic-naïve patients who had schizophrenia, Reynolds and colleagues [22] reported that the *5HTR2C* promoter polymorphism *(-759C/T)* was significantly associated with changes in PANSS negative and general psychopathology scores but not with changes in positive symptom scores during 10 weeks of treatment with risperidone or chlorpromazine.

5HTR6 *Single-nucleotide polymorphisms*

The influence of the *267T/C* polymorphism in the *5HTR6* receptor gene on risperidone efficacy was investigated by Lane and colleagues [33] in inpatients 123 who had acutely exacerbated schizophrenia. Compared with patients who had the *267T/C* genotype (n = 50), those who had a *T/T* genotype (n = 5) showed less severe PANSS positive symptoms ($P = .006$) and general psychopathology

($P = .005$). The *267T/C* polymorphism had no influence on PANSS negative symptoms. Patients who had the *C/C* (n = 68) and *T/C* genotypes had comparable performances. Therefore, the *5HTR6* gene variant may affect the response of positive symptoms and general psychopathology to risperidone (but not the response the response of negative symptoms). These findings support the implication from animal model studies that *5HTR6*s may mediate positive symptoms but not negative symptoms [10], anxiety response [34], or cognitive function [35].

5HTTLPR *polymorphisms*

Malhotra and colleagues [36] investigated whether polymorphisms in the promoter region of the serotonin transporter (*5HTTLPR*) are associated with rapid relapse of positive psychotic symptoms in antipsychotic-free patients who have schizophrenia or schizoaffective disorder. They studied 50 patients who underwent double-blind ratings while antipsychotic-free for approximately 4 weeks. Patients who had the *5HTTLPR ll* genotype (n = 19) had significantly higher Brief Psychiatric Rating Scale (BPRS) [37] ratings of thought disorder than patients with the *ls* (n = 25) or *ss* (n = 6) genotypes ($P = .003$). Inspection of individual items revealed a specific significant increase in intensity of hallucinations in patients who had the *5HTTLPR ll* genotype. This finding suggests that serotonin plays a role in the pathophysiology of hallucinations and rapid relapse of positive psychotic symptoms.

Association Studies of the Treatment Response to Second-Generation Antipsychotics with the Polymorphic P-glycoprotein Transporter Gene

P-glycoprotein (PGP) is an energy-dependent efflux transporter located on the blood–brain barrier and plays a role in transporting central-acting medications into the central nervous system (CNS) [38]. Clinically this drug transporter has been associated with differences in the pharmacokinetics of its substrates by limiting oral absorption and tissue penetration and promoting elimination [39]. PGP is the product of the polymorphic ATP-binding cassette subfamily B member 1 (*ABCB1*) gene, also known as the "multidrug resistance 1" (*MDR1*) gene, located on chromosome 7q21. There are three SNPs primarily associated with PGP activity and expression: *C1236T*, *G2677TA*, and *C3435T*. Among these SNPs, only *G2677TA* results in an amino acid change (Ala893Ser/Thr). Although *C3435T* is a synonymous SNP located within a wobble position, it has been linked to PGP expression and function and is a widely accepted marker for PGP activity [39]. Although the relationship between PGP expression and these polymorphisms is controversial, the majority of data to date suggests that the variant T alleles for these three SNPs are associated with reduced PGP activity leading to higher serum and, potentially, higher CNS concentrations of its substrates [39–42]. The relationship between olanzapine and PGP was tested by Wang and colleagues [43] using a PGP knockout mouse model. As part of this study, olanzapine concentrations were found to be threefold higher in the brain of PGP-deficient mice than in controls, indicating that olanzapine is a PGP substrate and that the distribution and elimination of this drug may be highly affected by PGP expression. Doran and colleagues [44] have shown that most CNS-active agents demonstrate at least some PGP-mediated transport that can affect brain concentrations. In their study, clozapine showed about a twofold difference in brain-to-plasma and area under plasma concentration curve (AUC) ratios, and risperidone and its active metabolite 9-hydroxyrisperidone showed a greater difference in brain-to-plasma and AUC ratios (10 and 17 respectively). In addition to olanzapine, other atypical antipsychotics (eg, risperidone and quetiapine [45]) have been shown to have a higher PGP affinity. Thus for schizophrenia and the use of SGAs, one would expect that the presence of the T allele would mean higher CNS concentrations of these medications, potentially leading to an enhanced response caused by reduced PGP activity on the blood–brain barrier. Patients that are C/C homozygotes at the *C3435T* position would have lower mean CNS concentrations of the SGAs and possibly poor clinical response. This possibility is consistent with the one human study that has determined an association between this polymorphism and clinical response to olanzapine [46]. Lin and colleagues [46] examined the relationship between three PGP polymorphisms (*C1236T*, *G2677T/A*, and *C3435T*) and response to olanzapine, including symptom reduction and changes in weight over 6 weeks. In looking at the relationship between percent change in BPRS score and the *3435* genotype, an interaction was found between the T allele and end-point serum concentrations of olanzapine. In subjects who were carriers of the T allele carrier, the serum olanzapine concentration alone was positively associated with percent change in BPRS score ($F = 6.19$; $df = 29$; $P = .02$), whereas this relationship was not seen for the *3435CC* group ($F = 0.32$; $df = 11$; $P = .58$), and there was a statistical interaction between the two genotype groups. After controlling for differences in the baseline BPRS scores, this model maintained its significance ($F = 2.59$; $df = 4$ 37; $P = .05$). In addition to positive scores, the T allele group was found to be associated with change in Scale for the Adjustment of Negative Symptoms (SANS scores), showing a similar interaction ($P = .03$). An analysis-of-variance model involving olanzapine serum concentrations, the *C3435T* genotype, and the interaction between these two variables did not find a statistically significant relationship, but a trend was seen ($F = 2.38$; $df = 3.38$; $P = .08$). No other relationships between change in BPRS or SANS scores and the other genotypes were found. These data suggest that PGP polymorphisms may affect the penetration of olanzapine into the CNS and that the *3435* genotype may help determine positive symptom reduction during olanzapine treatment.

PHARMACOGENETICS OF ANTIPSYCHOTIC ADVERSE EFFECTS
Association Studies of Antipsychotic-Related Weight Gain
There seems to be considerable variability among individuals with respect to the ability of an SGA to cause weight gain; that is, not all patients treated with agents such as olanzapine or clozapine gain weight. It is likely that the propensity to gain weight is determined by a combination of genetic and environmental factors. The genetic factors may include pharmacokinetic factors

(ie, factors involved in the metabolism and elimination of the drug from the body) as well as pharmacodynamic factors (ie, factors such as direct site of action of the drug within the body). Because of genetic variations in pharmacodynamic factors such as brain receptors, some patients may have receptors with higher affinity for the medication, and it might be possible to predict which patients are most likely to develop this side effect. Genetic differences in pharmacokinetic factors such as drug-metabolizing enzymes may subject some patients to less active enzymatic forms, resulting in higher plasma concentrations of the medication and possibly allowing a propensity for weight gain to be predicted. To date a number of studies have examined the relationship between genetic variations and the propensity of SGAs to produce weight gain in persons who have schizophrenia, but none of these studies has investigated the relationship with the metabolic effects. A genetic predisposition for SGA-induced weight gain has been suggested, and there is ample evidence demonstrating that body weight and feeding behavior are influenced by genetic factors.

Weight gain associated with SGAs is likely to be caused by a combination of disturbances and alterations in satiety control mechanisms, energy expenditure, metabolism, and lipogenesis, although research seeking to uncover the precise mechanisms is limited. A large body of research supports the role of the serotonin system in regulating feeding behavior. Studies in both animals and humans have shown that increasing 5HT results in decreased feeding and that decreasing 5HT increases feeding [47–49]. It has been shown that agonists of the 5HT1A family of receptors produce hyperphagia, and, conversely, antagonists of the 5HT2 family of receptors lead to hypophagia [50]. The *5HT2C* serotonin receptor became a target for pharmacogenetic research investigating weight gain accompanying the use of antipsychotic drugs because of the obesity and increased feeding noted in 5HT2C knockout mouse [51].

The peptide that exerts the most significant effects on feeding and weight regulation is leptin. Leptin is secreted by adipocytes in direct proportion to the amount of fat stored within that cell. It is believed to act at the level of the hypothalamus, where it initiates a cascade of events that lead to the regulation of appetite, energy expenditure, and satisfaction. It also is well established that histamine H1 receptor antagonism causes increased feeding and weight gain [52,53]. The SGAs such as clozapine and olanzapine bind to histamine H1 receptors as well as to *5HT2C* and *5HT1A* receptors, and the subsequent change in the action of these receptors within the hypothalamus may disrupt satiety control mechanisms, in turn resulting in weight gain. Genetic differences in these central brain receptors may predict a patient's propensity to gain weight while being treated with these agents.

Reynolds and colleagues [54] found an association between the -759C/T SNP and increase in body mass index at 6 and 10 weeks of hospitalization in first-episode Chinese Han patients who were antipsychotic naive and who were treated with chlorpromazine and risperidone. These findings were not substantiated in two independent studies involving patients treated with clozapine for

6 weeks [55] and 4 months [56]. Reynolds and colleagues [57] subsequently replicated their previous finding in 32 Chinese Han subjects treated with clozapine. Likewise, Ellingrod and colleagues [58] found that subjects without the -759T allele were at a higher risk of gaining weight during a 6-week trial with olanzapine than those who had the -759T allele. Miller and colleagues [59] also explored the association between -759C/T polymorphism of the 5-HT2C receptor and weight gain following 6 months of treatment with clozapine in a population of patients who had treatment-refractory schizophrenia. The authors found that subjects without the -759T allele of the 5HT2C receptor gained significantly more weight than the subjects who had the T allele. They concluded that the T-allele holders were at lesser risk of gaining weight than the subjects without this allele. The findings of an association between genetic variants of the -759C/T SNP are supported in a preclinical study by Buckland and colleagues [60], who found that the -759C allele of 5HT2C reduces its expression and mRNA expression and thus increases the susceptibility for weight gain from second-generation antipsychotics.

Addressing the role of the genetic variation of leptin genes in SGA-induced weight gain, Templeman and colleagues [61] investigated whether polymorphisms of the promoter regions of both the serotonin 5-HT2C receptor and the leptin genes are associated with antipsychotic-induced weight gain in a white first-episode psychosis and initially drug-naive population, following longer term treatment. Patients were genotyped for the 5-HT2C receptor -759C/T and leptin -2548A/G polymorphisms. Carriers of the -759T variant allele had significantly less weight gain than those without this allele. The -2548 leptin polymorphism was not associated with short-term weight gain but showed significant association with antipsychotic-induced weight gain at 9 months. The 5-HT2C -759 genotype was significantly associated with pretreatment plasma leptin levels.

A study by Basile and colleagues [62] found that variations in the histamine H1 and H2 receptor genes (H1R/H2R) were not associated with weight gain in patients treated with clozapine for 6 weeks.

TARDIVE DYSKINESIA

Tardive dyskinesia (TD) is an involuntary movement disorder of the musculature of the orofacial area, trunk, and/or extremities that occurs in 20% to 30% of patients with the chronic administration of antipsychotic medications. Why some patients develop TD and others do not is unknown. Clinical risk factors for TD that have been identified include age, duration of antipsychotic exposure, and exposure to conventional antipsychotics and anticholinergic medications [63]. These various factors predict only a small portion of the variance in the TD phenotype; thus a genetic component may contribute significantly to this variance and help identify patients who are more susceptible to developing TD. Although the precise mechanisms of TD are not fully understood, overactivity of the dopamine neurotransmission in the basal ganglia and increased expression of the dopamine D2 family of receptors (DRD2, DRD3, and *DRD4*) have been postulated to play a major role in its pathophysiology [64]. As a result, pharmacogenetic studies have focused primarily on the dopamine receptor genes, although there are also studies examining the serotonin receptor and hepatic isoenzyme genes.

Although the *DRD2* receptor has long been hypothesized to be the main target for antipsychotic medications, only a few polymorphisms in *DRD2* have been investigated for their potential association with TD. Zai and colleagues [65] investigated 12 polymorphisms spanning the *DRD2* gene and their association with TD in white European (n = 202) and African American (n = 30) samples. Genotype frequencies for a functional polymorphism, *C957T*, and the adjacent *C939T* polymorphism were found to be significantly associated with TD ($P = .013$ and $P = .022$, respectively). *DRD2* genotypes, however, were not significantly associated with TD severity as measured by the Abnormal Involuntary Movement Scale (AIMS) [66] with the exception of a trend for *C939T* ($P = .071$). Both TD and total AIMS scores were found to be significantly associated with two-marker haplotypes containing *C939T* and *C957T* ($P = .021$ and $P = .0087$, respectively). They concluded that *DRD2* may be involved in TD in the white population, although further research is needed.

Several studies have independently reported that the *Ser9Gly DRD3* gene variants with either the glycine/glycine genotype or the presence of a glycine allele increased the risk for TD [67–75]. This result was not found in studies by Inada and colleagues [76], Rietschel and colleagues [77], or Garcia-Barcelo and colleagues [78]. These discrepant findings probably are related to differences in study populations and study designs. In a subset of the patients reported by Basile and colleagues [69], Potkin and colleagues [79], using fluorodeoxyglucose positron emission tomography, found that patients with the glycine/glycine genotype who were treated with haloperidol had increased metabolism in the caudate nucleus and the putamen than patients who had the serine/serine or serine/glycine genotypes. The subjects who had increased brain activity in these regions had the most severe TD.

Srivastava and collaborators [80] performed a case-control study of 335 North Indian patients who had schizophrenia to evaluate the associations in polymorphisms of candidate genes from the dopaminergic pathway with TD. Of 24 markers from six genes, *DRD1, DRD2, DRD3, DRD4, DAT* (dopamine transporter), and *COMT*, there was a significant association of a 120-bp duplication allele of *DRD4* with TD and an association of the coding SNP 472 G>A (*Val158Met*) of the *COMT* gene with TD. The high-activity allele (Val) may be protective, and the low-activity allele may contribute to the susceptibility of TD.

Various investigators [81–83] explored the possibility that genetic variability in the *5-HT2A* receptor may influence the risk for TD in patients who have schizophrenia or schizoaffective disorder. These investigators found significant associations of the *5-HT2A* receptor with TD. This finding, however, was not replicated in a prospective study conducted by Basile and colleagues [84]. Lerer and colleagues [83] also reported that the *His425Tyr* genotype of the *5-HT2A* receptor was not associated with TD risk. Zhang and colleagues [85] found a significant association of the -607G/C promoter SNP of 5HT2C with TD in a sample of Chinese male patients who had schizophrenia chronically treated with antipsychotics.

There is a series of studies examining the association between TD and the cytochrome P450 genes CYP2D6 and CYP1A2, which are involved in the metabolism of many antipsychotic medications. One or more CYP 450 enzymes may contribute to the oxidative metabolism of a given drug (for example, aripiprazole is a substrate for CYP450 2D6 and 3A4, whereas risperidone is a major substrate for CYP450 2D6). CYP2D6 metabolizes approximately 25% of drugs biotransformed by cytochromes and contributes to the metabolism of many psychotropic drugs, including antipsychotics such as haloperidol, thioridazine, perphenazine, chlorpromazine, risperidone, and aripiprazole [86]. CYP2D6 is encoded by a gene located in chromosome 22 and has a high level of genetic polymorphism, including mutations, deletions, and duplications. There are more than 50 variants of CYP2D6, resulting in four phenotypes. Extensive metabolizers have one or two functional copies of the CYP2D6 gene and yield 2D6 substrates with a normal metabolic rate. Intermediate metabolizers have one nonfunctional allele and one low-activity 2D6 allele, yielding substrates with a lower-than-normal metabolic rate; in the presence of a CYP2D6 inhibitor they act like poor metabolizers. Poor metabolizers have two nonfunctional 2D6 alleles leading to very slow or no 2D6 activity and side effects. Ultrarapid metabolizers have three or more copies of the active 2D6 gene; they metabolize substrates rapidly and have limited clinical response at standard doses of drugs. All metabolizer groups have ethnic variability [87,88]. Three studies investigating the association between genetic variants of CYP2D6 found that mutations resulting in reduced 2D6 activity (and presumably in higher plasma concentrations of antipsychotic medications) were positively correlated with higher AIMS scores and the development of TD [89–91]. Cigarette smoking has been associated with TD in patients who have schizophrenia [92,93] and also is known to induce hepatic isoenzymes, increasing the metabolism of many antipsychotics [94]. Ellingrod and colleagues [95] investigated the relationships between cytochrome CYP 450 2D6 genotypes, antipsychotic drug exposure, abnormal involuntary movements, and cigarette smoking in a group of subjects who had schizophrenia. They reported a significant interaction between antipsychotic drug exposure, CYP2D6 genotype, and cigarette smoking in patients with the CYP2D6 *1/*3, *4 genotype. Seventy-eight percent of smokers with the CYP2D6 *1/*3, *4 genotype had TD, compared with 20% to 33% of the patients in other groups. They concluded that patients who have a CYP2D6 *3 or *4 allele may shunt antipsychotic metabolism through other pathways that are induced by cigarette smoke and that this induction may result in the formation of neurotoxic metabolites, leading to increased AIMS scores and a higher frequency of TD than seen in patients who do not have these alleles. Sachse and colleagues [96] found that the CYP2D6 polymorphisms did not predict TD but that the CYP1A2 polymorphisms were significantly associated with TD. Patients who were homozygous for the C allele of the *CYP1A2* gene had significantly higher AIMS scale scores in a study by Basile and colleagues [97]. This finding was not replicated in a study by Schulze and colleagues [98].

Numerous factors limit the clinical application of pharmacogenetics in schizophrenia. Many of the studies have not been replicated, possibly because the phenotypes chosen in various studies are not uniform and the sample size is too small to identify genes of modest effect [3]. In addition, polymorphisms have ethnic variability. For example, the Middle Eastern population has a high percentage of *CYP 450 2D6* gene duplications, so that 10% to 29% of the population has the ultrarapid metabolizer phenotype, versus 1% to 10% of whites and 2% of African Americans [87,88]. Serretti [99] suggested that placebo response might reduce the power to detect the effect of the gene variants on antidepressant response. This issue has not been addressed in investigations of the pharmacogenetics of antipsychotic response. Blasi and Bertolino [100] addressed the variability of phenotypes chosen in pharmacogenetics and proposed that choosing intermediate phenotypes that allow in vivo measurement of specific neuronal functions may help reduce potential confounds intrinsic to clinical measurements. Functional neuroimaging is suggested as a powerful strategy to investigate the relationships between behavior, brain function, genes, and individual variability in the response to treatment with antipsychotic drugs in schizophrenia. Authors cite a study of the interaction of *COMT Val^{158-Met}* genotype and treatment with olanzapine by Bertolino and colleagues [101]. Medication-naive patients who had schizophrenia received olanzapine for 8 weeks, and PANSS scores were measured at baseline, at 4 weeks, and at the end of treatment. Twenty of the 30 patients also had functional MRI during the number-back-working memory task at 4 and 8 weeks of treatment. The PANSS performance, the working memory performance, and the dorsolateral prefrontal cortical neuronal efficiency improved in Met-homozygous subjects compared with both heterozygous subjects and Val-homozygous subjects after 8 weeks of treatment. Finally, the cost of genetic testing, even if such testing were widely clinically available, might prohibit its assimilation in day-to-day practice. Limited but compelling data show that the cost of treating patients with extremes of *CYP2D6* (poor and ultrarapid metabolizers) is significantly higher than that of treating patients who are intermediate and extensive metabolizers [102]. Perlis and colleagues [103] assumed that a genetic test meant to predict clozapine efficacy already existed and studied its potential application in a modeled schizophrenia population comparing three groups of patients. The first was a "no-test" group. The second group had a genetic test negative for clozapine response. Both these groups received clozapine as third-line treatment. The third group, with a genetic test positive for clozapine response, received clozapine as first-line treatment. The authors, using a decision analytic model, showed that such testing might, at a cost, improve the quality-adjusted life expectancy in schizophrenia but acknowledged the methodologic limitations, including the practicality and financial affordability of such testing.

SUMMARY

This article suggests that there is strong evidence that genetic variation plays an important role in interindividual differences in response to medication and in toxicity. The rapidly evolving disciplines of pharmacogenetics and pharmacogenomics seek to uncover this genetic variation to predict treatment outcomes. The goal is individualized therapy—being able to select the drugs that have the greatest likelihood of benefit and the least likelihood of harm for an individual patient, based on the patient's genetic make-up. To the extent that the findings reviewed here become more widely verified and replicated, the field of psychiatry will move closer to having clinically meaningful tests that will be useful in deciding the best drug for each individual patient treated with antipsychotic medications. The authors recommend that, in the future, all large schizophrenia treatment studies include a genetic component to complement the clinical part of the study. This measure would allow the opportunity for replicating findings like the ones described in this article in large numbers of patients and in various ethnic populations.

References

[1] Craddock N, O'Donovan MC, Owen MJ. The genetics of schizophrenia and bipolar disorder: dissecting psychosis. J Med Genet 2005;42:193–204.

[2] Kirov G, O'Donovan M, Owen MJ. Finding schizophrenia genes. J Clin Invest 2005;115(6):1440–8.

[3] Lane HY, Lee CC, Liu YC, et al. Pharmacogenetic studies of response to risperidone and other newer atypical antipsychotics. Pharmacogenomics 2005;6(2):139–49.

[4] Malhotra AK, Murphy GM Jr, Kennedy JL. Pharmacogenetics of psychotropic drug response. Am J Psychiatry 2004;161(5):780–96.

[5] Kirchheiner J, Nickchen K, Bauer M, et al. Pharmacogenetics of antidepressants and antipsychotics: the contribution of allelic variations to the phenotype of drug response. Mol Psychiatry 2004;9:442–73.

[6] Bishop JR, Ellingrod VL. Neuropsychiatric pharmacogenetics: moving toward a comprehensive understanding of predicting risks and response. Pharmacogenomics 2004;5(5):463–77.

[7] Roses AD. Pharmacogenetics and drug development: the path to safer and more effective drugs. Nat Rev Genet 2004;5(9):645–56.

[8] Aitchison KJ, Basu A, McGuffin P, et al. Psychiatry and the "new genetics": hunting for genes for behaviour and drug response. Br J Psychiatry 2005;186:91–2.

[9] Lopez-Garcia P, Rodriguez JT, De Castro P, et al. Association between clozapine-induced agranulocytosis and HLA subtyping. J Clin Psychiatry 2006;67(10):1652–3.

[10] Pouzet B, Didriksen M, Arnt J. Effects of the 5-HT(6) receptor antagonist, SB-271046, in animal models for schizophrenia. Pharmacol Biochem Behav 2002;71(4):635–43.

[11] Jablensky A. Resolving schizophrenia's CATCH22. Nat Genet 2004;36(7):674–5.

[12] Meltzer HY. The role of serotonin in antipsychotic drug action. Neuropsychopharmacology 1999;21(Suppl 2):106–15.

[13] Itokawa M, Toru M, Ito K, et al. Sequestration of the short and long isoforms of dopamine D2 receptors expressed in Chinese hamster ovary cells. Mol Pharmacol 1996;49(3):560–6.

[14] Schafer M, Rujescu D, Giegling I, et al. Association of short-term response to haloperidol treatment with a polymorphism in the dopamine D(2) receptor gene. Am J Psychiatry 2001;158(5):802–4.

[15] Dubertret C, Gouya L, Hanoun N, et al. The 3' region of the DRD2 gene is involved in genetic susceptibility to schizophrenia. Schizophr Res 2004;67(1):75–85.

[16] Arinami T, Gao M, Hamaguchi H, et al. A functional polymorphism in the promoter region of the dopamine D2 receptor gene is associated with schizophrenia. Hum Mol Genet 1997;6(4):577–82.

[17] Jonsson EG, Nothen MM, Grunhage F, et al. Polymorphisms in the dopamine D2 receptor gene and their relationships to striatal dopamine receptor density of healthy volunteers. Mol Psychiatry 1999;4(3):290–6.

[18] Wu S, Xing Q, Gao R, et al. Response to chlorpromazine treatment may be associated with polymorphisms of the DRD2 gene in Chinese schizophrenic patients. Neurosci Lett 2005;376(1):1–4.

[19] Parsons M, Mata I, Beperet M, et al. Association of a D2 receptor gene polymorphism with schizophrenia and treatment response in the Basque and Spanish populations [abstract]. Am J Med Genet [B] 2004;130:164.

[20] Yamanouchi Y, Iwata N, Suzuki T, et al. Effect of DRD2, 5-HT2A, and COMT genes on antipsychotic response to risperidone. Pharmacogenomics J 2003;3(6):356–61.

[21] Kay SR, Fiszbein A, Opler LA. The Positive and Negative Syndrome Scale (PANSS) for schizophrenia. Schizophr Bull 1987;13(2):261–76.

[22] Reynolds GP, Yao Z, Zhang X, et al. Pharmacogenetics of treatment in first-episode schizophrenia: D3 and 5-HT2C receptor polymorphisms separately associate with positive and negative symptom response. Eur Neuropsychopharmacol 2005;15(2):143–51.

[23] Lencz T, Robinson D, Xu K, et al. DRD2 promoter region as a predictor of sustained response to antipsychotic medication in first episode schizophrenia patients. Am J Psychiatry 2006;163(3):529–31.

[24] Lane HY, Lee CC, Chang YC, et al. Effects of dopamine D2 receptor Ser311Cys polymorphism and clinical factors on risperidone efficacy for positive and negative symptoms and social function. Int J Neuropsychopharmacol 2004;7(4):461–70.

[25] Kapur S, Seeman P. Does fast dissociation from the dopamine D(2) receptor explain the action of atypical antipsychotics? A new hypothesis. Am J Psychiatry 2001;158(3):360–9.

[26] Arranz M, Collier D, Sodhi M, et al. Association between clozapine response and allelic variation in 5_HT2A receptor gene. Lancet 1995;346:281–2.

[27] Lane HY, Chang YC, Chiu CC, et al. Association of risperidone treatment response with a polymorphism in the 5-HT(2A) receptor gene. Am J Psychiatry 2002;159(9):1593–5.

[28] Polesskaya OO, Sokolov BP. Differential expression of the "C" and "T" alleles of the 5-HT2A receptor gene in the temporal cortex of normal individuals and schizophrenics. J Neurosci Res 2002;67(6):812–22.

[29] Ellingrod VL, Lund BC, Miller D, et al. 5-HT2A receptor promoter polymorphism, -1438G/A and negative symptom response to olanzapine in schizophrenia. Psychopharmacol Bull 2003;37(2):109–12.

[30] Ellingrod VL, Perry PJ, Lund BC, et al. 5HT2A and 5HT2C receptor polymorphisms and predicting clinical response to olanzapine in schizophrenia. J Clin Psychopharmacol 2002;22(6):622–4.

[31] Davies MA, Setola V, Strachan RT. Pharmacologic analysis of non synonymous coding h5-HT2A SNPs reveals alterations in atypical antipsychotics and agonist efficacies. Pharmacogenomics J 2006;6:42–51.

[32] Reynolds GP, Templeman LA, Zhang ZJ. The role of 5HT2C receptor polymorphisms in the pharmacogenetics of antipsychotic drug treatment. Prog Neuropsychopharmacol Biol Psychiatry 2005;29:1021–8.

[33] Lane HY, Lin CC, Huang CH, et al. Risperidone response and 5-HT6 receptor gene variance: genetic association analysis with adjustment for nongenetic confounds. Schizophr Res 2004;67(1):63–70.

[34] Otano A, Frechilla D, Cobreros A, et al. Anxiogenic-like effects and reduced stereological counting of immunolabelled 5-hydroxytryptamine6 receptors in rat nucleus accumbens by antisense oligonucleotides. Neuroscience 1999;92(3):1001–9.

[35] Meneses A. Effects of the 5-HT(6) receptor antagonist Ro 04-6790 on learning consolidation. Behav Brain Res 2001;118(1):107–10.

[36] Malhotra AK, Goldman D, Mazzanti C, et al. A functional serotonin transporter (5-HTT) polymorphism is associated with psychosis in neuroleptic-free schizophrenics. Mol Psychiatry 1998;3(4):328–32.

[37] Overall JE, Gorham DR. The brief psychiatric rating scale. Psychol Rep 1962;10: 799–812.

[38] Fromm MF. Importance of P-glycoprotein at blood-tissue barriers. Trends Pharmacol Sci 2004;25(8):423–9.

[39] Marzolini C, Paus E, Buclin T, et al. Polymorphisms in human MDR1 (P-glycoprotein): recent advances and clinical relevance. Clin Pharmacol Ther 2004;75(1):13–33.

[40] Hoffmeyer S, Burk O, von Richter O, et al. Functional polymorphisms of the human multidrug-resistance gene: multiple sequence variations and correlation of one allele with P-glycoprotein expression and activity in vivo. Proc Natl Acad Sci U S A 2000;97(7): 3473–8.

[41] Tanabe M, Ieiri I, Nagata N, et al. Expression of P-glycoprotein in human placenta: relation to genetic polymorphism of the multidrug resistance (MDR)-1 gene. J Pharmacol Exp Ther 2001;297(3):1137–43.

[42] Woodahl EL, Ho RJ. The role of MDR1 genetic polymorphisms in interindividual variability in P-glycoprotein expression and function. Curr Drug Metab 2004;5(1):11–9.

[43] Wang JS, Taylor R, Ruan Y, et al. Olanzapine penetration into brain is greater in transgenic Abcb1a P-glycoprotein-deficient mice than FVB1 (wild-type) animals. Neuropsychopharmacology 2004;29(3):551–7.

[44] Doran A, Obach RS, Smith BJ, et al. The impact of P-glycoprotein on the disposition of drugs targeted for indications of the central nervous system: evaluation using the MDR1A/1B knockout mouse model. Drug Metab Dispos 2005;33(1):165–74.

[45] Boulton DW, DeVane CL, Liston HL, et al. In vitro P-glycoprotein affinity for atypical and conventional antipsychotics. Life Sci 2002;71(2):163–9.

[46] Lin YC, Ellingrod VL, Bishop JR, et al. The relationship between P-glycoprotein (PGP) and response to olanzapine treatment in schizophrenia. Ther Drug Monit 2006;28(5): 668–72.

[47] Blundell JE. Serotonin and appetite. Neuropharmacology 1984;23:1537–51.

[48] Liebowitz MR, Hollander E, Schneier F, et al. Anxiety and depression: discrete diagnostic entities? J Clin Psychopharmacol 1990;10:61S–6S.

[49] Wurtman J, Wurtman R, Berry E, et al. Dexfenfluramine, fluoxetine, and weight loss among female carbohydrate cravers. Neuropsychopharmacology 1993;9:201–10.

[50] Davis R, Faulds D. Dexfenfluramine. An updated review of its therapeutic use in the management of obesity. Drugs 1996;52:696–724.

[51] Tecott LH, Sun LM, Akana SF, et al. Eating disorder and epilepsy in mice lacking 5-HT2C serotonin receptors. Nature 1995;374:542–6.

[52] Morimoto T, Yamamoto Y, Mobarakeh JI, et al. Involvement of the histaminergic system in leptin-induced suppression of food intake. Physiol Behav 1999;67:679–83.

[53] Baptista T. Body weight gain induced by antipsychotic drugs: mechanisms and management. Acta Psychiatr Scand 1999;100:3–16.

[54] Reynolds GP, Zhang ZJ, Zhang XB. Association of antipsychotic induced weight gain with a 5HT2 receptor gene polymorphism. Lancet 2002;359:2086–7.

[55] Basile VS, Masellis M, Meltzer HY, et al. Serotonin 2C receptor gene and clozapine-induced weight gain. Lancet 2002;360(9347):1790–1.

[56] Tsai SJ, Hong CJ, Yu YW-Y, et al. 759C/T genetic variation of 5HT2c receptor and clozapine-induced weight gain. Lancet 2002;360:1790.

[57] Reynolds GP, Zhang ZJ, Zhang XB. Clozapine-induced weight gain associated with a polymorphism of the promotor region of the 5-HT2C receptor gene. Am J Psychiatry 2003;160: 677–9.

[58] Ellingrod VL, Perry PJ, Ringold JC, et al. Weight gain associated with the -759 C/T polymorphism of the 5HT2C receptor and olanzapine. Am J Med Genet B Neuropsychiatr Genet 2005;134:76–8.

[59] Miller DD, Ellingrod VL, Holman TL, et al. Clozapine-induced weight gain associated with the 5HT2C receptor -759C/T polymorphism. Am J Med Genet B Neuropsychiatr Genet 2005;133(1):97–100.

[60] Buckland PR, Hoogendoorn B, Smith SK, et al. Low gene expression conferred by association of an allele of the 5HT2c receptor gene with antipsychotic-induced weight gain. Am J Psychiatry 2005;162(3):613–5.

[61] Templeman LA, Reynolds GP, Arranz B, et al. Polymorphisms of the 5-HT2C receptor and leptin genes are associated with antipsychotic drug-induced weight gain in Caucasian subjects with a first-episode psychosis. Pharmacogenet Genomics 2005;15(4):195–200.

[62] Basile VS, Masellis M, McIntyre RS, et al. Genetic dissection of atypical antipsychotic-induced weight gain: novel preliminary data on the pharmacogenetic puzzle. J Clin Psychiatry 2001;62:45–66.

[63] Miller DD, McEvoy JP, Davis S, et al. Clinical correlates of tardive dyskinesia in schizophrenia: baseline data from the CATIE schizophrenia trial. Schizophr Res 2005;80:33–43.

[64] Meshul CK, Casey DE. Regional, reversible ultrastructural changes in rat brain with chronic neuroleptic treatment. Brain Res 1989;489:338–46.

[65] Zai CC, Hwang RW, De Luca V, et al. Association study of tardive dyskinesia and twelve DRD2 polymorphisms in schizophrenia patients, . Int J Neuropsychopharmacol; Published online. Cambridge, UK: Cambridge University Press; September 7, 2006.

[66] Guy W. Abnormal involuntary movement scale. In: ECDEU assessment manual for psychopharmacology. Washington, DC: U.S. Public Health Service; 1976. p. 534–7.

[67] Badri F, Masellis M, Petronis A, et al. Dopamine and serotonin system genes may predict clinical response to clozapine. In: Proceedings of the 46th Annual Meeting of the American Society of Human Genetics. Am J Hum Genet 1996;59(Suppl):A247.

[68] Steen VM, Lovlie R, MacEwan T, et al. Dopamine D3-receptor gene variant and susceptibility to tardive dyskinesia in schizophrenic patients. Mol Psychiatry 1997;2: 139–45.

[69] Basile VS, Masellis M, Badri F, et al. Association of the MscI polymorphism of the dopamine D3 receptor gene with tardive dyskinesia in schizophrenia. Neuropsychopharmacology 1999;21:17–27.

[70] Segman R, Neeman T, Heresco-Levy U, et al. Genotypic association between the dopamine D3 receptor and tardive dyskinesia in chronic schizophrenia. Mol Psychiatry 1999;4:247–53.

[71] Liao DL, Yeh YC, Chen HM, et al. Association between the Ser9Gly polymorphism of the dopamine D3 receptor gene and tardive dyskinesia in Chinese schizophrenic patients. Neuropsychobiology 2001;44:95–8.

[72] Lovlie R, Daly AK, Blennerhassett R, et al. Homozygosity for the Gly-9 variant of the dopamine D3 receptor and risk for tardive dyskinesia in schizophrenic patients. Int J Neuropsychopharmacol 2000;3:61–5.

[73] Woo SI, Kim JW, Rha E, et al. Association of the Ser9Gly polymorphism in the dopamine D3 receptor gene with tardive dyskinesia in Korean schizophrenics. Psychiatry Clin Neurosci 2002;56:469–74.

[74] Lerer B, Segman RH, Fangerau H, et al. Pharmacogenetics of tardive dyskinesia. Combined analysis of 780 patients supports association with dopamine D3 receptor gene Ser9Gly polymorphism. Neuropsychopharmacology 2002;27:105–19.

[75] de Leon Jose, Susce MT, Pan RM, et al. Polymorphic variations in GSTM1, GSTT1, PgP, CYP2D6, CYP3A5, and dopamine D2 and D3 receptors and their association with tardive dyskinesia in severe mental illness. J Clin Psychopharmacol 2005;25(5):448–56.

[76] Inada T, Dobashi I, Sugita T, et al. Search for a susceptibility locus to tardive dyskinesia. Hum Psychopharmacol Clin Exp 1997;12:35–9.

[77] Rietschel M, Krauss H, Muller DJ, et al. Dopamine D3 receptor variant and tardive dyski-nesia. Eur Arch Psychiatry Clin Neurosci 2000;250:31–5.

[78] Garcia-Barcelo MM, Lam LC, Ungvari GS, et al. Dopamine D3 receptor gene and tardive dyskinesia in Chinese schizophrenic patients. J Neural Transm 2001;108:671–7.

[79] Potkin SG, Kennedy JL, Basile VS. Combining brain imaging and pharmacogenetics in un-derstanding clinical response in Alzheimer's disease and schizophrenia. In: Lerer B, editor. Pharmacogenetics of psychotropic drugs. Cambridge, UK: Cambridge University Press; 2002.

[80] Srivastava V, Varma PG, Prasad S, et al. Genetic susceptibility to tardive dyskinesia among schizophrenia subjects: IV role of dopaminergic pathway gene polymorphisms. Pharmaco-genet Genomics 2006;16:111–7.

[81] Segman RH, Heresco-Levy U, Finkel B, et al. Association between the serotonin 2A receptor gene and tardive dyskinesia in chronic schizophrenia. Mol Psychiatry 2001;6: 225–9.

[82] Tan EC, Chong SA, Mahendran R, et al. Susceptibility to neuroleptic-induced tardive dys-kinesia and the T102C polymorphism in the serotonin type 2A receptor. Biol Psychiatry 2001;50:144–7.

[83] Lerer B, Segman RH, Tan E-C, et al. Combined analysis of 635 patients confirms an age related association of serotonin 2A receptor gene with tardive dyskinesia and specificity for non-orofacial subtype. Int J Neuropsychopharmacol 2005;8:411–25.

[84] Basile VS, Ozdemir V, Masellis M, et al. Lack of association between serotonin-2A receptor gene (HTR2A) polymorphisms and tardive dyskinesia in schizophrenia. Mol Psychiatry 2001;6:230–4.

[85] Zhang ZJ, Zhang XB, Sha WW, et al. Association of a polymorphism in the promoter re-gion of the serotonin 5-HT2C receptor gene with tardive dyskinesia in patients with schizo-phrenia. Mol Psychiatry 2002;7(7):670–1.

[86] Ingelman-Sundberg M. Pharmacogenetics of cytochrome P450 and its applications to drug therapy: the past, the present and the future. Trends Pharmacol Sci 2004;25(4): 3–200.

[87] De Leon J, Armstrong SC, Cozza KL, et al. Clinical guidelines for psychiatrists for the use of pharmacogenetic testing for CYP450 2D6 and CYP450 2C19. Psychosomatics 2006;47(1):75–85.

[88] Bradford D. CYP2D6 allele frequency in European Caucasians, Asians, Africans and their descendants. Pharmacogenomics 2002;3(2):229–43.

[89] Kapitany T, Meszaros K, Lenzinger E, et al. Genetic polymorphism for drug metabolism (CYP2D6) and tardive dyskinesia in schizophrenia. Schizophr Res 1998;32:101–6.

[90] Ohmori O, Suzuki T, Kojima H, et al. Tardive dyskinesia and debrisoquine 4-hydroxylase (CYP2D6) genotype in Japanese schizophrenics. Schizophr Res 1998;32:107–13.

[91] Ellingrod VL, Schultz SK, Arndt S. Association between cytochrome P4502D6 (CYP2D6) genotype, antipsychotic exposure, and abnormal involuntary movement scale (AIMS) score. Psychiatr Genet 2000;10(1):9–11.

[92] Kirch DG, Alho AM, Wyatt RJ. Hypothesis: a nicotine dopamine interaction linking smok-ing with Parkinson's disease and tardive dyskinesia. Cell Mol Neurobiol 1988;8:285–90.

[93] Yassa R, Lal S, Korpassy A, et al. Nicotine exposure and tardive dyskinesia. Biol Psychiatry 1987;22:67–72.

[94] Miller DD, Kelly MW, Perry PJ, et al. The influence of cigarette smoking on haloperidol pharmacokinetics. Biol Psychiatry 1990;28:529–31.

[95] Ellingrod VL, Schultz SK, Arndt S. Abnormal movements and tardive dyskinesia in smokers and nonsmokers with schizophrenia genotyped for cytochrome P450 2D6. Pharmacother-apy 2002;22(11):1416–9.

[96] Sachse C, Brockmoller J, Baue S, et al. Cytochrome P450 2D6 variants in a Caucasian population: allele frequencies and phenotypic consequences. Am J Hum Genet 1997;60:284–95.

[97] Basile VS, Ozdemir V, Masellis M, et al. A functional polymorphism of the cytochrome P450 1A2 (CYP1A2) gene: association with tardive dyskinesia in schizophrenia. Mol Psychiatry 2000;5:410–7.

[98] Schulze TG, Schumacher J, Muller DJ, et al. Lack of association between a functional polymorphism of the cytochrome P450 1A2 (CYP1A2) gene and tardive dyskinesia in schizophrenia. Am J Med Genet 2001;105:498–501.

[99] Serretti A, Benedetti F, Zanardi R, et al. The influence of serotonin transporter polymorphism (SERTPR) and other polymorphisms of the serotonin pathway on the efficacy of antidepressant treatments. Prog Neuropsychopharmacol Biol Psychiatry 2005;29:1074–84.

[100] Blasi G, Bertolino A. Imaging genomics and response to treatment with antipsychotics in schizophrenia. NeuroRx 2006;3(1):117–30.

[101] Bertolino A, Caforio G, Blasi G, et al. Interaction of COMT Val108/158Met genotype and olanzapine treatment on prefrontal cortical function in patients with schizophrenia. Am J Psychiatry 2004;10:1798–805.

[102] Chou WV, Yan FX, de Leon J, et al. Extension of a pilot study: impact from the cytochrome P450 2D6 polymorphism on outcome and costs associated with severe mental illness. J Clin Psychopharmacol 2000;20(2):246–51.

[103] Perlis RH, Ganz DA, Avron J, et al. Pharmacogenetic testing in the clinical management of schizophrenia, a decision analytic model. J Clin Psychopharmacol 2005;25(5):427–34.

Antipsychotic Medication Adherence in Schizophrenia

Matthew J. Byerly, MD[a,*], Paul A. Nakonezny, PhD[b], Emmeline Lescouflair, MD[a]

[a]Department of Psychiatry, The University of Texas Southwestern Medical Center at Dallas, 6363 Forest Park Rd., Suite 651, Dallas, TX 75235-8828, USA
[b]Department of Biostatistics & Clinical Science, The University of Texas Southwestern Medical Center at Dallas, 6363 Forest Park Rd., Suite 651, Dallas, TX 75235-8828, USA

For any medication to have beneficial results, it must be taken. This observation is particularly relevant to individuals who have schizophrenia, whose adherence to medication is often poor and for whom stopping medication often has serious consequences. This article provides an update on recent literature regarding the frequency, clinical and social impact, and clinical correlates of nonadherence to antipsychotic medication in schizophrenia. The authors then review published trials of adherence interventions in schizophrenia.

NONADHERENCE TO ANTIPSYCHOTIC MEDICATION IS COMMON AMONG PERSONS WHO HAVE SCHIZOPHRENIA

The frequency and degree of nonadherence to antipsychotic medication has been studied in multiple prior studies in schizophrenia. The majority of these studies, however, have used subjective measures of adherence that rely on patient, family member, or clinician reports, all of which have been shown repeatedly to overestimate adherence [1] Only a few recent studies [2–6] have used an objective method—electronic monitoring [7]—to assess adherence to oral antipsychotic medication in outpatients who have schizophrenia.

A 1986 review of 26 studies, using varied definitions and traditional detection methods to evaluate antipsychotic medication adherence among persons who had schizophrenia, found a median nonadherence rate of 41% (range, 10%–76%) [8]. A 1997 review of 15 studies, which also used varied definitions of medication nonadherence as well as traditional adherence-assessment methods, reported a 1-month to 2-year median nonadherence rate of 55% (range, 24%–88%) [9]. Finally, a recent and extensive review of adherence

This work was supported by Grant No. 5 K23 MH064930 from the National Institute of Mental Health.

*Corresponding author. E-mail address: matt.byerly@utsouthwestern.edu (M.J. Byerly).

© 2007 Elsevier Inc. All rights reserved.
psych.theclinics.com

studies published since 1980 found that among 10 studies that used a "strict" definition of nonadherence ("regularly taking medication as prescribed") the weighted (by sample size) mean nonadherence rate was 41% (range, 20%–56%) [10]. In this same extensive review, in five studies that used a "stricter" definition of adherence ("taking medication as prescribed at least 75% of the time"), the weighted mean nonadherence rate was a bit higher (mean, 50%; range, 38%–56%) [10].

Several recent studies that used electronic monitoring to assess adherence to oral antipsychotic medication have extended the literature and understanding concerning the medication-taking behavior of outpatients who have schizophrenia [2–6]. Electronic monitoring is described increasingly as the objective reference standard for adherence-assessment methods [11]. In fact, a recently published review in the *New England Journal of Medicine* stated that electronic monitoring "provides the most accurate and valuable data on adherence in difficult clinical situations and in the setting of clinical trials and adherence research"[7]. Diaz and colleagues [2,3] have reported on two studies that used electronic monitoring. The first included 14 patients who had schizophrenia or schizoaffective disorder who were enrolled as inpatients and then monitored during a 6-month postdischarge period [2]. Mean monthly oral antipsychotic adherence rates ranged from 45% to 63%, but these rates were based on adherence data that were unavailable from 52% of the planned assessments. In the second study, Diaz and colleagues [3] reported on the electronically monitored adherence of 50 patients who had schizophrenia or schizoaffective disorder who were monitored in a 3-month postdischarge period. Fifty-five percent of the adherence data were missing in this study. When missing data were considered as zero adherence, the overall mean adherence was 37.5%. When it was assumed that the mean adherence during a period of missing data "was the same as during the time of measurement," however, overall mean adherence increased to 47%. In three recent trials of outpatients who had schizophrenia, in which more than 80% of planned electronically monitored adherence data were collected, mean adherence, which was estimated by omitting missing data [4] and by using mixed models of analysis to account for missing data [5,6], was considerably higher (78.2%, 69%–82%, and 64%–69%, respectively).

CONSEQUENCES OF NONADHERENCE TO ANTIPSYCHOTIC MEDICATION

Previous research suggests that nonadherence is associated with serious consequences, including exacerbation of psychotic symptoms, increased aggression toward self and others, worse prognosis [12,13], increased hospital and emergency room use [9,14], and high health care costs [15].

The most important consequence of nonadherence to antipsychotic medication in schizophrenia is the potential of psychotic symptom relapse. A summary of seven studies examining the relationship between nonadherence and future hospitalization found a 3.7 times greater odds of rehospitalization for nonadherent patients than for adherent patients over a 6- to 24-month period [9]. A subsequent study found that 75% of patients who stopped taking antipsychotic medication experienced a clinically meaningful symptom exacerbation over the course of a year [16]. Using California Medicaid pharmacy fill and medical claims data from 4325 outpatients who had schizophrenia, Weiden and colleagues [17] recently reported on the effect of patient gaps in antipsychotic medication-taking behavior on hospitalization risk. During a 1-year assessment period, gaps of 1 to 10 days (as opposed to no gaps) led to a twofold increased risk of hospitalization in patients taking antipsychotic medication. Gaps of 11 to 30 days and longer than 30 days led to approximately threefold and fourfold increased risks of hospitalization, respectively [17].

A relapse caused by nonadherence to medication can have other serious consequences. Relapse is associated with an increased risk of homelessness [14], the likelihood of aggression toward self and others, and damage to property [18]. Repeated psychotic relapses, particularly in early stages of the illness, may worsen the course and prognosis of the patient [12] and may result in resistance to antipsychotic medications and to the development of chronic psychotic symptoms [13]. Finally, psychotic relapse resulting from nonadherence to medication, increases health care costs associated with schizophrenia because of a greater need for hospitalization and emergency room care [14]. Research suggests that about 40% of the costs of hospitalization for persons who have schizophrenia are attributable to nonadherence to medication; the remaining 60% results from lost efficacy of antipsychotic medication [15].

Of the 250,000 patients who have multiple-episode schizophrenia (ie, $\geq$ two hospitalizations) who were discharged from inpatient psychiatric settings in the United States in 1986, the cost of schizophrenia-related readmission was approximately $2 billion [15]. Furthermore, of this $2 billion in the United States in 1986, the annual cost of psychiatric hospitalization directly attributable to nonadherence to antipsychotic medication by persons who had schizophrenia was about $800 million [15]. The portion of costs for inpatient care relative to the overall costs of care for schizophrenia probably has decreased since the 1986 estimate [19], but a 1999 estimate suggested that inpatient care still accounted for about 78% to 94% of the total health care costs associated with schizophrenia in the United States [20].

Improved interventions for managing nonadherence to antipsychotic medications may reduce psychiatric morbidity and costs of care considerably. These reductions could improve the welfare of persons who have schizophrenia; mitigate safety risks to themselves and others; and reduce the use of resources for acute psychotic episodes.

CORRELATES OF NONADHERENCE TO ANTIPSYCHOTIC MEDICATION AS POTENTIAL TARGETS FOR ADHERENCE INTERVENTIONS

To develop interventions that improve adherence to medication in schizophrenia, it may be necessary to understand the correlates of nonadherence. Many studies have evaluated factors correlated with nonadherence to antipsychotic medications in schizophrenia. In two systematic literature reviews of studies that used traditional adherence-assessment methods, Fenton and colleagues [9] and Lacro and colleagues [10] reported a relatively consistent set of correlates of nonadherence: poor insight, negative attitude or subjective response to medication, comorbid substance abuse, and poor therapeutic alliance.

Two recent studies that used electronic monitoring of adherence to antipsychotic medication [3,6], which is considered the reference standard of adherence assessment [7,11], provided quite different results regarding correlates of antipsychotic medication adherence (Table 1). Although one of the two studies that used electronic monitoring found an association between poorer adherence and worse symptoms (the other did not find an association between adherence and symptom severity), the same study found no association between adherence and poor insight, negative attitude or subjective response to medication, or substance abuse, all factors that consistently are associated with nonadherence when assessed by traditional methods. Moreover, the two studies that used electronic monitoring found a significant association between poor adherence and education level and nonwhite race, respectively [6], and between poor adherence and greater dose frequency and male gender, respectively [3]. These factors, which correlate with electronically monitored adherence, previously had been found not to correlate with adherence when adherence was assessed by traditional measures [9,10].

Although findings from electronically monitored adherence studies must be replicated before any definitive conclusions can be drawn, it seems plausible that the correlates of adherence might differ depending on the method of adherence assessment (particularly if bias were present in one or more of the methods being compared). A wealth of literature already exists about the tendency of patient and clinician ratings (the traditional methods most commonly used) to overestimate adherence [1]. In addition, clinician reports of adherence may be biased toward identifying correlates assumed to affect medication taking (eg, poor insight, concurrent drug use). Patient reports of adherence could be similarly biased. For example, patients who have better insight into their illness might provide overly optimistic reports of adherence in an attempt to please raters. Nonetheless, the finding in recent studies that correlates of adherence may vary depending on the chosen adherence-assessment method suggests that additional studies should be conducted using objective and direct measures of adherence [1]. Such studies may aid in identifying more appropriate targets for interventions to promote adherence in the patient populations most likely to benefit.

INTERVENTIONS FOR ADHERENCE TO ANTIPSYCHOTIC MEDICATION FOR PERSONS WHO HAVE SCHIZOPHRENIA
Psychosocial Interventions
Psychosocial interventions designed to improve adherence to antipsychotic medication in schizophrenia, although often multifaceted, generally can be

classified by the following treatment orientations: educational approaches, skills training, group therapy, family interventions, cognitive treatments, behavioral modification techniques, or a combination of psychosocial treatments [21].

Three previous systematic reviews of the literature have evaluated the effect of psychosocial interventions for adherence in schizophrenia (Table 2) [21–23]. Although the use of varied study-selection criteria resulted in the inclusion of different trials in these reviews, the findings across studies are quite consistent. All three reviews found that psychoeducational approaches, particularly when delivered only to patients, were generally ineffective [21–23]. In contrast, with "compliance therapy" (a brief cognitively based intervention that uses motivational interviewing techniques), behavioral approaches, and family interventions, benefit in adherence was largely consistent across the studies [21–23]. In addition, studies that provided more sessions, which were delivered over a longer period of time, and that used combination strategies tended to be more successful [21–23].

The authors performed a systematic literature review of adherence studies published since 2001 (the last year reviewed in the reports discussed previously). Selection criteria for this review included (1) nonpharmacologic intervention focused on improving adherence; (2) individual group sample sizes of 10 or more; (3) participants diagnosed as having schizophrenia-spectrum disorders; and (4) assessment of adherence to antipsychotic medication as a primary or secondary outcome. The review included English-language studies published between 2002 and January 2007. Two of the authors (EL and MB) reviewed all the extracted articles to confirm that they met selection criteria.

Results of the updated literature review are provided in Table 3. It is perhaps not surprising that, of the six studies meeting the selection criteria [5,24–28], five included strategies identified as "promising" in prior reviews [5,24–27]. Three of the trials [5,24,25], including a large, multisite trial, evaluated the effect of compliance therapy on patients who had schizophrenia or schizoaffective disorder and found a lack of benefit of compliance therapy on adherence and on other clinical outcomes. These negative findings are in contrast to the positive findings of the initial studies of compliance therapy, which were delivered to psychotic inpatients who had mixed diagnoses [29,30]. Several important design elements may have contributed to the inconclusive results of the two earlier and three later studies of compliance therapy. First, the three later trials of compliance therapy included only patients who had psychotic disorders [5,24,25], whereas earlier studies included patients who had both affective and psychotic disorders [29,30]. Thus, it is possible that patients who have affective disorders experience greater benefit with compliance therapy than those who have psychotic disorders. Also, in contrast to the two prior trials that used the same unvalidated four-point Likert-type scale to assess adherence [29,30], two of the three later trials used validated adherence assessments [5,25]. One used the Medication Adherence Questionnaire [31], and one used electronic monitoring of adherence [7]. Compared with unvalidated clinician ratings,

Table 1
Risk factors of nonadherence to antipsychotic medication in schizophrenia

Risk factor	Literature reviews of studies using traditional adherence assessment methods		Original studies using electronic monitoring to assess adherence	
	Fenton et al, 1997[a], [9]	Lacro et al, 2002[b], [10]	Nakonezny et al, 2006 [6] (N = 61)	Diaz et al, 2004 [3] (N = 50)
Patient-related risk factors				
Symptom severity	Yes[c]	No[d]	Yes	No
Poor insight	Yes	Yes	No	Not assessed
Negative attitude or subjective response to medication	Yes	Yes	No	Not assessed
Substance abuse comorbidity	Yes	Yes	No	Not assessed
Shorter illness duration	No	Yes	No	Not assessed
Previous nonadherence	Not assessed	Yes	Not assessed	Not assessed
Cognitive impairment	Not assessed	No	Not assessed	Not assessed
Age	No	No	No	No
Male gender	No	No	No	Yes
Ethnicity (nonwhite race)	No	No	Yes	Not assessed
Lower education level	No	No	Yes	Not assessed
Income level	No	Not assessed	Not assessed	Not assessed
Medication-related risk factors				
Severity of medication side effects	Yes	No	No	No

Subtherapeutic or excessively high dosages	Yes	No	No	Not assessed
Complexity of regimen (dose frequency)	No	No	No	Yes
Environmental-related risk factors				
Practical barriers such as lack of money or transportation	Yes	Too few studies to draw conclusion	Not assessed	Not assessed
Inadequate support or supervision	Yes	Yes	No	Not assessed
Clinician-related risk factors				
Poor therapeutic alliance	Yes	Yes	Not assessed	Not assessed

[a] Review of all available studies identified through such key words as "compliance, adherence, psychopharmacology, and schizophrenia."

[b] Review of 39 articles published after 1980, which were identified through such key words as "risk factor(s), compliance, antipsychotic, neuroleptic, schizophrenia, and psychosis." Reports with fewer than 40 subjects were excluded.

[c] "Yes" indicates a consistent finding in the literature reviews or significant finding in the original studies using electronic monitoring to assess adherence.

[d] "No" indicates a finding that is not consistent in the literature reviews or not in the original studies using electronic monitoring to assess adherence.

Table 2
Systematic literature reviews of psychosocial interventions intended to improve adherence to antipsychotic medication in schizophrenia

Review	Study selection criteria	Number of studies included	Findings
Zygmunt et al, 2002 [21]	Randomized, controlled trial Group sample size ≥ 10 Diagnosis of schizophrenia spectrum disorder Adherence measured as primary or secondary outcome Studies published between 1980 and 2000	39	Psychoeducation alone is generally ineffective. Interventions focused on nonadherence are more likely to be successful than more broadly based interventions. Problem-solving or motivational techniques were common features of successful programs. Models of community care (eg, assertive community treatment) and those based on motivational interviewing (eg, compliance therapy) are promising.
McDonald et al, 2002 [23]	Randomized, controlled trial Diagnosis of schizophrenia or acute psychosis Adherence and treatment outcome assessed At least 80% follow-up for each group For long-term studies, at least 6-month follow-up for studies with positive findings Studies published between 1967 and 2001	8	Psychoeducation alone is generally ineffective. Combination interventions and compliance therapy seemed to be effective for adherence and clinical outcomes. Family interventions were effective in some, but not all, studies.
Dolder et al, 2003 [22]	Randomized, controlled trial Total sample size ≥ 20 Majority diagnosed as having schizophrenia or schizoaffective disorder Adherence reported quantitatively Studies published between 1980 and 2001	21	Psychoeducation alone is generally ineffective. Interventions using combinations of educational, behavioral, and affective strategies produced the greatest improvement in adherence. Compliance therapy was considered a behavioral and affective intervention.) Longer interventions and an alliance with therapists seemed to be important.

which were used in early studies of compliance therapy [29,30], electronic measurement, in particular, may provide greater precision and sophistication in assessing the adherence of patients in general medical populations [11] and of those who have schizophrenia [4].

Consistent with prior reviews [21–23], this updated literature review found that providing psychoeducation to patients alone resulted in no benefit over standard care for adherence or clinical outcomes [5,24,25]. In contrast, one [27] of two [26,27] trials that extended psychoeducation delivery to family members plus patients found a superior outcome for adherence, rehospitalization, symptoms, and social functioning compared with standard care at 12- and 24-month follow-up. Although the second study of family plus patient psychoeducation found no benefit for adherence, this intervention produced findings superior to standard care for symptoms and social functioning [26].

In summary, although two early studies of compliance therapy were promising for adherence (as assessed by an unvalidated instrument) and clinical outcomes of psychotic patients who had mixed diagnoses, three later studies of patients who had schizophrenia or schizoaffective disorder (including two studies that used validated instruments of adherence assessment) indicate that compliance therapy is not of benefit for patients who have psychotic disorders. Two studies using family psychoeducation coupled with patient psychoeducation extend the findings that indicate that family interventions are helpful, although only one of the studies demonstrated improvement in adherence. An increasingly consistent picture is emerging about the lack of impact of psychoeducation delivered to patients alone. Earlier literature reviews indicate that complex and intensive interventions with a supportive and problems-solving focus (eg, assertive community treatment) are likely to improve adherence; however, the resources needed to deliver such treatments limit their applicability. Thus, there remains a need to identify psychosocial interventions with demonstrated feasibility for widespread use and with proven effectiveness for clinical outcomes and for reducing the nonadherence to antipsychotic medication of persons who have schizophrenia or schizoaffective disorder.

Interventions to Improve Adherence to Pharmacologic Medication

Second-generation oral antipsychotics

Studies of medication type and adherence to antipsychotic medication in schizophrenia have proliferated in recent years [32]. One of the important lines of investigation, based on the supposition that the improved tolerability of second-generation antipsychotics might lead to improved adherence with these agents, has led to seven published studies comparing adherence associated with first- versus second-generation agents [3,14,32–36]. Of the four retrospective studies [32,34–36], two found significantly greater adherence among patients taking second-generation antipsychotics [32,36], one study found greater adherence among patients taking first-generation antipsychotics [35], and one study found no differences in adherence [34]. Moreover, one of the two retrospective studies that found greater adherence with second-generation

Table 3
Recent studies testing interventions to promote adherence with psychosocial medication schizophrenia

Study	Study design	Interventions	Adherence measurement	Number of sessions and Time/session	Study duration (months)	Outcome
Studies of compliance therapy						
O'Donnell, 2003 [24]	RCT Blinded adherence ratings	Compliance therapy (n = 28) versus nonspecific therapy (n = 28)	Four-point Likert scale	Five sessions, 30–60 minutes each (both groups)	24	No difference between groups in adherence, symptoms, insight, attitudes to treatment, level of functioning, or quality of life
Byerly, 2005 [5]	No control group Blinded adherence ratings	Compliance therapy (n = 30)	Electronic monitoring	Four to six sessions, 30–60 minutes each	6	No improvement in adherence, symptoms, insight, or attitudes to treatment
Gray, 2006 [25]	RCT Multicenter Blinded adherence ratings	Compliance "adherence" therapy (n = 204) versus didactic health education (n = 205)	Medication adherence questionnaire	Up to eight sessions, 30–50 minutes each (both groups)	18	No differences between groups in adherence, symptoms, or quality of life
Studies of patient plus family psychoeducation						
Li, 2005 [26]	RCT Unblinded adherence ratings	Psychoed for patients and their families (n = 46) versus standard care (n = 55)	Four-point Likert scale	Separate psychoeducation for patients, 8 hours total; Separate psychoeducation for family, 36 hours total (inpatient phase), then 2 hours/month with patient and family together for 3 months	9	No differences between groups in adherence or rehospitalization rate Patient plus family psychoeducation superior to standard care for symptoms and social functioning at 9 (but not at 3) months

Pitschel-Walz, 2006 [27]	RCT Multicenter Blinded adherence ratings	Separate psychoeducation groups for patients and families (n = 125) versus standard care (n = 92)	Four-point Likert scale validated by plasma drug levels	Patient psychoeducation: four sessions weekly, then four sessions monthly, 60 minutes each Family psychoeducation: eight sessions biweekly, 90 minutes each	24	Patient plus family psychoeducation superior to standard care at 12 and 24 months for adherence, rehospitalization rate, symptoms, and social functioning
Study of patient psychoeducation alone						
Vreeland, 2006 [28]	RCT Blinded adherence ratings	Intensive psychoeducation (n = 40) versus standard care (n = 34)	Treatment compliance interview	96 sessions, 60 minutes each	6	No differences between groups in adherence, symptoms, or social functioning

Abbreviations: Psychoed, adherence intervention with psychoeducational focus; RCT, randomized, controlled trial.

antipsychotics than with first-generation agents reported such small differences in adherence that the authors stated that the difference in adherence did "not appear to be clinically important" [36]. Three recent trials have prospectively evaluated patients' adherence associated with first- versus second-generation antipsychotics; none of the three studies found a difference in adherence between first- and second-generation agents [14,33,35]. One of the prospective trials that demonstrated no advantage in adherence among patients taking second-generation agents [3] used electronic monitoring to measure adherence with antipsychotic medication in 50 newly discharged patients who had schizophrenia and schizoaffective disorder. A second recent trial that used electronic monitoring to assess adherence also found no advantage in adherence for second-generation antipsychotics in a sample of 61 outpatients who had schizophrenia and schizoaffective disorder [6]. Growing evidence thus suggests that second-generation oral antipsychotics generally do not provide meaningful benefits in adherence over first-generation oral antipsychotics.

Long-acting injectable antipsychotic medications

Although current treatment guidelines in schizophrenia primarily recommend the use of long-acting injectable antipsychotics (LAIs) for patients who are assumed to be nonadherent to oral antipsychotic medication [37–39], surprisingly little research exists on the effect of LAIs on adherence. The authors were unable to find a single randomized, controlled trial that compared the adherence to LAI with the adherence to oral antipsychotic medications in outpatients who had schizophrenia. Thus empiric evidence is lacking despite the publication of six randomized, controlled trials that focused on the relapse rates associated with LAI versus those associated with oral antipsychotics [40–45]. Three studies have provided limited information even though they compared the adherence of schizophrenic outpatients receiving depot versus oral antipsychotics [46–48]. In all three studies, the choice of treatment choice was made as part of usual clinical care (ie, allocation was nonrandom). In one study, patients who received depot antipsychotic injections (n = 22) reported statistically significantly higher adherence during the 3 months before adherence assessment than those who received oral antipsychotic medication (n = 48) ($P < .01$) [48]. Two other studies, one using injection records as measures of adherence for patients receiving depots (n = 22) and urine drug tests for patients receiving oral antipsychotics (n = 11) [46], and the other using a structured interview and five-point Likert scale of antipsychotic adherence in 202 patients (78% taking oral medication, 22% taking depots) [47], found no significant difference in group adherence rates.

In the only study focusing on the adherence with depot versus oral forms of medication, Weiden and colleagues [49] evaluated the effect of converting inpatients who had schizophrenia to LAI (n = 40) or continuing with oral (n = 53) antipsychotic treatment (with type of medication treatment chosen as part of routine care) on outpatient adherence to antipsychotic medication. In this nonrandom design and with adherence raters who were aware of the route of drug delivery (ie, with unblinded raters), antipsychotic adherence ratings with the treatment compliance interview (a composite interview of patients, family, and outpatient clinicians) [49] revealed significantly greater adherence in the depot group at the 1-month postdischarge visit. This advantage waned, however, because as no adherence differences were found at the 6- and 12-month postdischarge visits [49].

If depot agents are assumed to be associated with greater adherence than oral agents, then the supposition is that this advantage in adherence should translate into improved clinical outcomes. Two meta-analyses of randomized, controlled trials comparing the clinical impact of oral versus LAIs among patients who have schizophrenia have been published. One of these studies, reported by Davis and colleagues [50], found that LAIs were superior in reducing risk of relapse. Another recent meta-analysis by Adams and colleagues [51] of the Cochrane Schizophrenia Group found LAIs to have a significant advantage over traditional oral agents on global change but saw no differences for relapse or study attrition. The Cochrane Schizophrenia Group emphasized, however, that these studies did not focus on patient populations in which LAIs might be most beneficial, specifically, patients who are nonadherent to antipsychotic medication [51]. Thus, it is possible that the advantages realized with LAIs in the general schizophrenia population will be magnified in persons who have schizophrenia and who are nonadherent to their antipsychotic medication.

Despite the lack of empiric evidence regarding the effect of LAIs on adherence to antipsychotic medication, an important clinical advantage of these agents remains: treating clinicians can identify immediately patients who fail to receive a scheduled injection. In contrast, nonadherence to oral antipsychotics can go undetected for weeks or months, often leading to an exacerbation of symptoms before the nonadherence problem can be addressed [52]. Thus, in theory, providing outreach services to patients who miss clinic appointments for LAIs could improve adherence to medication. One study that used intensive outreach for missed appointments for LAI injection found a 96% adherence rate when adherence was defined as receiving an injection within 4 days of the scheduled appointment [53].

SUMMARY

Although there is considerable research regarding the medication-taking behavior of persons who have schizophrenia, many unanswered questions remain about the frequency, correlates, consequences, and solutions to address nonadherence to antipsychotic medication. Recent studies using electronic monitoring of medication adherence now suggest that prior studies, which were based largely on subjective methods of assessing adherence, may have overestimated patients' adherence to antipsychotic medication. In addition, limited (and inconclusive) findings exist concerning the prevalence and correlates of nonadherence to antipsychotic medication and the individual patient characteristics that are most strongly associated with important clinical outcomes, such as symptom severity, symptom relapse, and rehospitalization.

Unfortunately, interventions to promote adherence that are feasible for delivery in the community have not been proven to be effective. Early positive studies of compliance therapy, a brief psychosocial intervention that seemed to be effective in two trials involving groups of psychotic inpatients who had mixed diagnoses, were not confirmed by three later studies in which compliance therapy was delivered to patients who had psychotic disorders. Although nonpharmacologic interventions with family or behavioral components and those involving intensive community support (eg, assertive community treatment) seem promising, none currently meet the full criteria necessary for widespread use in usual community care. The main difficulty associated with most of the current psychosocial interventions lies in the vast resources and patient (or family) involvement needed to deliver these treatments.

A growing body of literature regarding intervention approaches for medication adherence suggests that persons who have schizophrenia are not more adherent to second-generation antipsychotic medications than to first-generation oral antipsychotic medications. Additionally, the few studies that have investigated the adherence of patients taking depot antipsychotic preparations, which are recommended for use in nonadherent patients by all major schizophrenia treatment guidelines, generally have found depot medication to have little or no sustained advantage in adherence over oral antipsychotic medications.

To date, attempts to address the challenges associated with measuring the ongoing antipsychotic medication-taking behavior of patients who have schizophrenia in the community have been hindered by a lack of objective, valid, and reliable methods of assessing adherence. The recent availability of electronic monitoring devices, however, may provide the opportunity to address these challenges feasibly in real-world, community-based populations.

References

[1] Velligan DI, Lam YW, Glahn DC, et al. Defining and assessing adherence to oral antipsychotics: a review of the literature. Schizophr Bull 2006;32(4):724–42.

[2] Diaz E, Levine HB, Sullivan MC, et al. Use of the medication event monitoring system to estimate medication compliance in patients with schizophrenia. J Psychiatry Neurosci 2001;26(4):325–9.

[3] Diaz E, Neuse E, Sullivan MC, et al. Adherence to conventional and atypical antipsychotics after hospital discharge. J Clin Psychiatry 2004;65(3):354–60.

[4] Byerly M, Fisher R, Whatley K, et al. A comparison of electronic monitoring vs. clinician rating of antipsychotic adherence in outpatients with schizophrenia. Psychiatry Res 2005;133(2–3):129–33.

[5] Byerly MJ, Fisher R, Carmody T, et al. A trial of compliance therapy in outpatients with schizophrenia or schizoaffective disorder. J Clin Psychiatry 2005;66(8):997–1001.

[6] Nakonezny PA, Byerly MJ. Electronically monitored adherence in outpatients with schizophrenia or schizoaffective disorder: a comparison of first- vs. second-generation antipsychotics. Schizophr Res 2006;82(1):107–14.

[7] Osterberg L, Blaschke T. Adherence to medication. N Engl J Med 2005;353(5):487–97.

[8] Young JL, Zonana HV, Shepler L. Medication noncompliance in schizophrenia: codification and update. Bull Am Acad Psychiatry Law 1986;14(2):105–22.

[9] Fenton WS, Blyler CR, Heinssen RK. Determinants of medication compliance in schizophrenia: empirical and clinical findings. Schizophr Bull 1997;23(4):637–51.

[10] Lacro JP, Dunn LB, Dolder CR, et al. Prevalence of and risk factors for medication nonadherence in patients with schizophrenia: a comprehensive review of recent literature. J Clin Psychiatry 2002;63(10):892–909.
[11] Farmer KC. Methods for measuring and monitoring medication regimen adherence in clinical trials and clinical practice. Clin Ther 1999;21(6):1074–90 [discussion: 1073].
[12] Wyatt RJ. Neuroleptics and the natural course of schizophrenia. Schizophr Bull 1991;17(2):325–51.
[13] Lieberman JA, Sheitman B, Chakos M, et al. The development of treatment resistance in patients with schizophrenia: a clinical and pathophysiologic perspective. J Clin Psychopharmacol 1998;18(2 Suppl 1):20S–4S.
[14] Olfson M, Mechanic D, Hansell S, et al. Predicting medication noncompliance after hospital discharge among patients with schizophrenia. Psychiatr Serv 2000;51(2):216–22.
[15] Weiden PJ, Olfson M. Cost of relapse in schizophrenia. Schizophr Bull 1995;21(3): 419–29.
[16] Ayuso-Gutierrez JL, del Rio Vega JM. Factors influencing relapse in the long-term course of schizophrenia. Schizophr Res Dec 19, 1997;28(2–3):199–206.
[17] Weiden PJ, Kozma C, Grogg A, et al. Partial compliance and risk of rehospitalization among California Medicaid patients with schizophrenia. Psychiatr Serv 2004;55(8):886–91.
[18] Steadman HJ, Mulvey EP, Monahan J, et al. Violence by people discharged from acute psychiatric inpatient facilities and by others in the same neighborhoods. Arch Gen Psychiatry 1998;55(5):393–401.
[19] Leslie DL, Rosenheck R. Shifting to outpatient care? Mental health care use and cost under private insurance. Am J Psychiatry 1999;156(8):1250–7.
[20] Mauskopf JA, David K, Grainger DL, et al. Annual health outcomes and treatment costs for schizophrenia populations. J Clin Psychiatry 1999;60(Suppl 19):14–9 [discussion: 20–2].
[21] Zygmunt A, Olfson M, Boyer CA, et al. Interventions to improve medication adherence in schizophrenia. Am J Psychiatry 2002;159(10):1653–64.
[22] Dolder CR, Lacro JP, Leckband S, et al. Interventions to improve antipsychotic medication adherence: review of recent literature. J Clin Psychopharmacol 2003;23(4):389–99.
[23] McDonald HP, Garg AX, Haynes RB. Interventions to enhance patient adherence to medication prescriptions: scientific review. JAMA 2002;288(22):2868–79.
[24] O'Donnell C, Donohoe G, Sharkey L, et al. Compliance therapy: a randomised controlled trial in schizophrenia. BMJ 2003;327(7419):834.
[25] Gray R, Leese M, Bindman J, et al. Adherence therapy for people with schizophrenia. European multicentre randomised controlled trial. Br J Psychiatry 2006;189:508–14.
[26] Li Z, Arthur D. Family education for people with schizophrenia in Beijing, China: randomised controlled trial. Br J Psychiatry 2005;187:339–45.
[27] Pitschel-Walz G, Bauml J, Bender W, et al. Psychoeducation and compliance in the treatment of schizophrenia: results of the Munich Psychosis Information Project Study. J Clin Psychiatry 2006;67(3):443–52.
[28] Vreeland B, Minsky S, Yanos PT, et al. Efficacy of the team solutions program for educating patients about illness management and treatment. Psychiatr Serv 2006;57(6):822–8.
[29] Kemp R, Hayward P, Applewhaite G, et al. Compliance therapy in psychotic patients: randomised controlled trial. BMJ 1996;312(7027):345–9.
[30] Kemp R, Kirov G, Everitt B, et al. Randomised controlled trial of compliance therapy. 18-month follow-up. Br J Psychiatry 1998;172:413–9.
[31] Morisky DE, Green LW, Levine DM. Concurrent and predictive validity of a self-reported measure of medication adherence. Med Care 1986;24(1):67–74.
[32] Dolder CR, Lacro JP, Dunn LB, et al. Antipsychotic medication adherence: is there a difference between typical and atypical agents? Am J Psychiatry 2002;159(1):103–8.
[33] Rosenheck R, Chang S, Choe Y, et al. Medication continuation and compliance: a comparison of patients treated with clozapine and haloperidol. J Clin Psychiatry 2000;61(5): 382–6.

[34] Cabeza IG, Amador MS, Lopez CA, et al. Subjective response to antipsychotics in schizo-phrenic patients: clinical implications and related factors. Schizophr Res 2000;41(2): 349–55.

[35] Grunebaum MF, Weiden PJ, Olfson M. Medication supervision and adherence of persons with psychotic disorders in residential treatment settings: a pilot study. J Clin Psychiatry 2001;62(5):394–9 [quiz: 400–1].

[36] Gianfrancesco FD, Rajagopalan K, Sajatovic M, et al. Treatment adherence among patients with schizophrenia treated with atypical and typical antipsychotics. Psychiatry Res 2006;144(2–3):177–89.

[37] Lehman AF, Lieberman JA, Dixon LB, et al. Practice guideline for the treatment of patients with schizophrenia, second edition. Am J Psychiatry 2004;161(2 Suppl):1–56.

[38] Miller AL, Hall CS, Buchanan RW, et al. The Texas Medication Algorithm Project antipsy-chotic algorithm for schizophrenia: 2003 update. J Clin Psychiatry 2004;65(4):500–8.

[39] Kane JM, Leucht S, Carpenter D, et al. Expert consensus guideline series. Optimizing phar-macologic treatment of psychotic disorders. Introduction: methods, commentary, and sum-mary. J Clin Psychiatry 2003;64(Suppl 12):5–19.

[40] Crawford R, Forrest A. Controlled trial of depot fluphenazine in out-patient schizophrenics. Br J Psychiatry 1974;124:385–91.

[41] del Giudice J, Clark WG, Gocka EF. Prevention of recidivism of schizophrenics treated with fluphenazine enanthate. Psychosomatics 1975;16(1):32–6.

[42] Rifkin A, Quitkin F, Rabiner CJ, et al. Fluphenazine decanoate, fluphenazine hydrochloride given orally, and placebo in remitted schizophrenics. I. Relapse rates after one year. Arch Gen Psychiatry 1977;34(1):43–7.

[43] Falloon I, Watt DC, Shepherd M. A comparative controlled trial of pimozide and fluphen-azine decanoate in the continuation therapy of schizophrenia. Psychol Med 1978;8(1): 59–70.

[44] Hogarty GE, Schooler NR, Ulrich R, et al. Fluphenazine and social therapy in the aftercare of schizophrenic patients. Relapse analyses of a two-year controlled study of fluphenazine decanoate and fluphenazine hydrochloride. Arch Gen Psychiatry 1979;36(12):1283–94.

[45] Schooler NR, Levine J, Severe JB, et al. Prevention of relapse in schizophrenia. An evalua-tion of fluphenazine decanoate. Arch Gen Psychiatry 1980;37(1):16–24.

[46] Buchanan A. A two-year prospective study of treatment compliance in patients with schizo-phrenia. Psychol Med 1992;22(3):787–97.

[47] Nageotte C, Sullivan G, Duan N, et al. Medication compliance among the seriously mentally ill in a public mental health system. Soc Psychiatry Psychiatr Epidemiol 1997;32(2):49–56.

[48] Garavan J, Browne S, Gervin M, et al. Compliance with neuroleptic medication in outpa-tients with schizophrenia; relationship to subjective response to neuroleptics; attitudes to medication and insight. Compr Psychiatry 1998;39(4):215–9.

[49] Weiden P, Rapkin B, Zygmunt A, et al. Postdischarge medication compliance of inpatients converted from an oral to a depot neuroleptic regimen. Psychiatr Serv 1995;46(10): 1049–54.

[50] Davis JM, Matalon L, Watanabe MD, et al. Depot antipsychotic drugs. Place in therapy. Drugs 1994;47(5):741–73.

[51] Adams CE, Fenton MK, Quraishi S, et al. Systematic meta-review of depot antipsychotic drugs for people with schizophrenia. Br J Psychiatry 2001;179:290–9.

[52] McEvoy JP. Risks versus benefits of different types of long-acting injectable antipsychotics. J Clin Psychiatry 2006;67(Suppl 5):15–8.

[53] Heyscue BE, Levin GM, Merrick JP. Compliance with depot antipsychotic medication by patients attending outpatient clinics. Psychiatr Serv 1998;49(9):1232–4.

Reaching for Wellness in Schizophrenia

Deanna L. Kelly, PharmD, BCPP*,
Douglas L. Boggs, PharmD, MS,
Robert R. Conley, MD

Maryland Psychiatric Research Center, University of Maryland School of Medicine, Box 21247,
Baltimore, MD 21228, USA

Overwhelming evidence illustrates that people who have schizophrenia have increased rates of physical illness compared with the general population. Recent data suggest that approximately 70% of people who have schizophrenia suffer from at least one medical comorbidity, and 33% suffer from three or more comorbid health disorders [1]. Common medical comorbidities include hypertension, chronic obstructive pulmonary disease, and diabetes; all of which may contribute to the risk of cardiovascular disease and associated mortality [1,2].

Early mortality is more than fivefold higher in people who have schizophrenia than in the general population [3]. In fact schizophrenia is considered to be a life-shortening illness [4]. Currently, the life expectancy for the general population in the United States is approximately 76 years, but people who have schizophrenia have about a 20% lower life expectancy of about 61 years [2]. Early studies reported that increased mortality resulted from a high rate of suicide [5–7]. Even after controlling for the increase in suicide (approximately 10%), life expectancy is still much lower than in the general population. The majority of excess mortality seems to be caused by cardiovascular complications, notably coronary heart disease (CHD) [3]. The 10-year risk of developing CHD is significantly greater in both men and women who have schizophrenia than in the general population (9.4% versus 7.0% and 6.3% versus 4.2%, respectively) [8].

The problem of medical comorbidities and mortality relating to CHD is particularly troubling at a time when much progress has been made in pharmacologic treatments and the rehabilitation of people who suffer from schizophrenia. Treatment has moved beyond the challenges of neuroleptic-related extrapyramidal symptoms and tardive dyskinesia to address more long-term

This work was supported by grant number P50 MH40279 (Advanced Center for Intervention and Services Research) from the National Institutes of Mental Health.

*Corresponding author. E-mail address: dkelly@mprc.umaryland.edu (D.L. Kelly).

0193-953X/07/$ – see front matter
doi:10.1016/j.psc.2007.04.003
© 2007 Elsevier Inc. All rights reserved.
psych.theclinics.com

outcome-orientated treatments and quality of life. Medical comorbidity associated with metabolic risk and CHD-related morbidity and mortality are among the least improved illness domains associated with schizophrenia. The risk of CHD now represents one of the greatest unmet challenges of the current treatment of schizophrenia.

RISK FACTORS AND BARRIERS TO TREATMENT FOR MORBIDITY AND MORTALITY RELATED TO CORONARY HEARD DISEASE

Risk Factors

Somatic illness is increased for people who have schizophrenia for a variety of reasons including poor lifestyle decisions, effects of medication treatment, and possible genetic predispositions that intrinsically add to the risk of CHD. People who have schizophrenia generally have a diet with a higher fat content and lower intake of fiber than the general population [9]. Most people who have schizophrenia have sedentary lifestyles and engage in very little physical activity for various reasons including sedating side effects of medications and poor economic backgrounds [10,11]. People who have schizophrenia tend to eat less fruits and vegetables, less dairy products, more carbohydrates, and more fast food than do age-matched controls in the general population [12,13]. A lack of knowledge about nutrition and healthy diets probably contributes to poor choices in food selection. Also, people who have schizophrenia may have difficulty with satiety and reward function as part of the pathophysiology of their disorder [14].

Comorbid substance use also is common in schizophrenia, with almost 50% of patients suffering from co-occurring substance abuse or dependence. Alcohol and marijuana are usually the drugs of choice for people who have schizophrenia. Cocaine, heroin, and amphetamines also are used by some who suffer from this illness [15]. Substance abuse is known to increase greatly the risk of several medical disorders, including CHD [16]. Several classes of commonly used psychotropic medications including mood stabilizers, antidepressants, and antipsychotics also are associated with side effects that may contribute to CHD [17]. Medication effects may worsen the risk of CHD by causing weight gain, glucose dysregulation, and hyperlipidemia. Thus, many of the risk factors for CHD in people who have schizophrenia are potentially modifiable. Several of these disease-related risks are discussed in this article.

Barriers to Treatment

Despite a growing recognition of concerns related to physical health, people who have schizophrenia have several barriers to receiving comprehensive treatment, including fewer medical visits, less-documented medical problems, fewer full physical examinations, and a lower likelihood of being told they have a somatic illness [18,19]. Because of these barriers, patients often do not receive treatment until their medical illness is painful, severe, or life threatening [20]. Many current health care systems for psychiatric and somatic care remain fragmented, and obtaining care from different providers in a multitude of systems is extremely challenging for individuals who at the core of their illness suffer from reality distortions, paranoia, and cognitive disturbances.

Nevertheless, there is a notable lack of comprehensive health care in the physical health domains for people who have schizophrenia. Lack of physician awareness does not account for the underrecognition and undertreatment of physical health. In fact, most psychiatrists are aware of the substantial risk of metabolic symptoms present in people who have schizophrenia [21]. Despite this understanding, appropriate treatment of physical illness in people who have schizophrenia continues to be a problem. Buckley and colleagues [22] reported that more than 60% of psychiatrists do not monitor fasting lipids or glucose routinely. A cross-sectional study of 103 patients who had schizophrenia found that although 26% had elevated total fasting cholesterol levels, and 55% had elevated fasting triglycerides levels, only 2.9% were receiving lipid-lowering therapy [23]. The recent Clinical Antipsychotic Trials of Intervention Effectiveness (CATIE) study evaluated baseline treatment for somatic diseases. The percentages of people having schizophrenia and not being treated for the following identified disorders were 30.2% for diabetes, 62.4% for hypertension, and 88.0% for dyslipidemia [24]. Even when metabolic abnormalities are recognized, appropriate follow-up and treatment interventions often are delayed. A study of 408 patients who had schizophrenia in the Veterans Affairs Medical Center (1999–2003) reported that although 85% of the individuals had a least one measurement of serum lipids during a 4-year period, the median follow-up for a repeat measurement, when clinically indicated, was 10 months [25]. Others have found that in patients who have diabetes, those who also have severe mental illness are significantly less likely than those in the general population to receive appropriate pharmacologic treatment, and only about one third of patients who have schizophrenia and comorbid chronic obstructive pulmonary disease receive treatment for this respiratory ailment [26,27].

CARDIOVASCULAR RISK FACTORS
Cigarette Smoking and Respiratory Disorders

In the United States between 70% and 90% of people who have schizophrenia smoke cigarettes and are considered nicotine dependent [28]. This trend is seen worldwide. A meta-analysis by de Leon and Diaz [29] of 42 studies in 20 countries found the odds ratio (OR) of cigarette smoking to be 5.3 times higher in people who have schizophrenia than in the general population. Although smoking is increased among persons who have most mental disorders, the risk is still doubled for those who have schizophrenia [29]. Reasons for more frequent smoking in schizophrenia remains unknown, but it has been suggested that some of the craving for nicotine arises from self-medicating effects, perhaps because of cognitive improvement from agonism of the $\alpha 7$ nicotinic receptor [30]. Despite the potential benefits of nicotine in schizophrenia, the effects of cigarette smoking are undoubtedly deleterious to the physical health of patients.

Most studies of medical morbidity and mortality in schizophrenia have reported a high rate of respiratory complications associated with this illness.

Some have reported respiratory ailments to be one of the primary causes of excess mortality [31,32]. A study of 200 subjects, controlled for age, reported that the prevalence of chronic obstructive pulmonary disease was 22.6% in people who had severe mental illness as compared with 5% in the general population [26]. This study also found a higher incidence of chronic bronchitis (OR, 3.75; 95% confidence interval [CI], 2.53–5.55) and emphysema (OR, 5.69; 95% CI, 2.53–5.55) than in the general population. In a study by the Health Surveys for England, Filik and colleagues [33] compared the lung function of 407 subjects who had schizophrenia with that in the general population. They found that a higher proportion of people who had schizophrenia had a lower predicted forced expiratory volume in 1 second (FEV_1) than in the general population (89.6% versus 47%). Using the same metric, they found 41.9% of people who had schizophrenia had below-average lung function, compared with 9% of the population, more than 1.64 SD below the predicted value. Reduced FEV_1 is as strong a predictor of mortality and has been compared with the risk of high cholesterol and its relationship to ischemic heart disease [34].

Cigarette smoking also is a major risk factor for several types of cancers and accounts for around 90% of lung cancer deaths [35]. The risk of mortality from lung cancer in people who have schizophrenia remains controversial, and discrepant findings have been reported with likely differences by age, race, and geographic location of the subjects. Lower lung cancer rates in people who have schizophrenia actually have been reported, but these data may be an artifact because people who have schizophrenia tend to die at a younger age [36]. Morbidity and mortality from respiratory disorders in persons who have schizophrenia may not result entirely from cigarette smoking. Sokal and colleagues [37] recently reported that the odds of developing respiratory disease are increased in people who have schizophrenia even after controlling for cigarette smoking; thus this population is at an even greater risk of morbidity and mortality from respiratory ailments.

It is noteworthy that cigarette smoking is a risk factor for CHD independent of its risk for morbidity and mortality associated with respiratory disorders. Cigarette smoking is undoubtedly a significant and modifiable risk factor for CHD. Cigarette smoking contributes to both CHD and peripheral arterial disease. Smoking-induced inflammation along with dyslipidemia cause vascular damage through oxidative stress. Smoking also is associated with many alterations in lipids and lipoproteins [38]. A recent literature review reported that the combined results of 20 publications illustrate a 36% crude relative risk reduction of mortality from CHD in smokers who quit compared with those who continued smoking. This risk reduction seems to be consistent regardless of age, sex, previous cardiac event, country, or year of study [39]. One would expect similar risk reductions with smoking cessation for people who have schizophrenia as well.

Obesity

Energy balance in the human body has two components, energy intake (ie, feeding) and energy expenditure. Sociologic changes have led to increased energy intake and decreased exercise, causing obesity to become an epidemic in many countries. In the United States and Europe, the majority of adults are above normal weight, and at least 30% of both populations are obese [40]. Obesity increases the risk of several other diseases including hypertension, diabetes, cancer, hyperlipidemia, gallbladder disease, osteoarthritis, and CHD [41]. Abdominal (visceral) adiposity in particular increases risk for diabetes and CHD [42,43]. Risks for CHD-related mortality are most significant with body mass indices greater than 25.0 kg/m^2 in women and 26.5 kg/m^2 in men [44].

Although the prevalence of obesity in the general population is estimated to be 30%, the rate of obesity among persons who have schizophrenia is estimated to be between 40% and 60% [45,46]. Obesity in people who have schizophrenia was reported in the literature before the introduction of antipsychotic medications, but much of the overweight and obesity noted in current patients who have schizophrenia is believed to be secondary to antipsychotic medications [47].

The mechanism for antipsychotic weight gain is not well understood, but antagonism of various monoaminergic receptors has been implicated in weight gain. The two most commonly implicated are the serotonin (5-HT_{2c}) and histamine (H_1) receptors. All second-generation antipsychotics have some affinity for the 5-HT_{2c} receptor at clinical doses [48]. Mice with a knockout mutation of the 5-HT_{2c} receptor are obese, suggesting mechanism could contribute to obesity [49]. Wirshing and colleagues [50] demonstrated a logarithmic relationship between H_1 receptor affinity and weight gain. Animal data also have shown orexigenic effects stimulated by H_1 activation of hypothalamic AMP-kinase [51]. Other receptors implicated in weight control include the adrenergic α_{1A}, and 5-HT_6 receptors [52]. Receptor binding is one of many proposed mechanisms of weight gain. Prolactin elevation, changes in insulin sensitivity, and decreased activity caused by sedation are other possible explanations of weight gain [53].

Among the available second-generation antipsychotics clozapine and olanzapine are associated with the most significant degree of weight gain (4–4.5 kg over 10 weeks) [54]. In a prospective 5-year follow-up of 89 outpatients prescribed clozapine, Henderson and colleagues [55] reported a mean gain of 14 kg that did not plateau until the fourth year. Olanzapine treatment is associated with a mean gain in weight of approximately 6 to 7 kg within the first year of treatment [56]. Risperidone and quetiapine also contribute to weight gain, albeit to a lesser degree. Some drugs such as ziprasidone and aripiprazole have been associated with very little change in weight even in 1-year studies (1 kg) [47]. In the CATIE trial average weight changes in the 18 months ranged from −0.9 kg to more than 4 kg in the different drug groups, demonstrating the highly variable penetrance of this side effect among antipsychotics. Significant weight gain (> 7%) occurred in 30% of subjects taking olanzapine, 16% of subjects taking quetiapine subjects, 14% of subjects taking risperidone, 12% of subjects taking perphenazine, and 7% of subjects taking ziprasidone treatment [57].

The risk of weight gain may be more profound in the first episode and in younger patients than in the older and chronic populations. Zipursky and colleagues [58] reported that gains of more than 15 kg over 2 years were noted among subjects newly treated with olanzapine compared with gains of approximately 7 kg in those treated with haloperidol. With risperidone weight gains of 7.0 kg over 5 months [59] and of 8.6 kg over 6 months [60] have been reported. Weight gain of 4.1 kg has been reported during 8 weeks of quetiapine treatment in adolescents [61]. All these studies demonstrate significantly higher weight gain with a variety of antipsychotics in younger or first episode patients as compared to older adults.

Diabetes Mellitus

Diabetes mellitus is a metabolic disorder caused by a deficit of insulin secretion, insulin activity, or a combination of the two, resulting in a persistent hyperglycemic state. There are several types of diabetes; but 90% to 95% of all diagnosed cases are type 2 diabetes. Having diabetes confers a significant risk of developing CHD and often occurs with other CHD risk factors such as hyperlipidemia, obesity, or hypertension [62]. The risk of stroke and CHD is two to four times higher for people who have diabetes than for adults who do not have diabetes.

Diabetes is a worldwide epidemic. More than 20 million people in the United States and 246 million people worldwide have diabetes mellitus, and the incidence is expected to continue increasing. By the year 2025, it is predicted that 380 million people will have diabetes mellitus [63,64]. Because of the worldwide obesity crisis, the rising prevalence of diabetes is not surprising. The risk of diabetes increases dramatically with increasing body mass index [65,66], although abdominal obesity may be a better predictor of diabetes than the body mass index itself [43]. Even among individuals who are not obese, inactivity increases the risk of developing diabetes [67].

Cross-sectional studies have found the prevalence of diabetes in people who have schizophrenia to be two to three times higher than in the general population [68,69]. People who have schizophrenia tend to have many of the traditional risk factors for developing diabetes such as obesity and lack of exercise. The risk for developing diabetes may be related to the pathophysiology or genetic liability of schizophrenia itself. Even before treatment with antipsychotics, fasting glucose levels have been found to be significantly higher in people who have schizophrenia than in the general population [70,71]. Also, diabetes is more prevalent in family members of people who have schizophrenia than in the general population [68,72,73].

Second-generation antipsychotics also have been implicated in the development of diabetes. Although the studies are not unequivocal, most pharmacoepidemiologic evidence suggests that the highest rate of diabetes may occur with clozapine and olanzapine treatment [74–78]. Evidence with long-term clozapine use has suggested that it is associated with a 7% annual risk of new-onset diabetes [55]. Recent pharmacoepidemiologic studies also report an increased risk of diabetes with other antipsychotic agents such as risperidone and quetiapine [79–81].

Direct prospective comparative studies are difficult to undertake, and data are lacking because it may take years for a prediabetic person to show overt signs of diabetes and to manifest actual increases in fasting glucose level. To compensate for insulin resistance, the beta cells in the pancreas increase production of insulin. Data suggest that, after 7 to 10 years of hyperinsulinemia, secretion by the beta cells begins to fail, resulting in a cascade of factors resulting in diabetes [82]. During the CATIE trial, there were no significant differences in fasting serum glucose levels among antipsychotic treatments (olanzapine, 13.7 ± 2.5 mg/dL; quetiapine, 7.5 ± 2.5 mg/dL; risperidone, 6.6 ± 2.5 mg/dL; ziprasidone, 2.9 ± 3.4 mg/dL; perphenazine, 5.4 ± 2.8 mg/dL) [57], but the change in glycosylated hemoglobin was 4 to 10 times greater with olanzapine than with the other antipsychotic medications.

Hyperlipidemia

Hyperlipidemia is a risk factor for the development of CHD. Elevated total cholesterol and low-density lipoprotein (LDL) levels are strong independent risk factors for CHD [83]. Hypertriglyceridemia also contributes to a greater risk [84]. In fact, increased risk for heart disease begins at a total cholesterol level of 160 mg/dL, well below the average level in the United States. Hyperlipidemia is a frequently overlooked problem in patients who have schizophrenia. More than 85% of patients who have elevated lipids are untreated, representing a serious gap in management [24].

The primary lipid abnormality caused by antipsychotic agents is hypertriglyceremia, although other abnormalities, such as increases in total cholesterol and LDL levels along with decreases in high-density lipoproteins (HDL) levels, can occur [85]. The propensity for lipid involvement varies among antipsychotic agents. Increases in plasma lipid levels were noted with the phenothiazines (ie, chlorpromazine, thioridazine) [86–88], but negligible effects on lipids have occurred with the higher-potency agents such as haloperidol [89,90]. Early on, clozapine was noted to cause a profound increase in serum triglycerides as well as a small increase in total cholesterol levels. The dibenzodiazepines (clozapine, olanzapine, and quetiapine) are the second-generation antipsychotics most commonly associated with hyperlipidemia, although quetiapine causes less hypertriglyceremia than either clozapine or olanzapine [57,91,92]. Risperidone has a favorable lipid profile especially when compared with olanzapine [92,93]. The two newer antipsychotic agents ziprasidone and aripiprazole are associated with little-to-no change in serum lipids and actually are associated with a decrease in lipid levels during monotherapy [94,95]. A recent matched case-control study using California Medicaid data reported that people who have schizophrenia treated with most second-generation antipsychotic agents (except aripiprazole) have greater risk of hyperlipidemia during treatment than persons not treated with antipsychotic medication [96].

The underlying causes of hyperlipidemia are not well known, but elevated body mass index at baseline and weight gain during treatment are risk factors for associated elevations in lipids [41,97,98]. Some studies note that weight gain is not correlated to changes in serum triglycerides [99,100]. It has been proposed that hyperlipidemia results from an increase in insulin resistance from antipsychotic treatment [82]. Insulin resistance enhances lipolysis, increasing free fatty acids along with the production of triglycerides. The resulting changes in lipid metabolism may lead to the production of smaller, denser HDL particles that have an increased clearance through the kidney. This mechanism might explain why the low-potency antipsychotic agents, and dibenzodiazepines specifically, are associated with hypertriglyceremia [85].

Hypertension

Hypertension is a major contributor to cardiovascular diseases including CHD, stroke, renal disease, and heart failure [101]. Hypertension results in the relatively late-developing component of a cluster of pathologic changes that includes a decrease in vascular elasticity, obesity, abnormal lipid metabolism, insulin resistance, and renal disease [56]. Hypertension is defined as a systolic blood pressure greater than 140 mm Hg or a diastolic blood pressure greater than 90 mm HG. The risk of CHD, beginning at 115/75 mm Hg, doubles with each increment of 20/10 mm Hg [101]. From the baseline data in the CATIE trial approximately one third of all people who have schizophrenia are diagnosed as having hypertension, compared with less than 20% in the general population [8]. Currently, however, more than 60% of people who have schizophrenia and who have hypertension are not being treated [24].

Very few data support clinically important changes in blood pressure during clinical and observational trials of antipsychotic medications, but study follow-up may not be long enough to capture changes over the long term. One retrospective review of 82 patients found that patients treated with clozapine over 5 years (1987–1992) had a significant increase in systolic and diastolic blood pressure [102]. The same study reported that treatment with antihypertensive medications was started more frequently in patients taking clozapine (27%) than in patients taking first-generation antipsychotics (4%) or other second-generation antipsychotics (9%).

Metabolic Syndrome

The metabolic syndrome, historically referred to as "syndrome X," [103] is a cluster of symptoms that increases the risk of diabetes mellitus [104] and CHD [105]. The metabolic syndrome has been found to be an independent predictor of all-cause mortality [106]. Although each of the individual components may be a risk factor for cardiovascular morbidity and mortality, the existence of several of these abnormalities together poses a risk that may be synergistic. The criteria for the metabolic syndrome are listed in Table 1 [62,107].

In the United States, the metabolic syndrome is present in approximately 22% of the general population more than 20 years old [108]. In people who have schizophrenia the prevalence of the metabolic syndrome is approximately 30% to 60% [109–112]. Baseline data from the CATIE study reported that approximately 43% of the enrolled subjects met criteria for the metabolic syndrome. Both sexes had a significantly greater prevalence of the metabolic syndrome than age- and gender-matched controls [113].

The prevalence of the metabolic syndrome in people who have schizophrenia may be higher in the United States than in other countries, specifically in Europe.

Table 1
Criteria for the metabolic syndrome[a]

Risk Factor	Defining Level
Abdominal obesity (waist circumference)	
Men	> 102 cm (> 40 in)
Women	> 88 cm (> 35 in)
Triglycerides	≥ 150 mg/dL
High-density lipoprotein cholesterol	
Men	< 40 mg/dL
Women	< 50 mg/dL
Blood pressure	≥ 130/≥ 85 mm Hg
Fasting glucose[b]	≥ 100 mg/dL

[a]Three of the five criteria must be meet to meet the classification.
[b]The American Heart Association recommendation.
Data from: Grundy SM, Cleeman JI, Daniels SR, et al. Diagnosis and management of the metabolic syndrome: an American Heart Association/National Heart, Lung, and Blood Institute scientific statement. Circulation 2005;112(17):2735–52.
   Data from Expert Panel on Detection, Evaluation, and Treatment of High Blood Cholesterol in Adults. Executive summary of the third report of the National Cholesterol Education Program (NCEP) Expert Panel on Detection, Evaluation, and Treatment of High Blood Cholesterol in Adults (Adult Treatment Panel III). JAMA 2001;285(19):2486–97.

In Spain, a large collaborative study reported that the prevalence of the metabolic syndrome in 1452 outpatients who had schizophrenia was about 24% [114]. Unlike the CATIE study, however, this study based the definition of metabolic syndrome on a fasting glucose level of 110 mg/dL or higher, in accordance with the National Cholesterol Education Program (NCEP) guidelines, rather than 100 mg/dL or higher, per the American Heart Association guidelines [62,107], decreasing the reported prevalence. When the NCEP criteria were used to evaluate CATIE subjects, 40.9% met criteria for the metabolic syndrome. This prevalence is still greater than in European studies. Two small studies in Finland enrolling 31 [115] and 35 [116] subjects, respectively, reported the prevalence of the metabolic syndrome to be 19% and 37% in their respective populations, a two- to fourfold increase in metabolic syndrome compared with the prevalence in the general population. After considering baseline differences in the prevalence of metabolic syndrome in the general population and in persons who have schizophrenia in the United States and Europe, schizophrenia seems to confer an independent risk in the population studied. Few data exist, however, to determine the prevalence of the metabolic syndrome in the absence of antipsychotic medications. Nevertheless, the antipsychotic agents that cause the greatest weight gain and lipid changes probably would entail the greatest risk of the metabolic syndrome in people who have schizophrenia [117].

PHYSICAL HEALTH MONITORING AND INTERVENTIONS
Smoking Cessation
A combination of pharmacologic and behavioral interventions is recommended for the treatment of nicotine dependence [118]. Nicotine replacement therapy was

the first treatment approved in the United States for smoking cessation. Multiple studies have assessed the efficacy of nicotine replacement therapy for people who have schizophrenia [119–125]. Some success has been achieved in short-term trials, but long-term abstinent rates to date for people who have schizophrenia are very low. Reducing smoking behavior in the short term may increase the likelihood of long-term cessation, however [126]. Bupropion studies have shown some initial success, but sample sizes have been low. Seven-day abstinence rates have ranged from 36% to 50% and were significantly greater than with placebo [127,128]. Abstinence rates for longer-term data are available only for samples of fewer than 10 patients, however, and do not seem to be very great even with the addition of supportive therapy [126,129].

Varenicline is the newest agent approved by the Food and Drug Administration for smoking cessation. This agent is a partial agonist at the α4β2 nicotinic acetylcholine receptor [130]. It has demonstrated 4-week abstinence rates of almost 50%, compared with rates of 17% and 33% with placebo and bupropion, respectively [131]. Although no published work is currently available for patients who have schizophrenia, several studies are underway. This drug may represent a promising pharmacologic option for the large population of persons who have schizophrenia and who smoke.

Several attempts at quitting are commonly required before long-term abstinence from tobacco dependence is achieved [126]. Clinicians should make an effort to address the consequences of smoking and the benefits of smoking cessation. A social support system should be bolstered if the patient is willing to attempt stopping tobacco use. The patient and caregivers should be educated about nicotine withdrawal symptoms, such as irritability, that can mimic early signs and symptoms of illness relapse. People who have schizophrenia should be monitored closely for changes in symptoms. Also, because cigarette smoking changes the pharmacokinetics of medications metabolized by the P450 1A2 enzyme, dose changes may be needed, particularly for olanzapine or clozapine [132].

Weight Reduction

Treatment for obesity requires lifestyle and behavioral changes and may include possible pharmacologic interventions. A recent meta-analysis of behavioral interventions for weight loss for people who have schizophrenia found that more than 80% (19/23) reported weight loss [133]. The authors raised methodologic concerns for several studies and acknowledged that many of the studies had a high dropout rate. Five randomized, controlled trials have evaluated treatment as usual versus weight loss programs that educate patients about diet and exercise [134–138]. Three of the studies reported a significant difference between the intervention group and treatment as usual in terms of weight loss (mean difference between groups was 2.5–8 kg) [134,135,137]. The studies ranged from 12 to 16 weeks with dropout rates ranging from zero to 33%. Although it is unknown if the results from educational programs extend to patients in the real world or if the results would persist after the education concluded, education nonetheless is a valuable component in the rehabilitation of people who have schizophrenia, and clinicians should make an effort to talk to patients about their diet and daily activity. Patients should be encouraged to engage in exercise and make better food choices, including smaller portions and healthier selections.

Pharmacologic interventions have focused on switching patients to antipsychotic medications with less propensity for causing weight-gain and the adjunctive use of agents promoting weight loss. Because olanzapine and clozapine have the highest liability for weight gain, switching to agents with neutral weight and metabolic profiles has been efficacious and safe. The most data are available for ziprasidone and aripiprazole [139–141]. Switching from olanzapine to either quetiapine [142] or risperidone [143] also has shown metabolic benefits, including weight loss. Changing a patient who is stable while taking one antipsychotic to another antipsychotic may lead to a worsened clinical outcome, however [144]. Therefore the clinician should consider the advantages and disadvantages of switching medications and the timing of the switch, titrating the antipsychotics over at least a 2- to 4-week period.

Multiple adjunctive medications have been evaluated to treat weight gain associated with antipsychotic therapy, including sibutramine [145,146], topiramate [147,148], roboxetine [149,150], amantadine [151,152], metformin ([153,154], nizatidine [155–158], fluoxetine [159,160], and famotidine [161]. Most studies were small and of short duration. Thus, no current recommendations are available to guide adjunctive treatment for weight loss. Fluoxetine is not a good option, because two randomized, controlled trials failed to find any weight loss [159,160]. Orlistat is another pharmacologic option for weight loss; however, no data are available to support its efficacy in people who have schizophrenia. Another drug on the horizon is rimonabant, a cannabinoid CB1 antagonist. Phase III clinical trials have shown a 6- to 7-kg weight reduction over 1 year in overweight individuals in conjunction with a behavioral program [162,163]. Currently, rimonabant is not approved in the United States, but it may be marketed in late 2007 or early 2008. A concern of rimonabant is melancholic or depressive symptoms that can occur with blockade of the endocannabinoid system [164]. Since the results for rimonabant are similar to other medications marketed for weight loss [165], the risk to benefit ratio has not been determined for the public or for people with mental illness.

Diabetes

Guidelines for diabetes monitoring have been developed. Table 2 lists the recommendations from United States guidelines for patients who have schizophrenia. Baseline fasting glucose should be measured when a patient starts taking or switches antipsychotic medications. Follow-up fasting glucose levels should be drawn 3 to 4 months after treatment is initiated and at least annually thereafter. A recent addition to diabetes care has been the incorporation of the condition prediabetes. Prediabetes is defined as either an impaired fasting glucose level (fasting blood glucose level between 100 and 125 mg/dL) or an impaired glucose tolerance (a 2-hour plasma glucose level between 140 and 199 mg/dL).

Table 2
A comparison of United States guidelines for monitoring metabolic symptoms during antipsychotic therapy

Measure and Publishing Agency	Baseline	Maintenance
Bodyweight/height/body mass index		
APA[a]	X	Every visit for first 6 months; quarterly thereafter
ADA[b]	X	4, 8, 12 weeks; quarterly thereafter
Mt. Sinai	X	Every visit for first 6 months; at least quarterly thereafter
Waist circumference		
APA[a]	–	–
ADA[b]	X	Annually
Mt. Sinai[c]	X	Every visit for first 6 months; at least quarterly thereafter
Blood pressure		
APA[a]	X	As clinically indicated, particularly as doses are titrated
ADA[b]	X	12 weeks; then annually
Mt. Sinai[c]	–	–
Lipid panel		
APA[a]	X	At least every 5 years
ADA[b]	X	12 weeks; then every 5 years
Mt. Sinai[c]	X	At least every 2 years when LDL is normal; every 6 months when LDL is > 130 mg/dL
Fasting plasma glucose		
APA[a]	X	4 months after medication initiation or change; then yearly
ADA[b]	X	12 weeks after medication initiation or change; then yearly
Mt. Sinai[c]	X	For patients with risk factors for diabetes: 4 months after starting, then yearly

Abbreviations: ADA, American Diabetes Association; APA, American Psychiatric Association; LDL, low-density lipoproteins.

[a]American Psychiatric Association guidelines for the treatment of schizophrenia (2nd edition). *From:* Lehman AF, Lieberman JA, Dixon LB, et al. Practice guideline for the treatment of patients with schizophrenia, second edition. Am J Psychiatry 2004;161(2 Suppl):1–56.

[b]American Diabetes Association, American Psychiatric Association, American Association of Clinical Endocrinologists, North American Association for the Study of Obesity. Consensus development conference on antipsychotic drugs and obesity and diabetes. Diabetes Care 2004;27(2):596–601.

[c]Mount Sinai guidelines for schizophrenia. Marder SR, Essock SM, Miller AL, et al. Physical health monitoring of patients with schizophrenia. Am J Psychiatry 2004;161(8):1334–49.

From Buckley PF, Miller DD, Singer B, et al. Clinicians' recognition of the metabolic adverse effects of antipsychotic medications. Schizophr Res 2005;79(2–3):281–8.

Initial interventions for glycemic control in people who have diabetes generally include diet and exercise. Even in people who have an impaired fasting glucose level, diet and exercise modifications have prevented the progression to a full-blown diabetes presentation [166,167]. The American Diabetes Association has guidelines and recommendations for nutrition and physical activity that could be helpful for decreasing weight as well as improving glycemic control [168–170]. If lifestyle modifications do not reduce the glycosylated hemoglobin (HgA1c) level below 7% in 3 months, pharmacologic interventions are recommended. In people who are unlikely to make lifestyle modifications, pharmacologic treatment may be initiated earlier. Thus, people who have schizophrenia may more likely to comply with less stringent treatment goals than would be recommended for people without mental illness [169,170]. Current recommendations for tight control include an HgA1c level below 7.0%, blood pressure below 130/80 mm Hg, LDL level below 100 mg/dL, triglycerides level below 150 mg/dL, and HDL level above 40 mg/dL [171–174].

There have been reports of people recovering from new-onset diabetes after withdrawal of olanzapine and clozapine [175,176]. Switching patients to quetiapine, aripiprazole, ziprasidone, or risperidone may have positive effects on weight and glucose homeostasis, but few data are available for sequential use or the global clinical effects of switching antipsychotic medications. In addition, there are no specific guidelines or recommendations for pharmacologic treatment of glycemic control in patients who have schizophrenia. The greatest problem, however, lies in recognition of the problem, because people who have schizophrenia and diabetes seem to respond very well to fairly routine care [70].

Several pharmacologic options for diabetes treatment are available. Sulfonyureas (ie, glyburide, glipizide, and glimepiride) work by increasing endogenous insulin. Metformin acts by decreasing hepatic glucose production, decreasing glucose absorption, and increasing glucose uptake into skeletal muscle. The thiazolidinedione class (ie, rosiglitazone and pioglitazone) work by stimulating the peroxisome-proliferative insulin-activated receptor gamma receptor, which causes insulin-sensitizing effects on skeletal muscle and adipose tissue and inhibits hepatic gluconeogenesis. Repaglinide and nateglinide (the meglitinides) act similarly to sulfonylureas to stimulate pancreatic insulin secretion but differ from this class in their rapid onset and short duration of action in lowering postprandial glucose. Last, the alpha-glucosidase inhibitors (ie, acarbose, miglitol) act by inhibiting the action of alpha-glucosidase enzymes at the brush border of the intestine. The inhibition slows the breakdown of dietary oligosaccharides and disaccharides. The delayed digestion of carbohydrates decreases postprandial glucose concentrations [177].

Prevention of the cardiovascular consequences of diabetes also is recommended as part of the diabetes treatment. People who have diabetes should receive aspirin (unless contraindicated), should maintain good blood pressure control, and should try to quit smoking. The risk of developing kidney disease is high in people who have diabetes; thus routine use of angiotensin-converting enzyme inhibitors (ACEI) or angiotensin receptor blockers (ARB) reduces the incidence of renal complications [178,179]. 3-Hydroxy-3-methylglutaryl coenzyme A (HMG CoA) reductase inhibitors (statins) are recommended in people who have diabetes regardless of their baseline lipid values [180]. All patients diagnosed as having diabetes should have a comprehensive eye examination routinely, should have their urine screened for microalbumin levels at least annually, and should have routine foot care.

Hyperlipidemia

Treatments for hyperlipidemia specifically for patients who have schizophrenia have not been characterized extensively, but some recommendations have been created for lipid monitoring (see Table 2). Current treatments are guided by recommendations from the NCEP Adult Treatment Panel III (ATPIII) guidelines (Table 3) [62]. Patients who have elevated cholesterol and triglycerides but have no other cardiac risk factors often can be managed with lifestyle modifications, including diet and exercise. In patients who have schizophrenia, however, lifestyle changes are difficult without an educational program and support, so pharmacologic treatments often are initiated.

Omega-3 fatty acids have been found to be effective in an open-label clozapine study, reducing triglyceride levels by 22% in 4 weeks [181]. Another recent study reported that rosuvastatin was effective in reducing triglycerides, total cholesterol, LDL, and non-HDL cholesterol after 3 months in patients who had schizophrenia and who had severe dyslipidemia at baseline [182].

Table 3

Low-density lipoprotein (LDL) goals and cut points for therapeutic lifestyle changes and drug therapy for different risk categories

Risk Category	LDL Goal (mg/dL)	LDL Level at Which to Initiate Therapeutic Lifestyle Changes (mg/dL)	LDL Level at Which to Consider Drug Therapy (mg/dL)
CHD or CHD risk equivalents (10-year risk > 20%[a])	< 100 (optional: < 70 for very high risk patients)	≥ 100	≥ 100
Two or more risk factors[b] (10-year risk 10%–20%[a])	< 130 (optional: < 100)	≥ 130	≥ 130 (100–129: LDL-lowering drug optional)
Two or more risk factors (10-year risk < 10%)	< 130	≥ 130	≥ 160
0–1 risk factors	< 160	≥ 160	≥ 190 (160–189: LDL-lowering drug optional)

Abbreviation: CHD, coronary heart disease.

[a]Ten-year risk assessment calculated using Framingham scoring. Available at: http://www.nhlbi.nih.gov/about/framingham/riskabs.htm. Accessed March 15, 2007.

[b]Risk factors include cigarette smoking; hypertension (blood pressure ≥ 140/90 mm Hg or an antihypertensive medication); low high-density lipoprotein cholesterol (< 40 mm/dL; if ≥ 60 mm/dL remove a risk factor); family history of premature CHD (CHD in male first-degree relative aged < 55 years; CHD in female first-degree relative aged < 65 years); age (men ≥ 45 years, women ≥ 55 years).

Data from Executive summary of the third report of the National Cholesterol Education Program (NCEP) Expert Panel on Detection, Evaluation, and Treatment of High Blood Cholesterol in Adults (Adult Treatment Panel III). JAMA 2001;285(19):2486–2497, and Grundy SM, Cleeman JI, Merz CNB, et al. Implications of recent clinical trials for the National Cholesterol Education Program Adult Treatment Panel III guidelines. Circulation 2004;110(2):227–239.

Another recent study also found beneficial effects of statin therapy in patients who had schizophrenia, suggesting that statin use is an effective first-line treatment for hyperlipidemia in patients who have schizophrenia [183].

Hypertension

Dietary and exercise approaches often are effective for reducing blood pressure. Recommendations to patients should include increasing the intake of vegetables, fruits, and low-fat diary products in conjunction with lowering the intake of saturated fats, sweets, and sugar-containing beverages [184]. As mentioned previously, however, people who have schizophrenia often have less motivation for change, and behavioral modifications alone may not be effective. Current recommendations for treatment of hypertension follow the guidelines from the Joint National Committee on Prevention, Detection, Evaluation and Treatment of High Blood Pressure (Table 4) [101].

The selection of pharmacologic agents for treatment of hypertension should focus on the individual because several classes of antihypertensive medications are available. The appropriate treatment for hypertension often is related to comorbid medical conditions [185]. Some antihypertensive medications such as thiazide-type diuretics and beta-antagonists may contribute to changes in lipids and glucose [186,187]. Lipid-soluble beta-antagonists may cause depressive symptoms; therefore, patients who have schizophrenia and who have with pre-existing depressive symptoms should not be treated with these agents.

Monitoring Guidelines

In the last several years, many attempts have been made to develop specific guidelines for monitoring the physical health of people who have schizophrenia. These attempts acknowledge the dire importance of monitoring for and preventing weight gain and metabolic complications during treatment. In 2004, three sets of guidelines were published in the United States recommending monitoring parameters for physical health with a focus on metabolic-related parameters. These guidelines are the American Psychiatric Association practice guidelines for the treatment of schizophrenia (second edition) [188], the joint American Diabetes Association/American Psychiatric Association antipsychotic obesity and diabetes guidelines [189], and the Mount Sinai guidelines for schizophrenia (see Table 2) [190]. Other guidelines are available, such as those from the United Kingdom [191], Canada [192], and Australia [193]. There is considerable consensus in some areas in the published guidelines; however, areas of dissent include which patients should be monitored, the usefulness of the glucose tolerance test, and the point at which to consider switching medications [194]. Because of the inconsistencies among guidelines and absence of a clear indication as to which guidelines are ideal, it remains somewhat difficult for the practicing clinician to know how and when to monitor weight, cardiovascular function, and metabolic parameters and, more importantly, how to proceed in treatment. Furthermore, recent evidence suggests that, with the current guidelines, screening for glucose dysregulation does not detect diabetes sufficiently in people who have schizophrenia [111,195]. Nevertheless,

Table 4
Classification and management of blood pressure in adults 18 years and older

Blood Pressure Classification			Initial Drug Therapy		
	Systolic Blood Pressure (mm Hg[a])	Diastolic Blood Pressure (mm Hg[a])	Lifestyle Modification	Without Compelling Indications	With Compelling Indications[d]
Normal	< 120	and < 80	Encourage	-	-
Prehypertension	120–139	or 80–89	Yes	No antihypertensive drug indicated	Drug(s) for the compelling indications[b]
Stage 1 hypertension	140–159	or 90–99	Yes	TTD for most; may consider ACEI, ARB, β-blocker, CCB, or combination	Drug(s) for the compelling indications. Other antihypertensive drugs (diuretics, ACEI, ARB, β-blocker, CCB) as needed
Stage 2 hypertension	≥ 160	or ≥ 100	Yes	Two-drug combination for most (usually TTD and ACEI or ARB or β-blocker or CCB)[c]	Drug(s) for the compelling indications. Other antihypertensive drugs (diuretics, ACEI, ARB, β-blocker, CCB) as needed

Abbreviations: ACEI, angiotensin-converting enzyme inhibitor; ARB, angiotensin-receptor blocker; CCB, calcium channel blocker; TID< three times daily; TTD, thiazide-type diuretic.

[a] Treatment determined by highest blood-pressure classification.

[b] Treat patients who have chronic kidney disease to blood pressure goal of < 130/80 mm Hg.

[c] Initial combined therapy should be used cautiously in those at risk for orthostatic hypotension.

[d] Disease states with medication indications: chronic kidney disease (ACEI, ARB); diabetes (diuretic, β-blocker, ACEI, ARB, CCB); heart failure (diuretic, β-blocker, ACEI, ARB, CCB, aldosterone antagonist); high coronary disease risk (diuretic, β-blocker, ACEI, CCB); postmyocardial infarction (β-blocker, ACEI, aldosterone antagonist); recurrent stroke prevention (diuretic, ACEI).

From Chobanian AV, Bakris GL, Black HR, et al. The seventh report of the Joint National Committee on Prevention, Detection, Evaluation, and Treatment of High Blood Pressure: the JNC 7 report. JAMA 2003;289(19):2560–72; with permission.

clinicians should adopt a structured system for monitoring and recording data pertaining to their patients' physical health and should develop means of collaborating with other health care specialists as needed to facilitate appropriate comprehensive care promoting patients' physical and mental well being [194,196].

SUMMARY

Literature review shows that the association between mental and physical illness has been the objective of scientific studies since the beginning of the twentieth century. There is also no question that people who have schizophrenia have excessive rates of physical problems. Strategies to improve physical illness have not yet been sufficient, however, and it is entirely possible that long-term health outcomes related to the increased risk of CHD in people who have schizophrenia actually may merit more concern than in the past.

For a variety of reasons, physical and mental health care have remained fragmented, and physical health treatment often is overlooked in people who have schizophrenia. Indeed these patients may not have sufficient access to medical treatment. Also, as clinicians, psychiatrists may not be doing a sufficient job looking "below the neck" of their patients [197]. The good news, however, is that the disorders and risk factors discussed in this article are generally modifiable. Thus, psychiatrists have an opportunity as treatment providers to decrease the risk of morbidity and mortality in people who have schizophrenia by providing more comprehensive clinical care to their patients.

The optimal mode of medical health delivery in people who have schizophrenia is unclear. Integrated clinics have been created to improve communication between mental health and medical personnel [198]. Although beneficial results have been achieved without increasing costs, this model of service will not occur in routine settings in the near future. Regardless of the system of care, psychiatric clinicians often must assume a primary role for treating both mental and physical health of their patients. Assessing the quality of medical care that patients receive, arranging for preventive care and monitoring, and providing education and support for health and lifestyle decisions should be included in the routine care of patients who have schizophrenia. Collaboration and communication with other medical caregivers is an essential part of providing optimal care [56].

Thus, although treatment recommendations and monitoring parameters continue to develop, and optimal identification and treatment for CHD and metabolic risk factors are still far from ideal, attempts should be made to strive for greater wellness in patients whom psychiatrists treat to improve their long-term outcomes and increase their healthy lifespan. Metabolic and cardiac vulnerability is part of the schizophrenia syndrome. The standard of care in psychiatry should be holistic treatment of these patients.

References

[1] Carney CP, Jones L, Woolson RF. Medical comorbidity in women and men with schizophrenia: a population-based controlled study. J Gen Intern Med 2006;21(11):1133–7.

[2] Newman SC, Bland RC. Mortality in a cohort of patients with schizophrenia: a record linkage study. Can J Psychiatry 1991;36(4):239–45.

[3] Hennekens CH, Hennekens AR, Hollar D, et al. Schizophrenia and increased risks of cardiovascular disease. Am Heart J 2005;150(6):1115–21.

[4] Lambert TJ, Velakoulis D, Pantelis C. Medical comorbidity in schizophrenia. Med J Aust 2003;178(Suppl):S67–70.

[5] Allebeck P. Schizophrenia: a life-shortening disease. Schizophr Bull 1989;15(1):81–9.

[6] Allebeck P, Wistedt B. Mortality in schizophrenia. A ten-year follow-up based on the Stockholm County inpatient register. Arch Gen Psychiatry 1986;43(7):650–3.

[7] Black DW, Warrack G, Winokur G. Excess mortality among psychiatric patients. The Iowa Record-Linkage Study. JAMA 1985;253(1):58–61.

[8] Goff DC, Sullivan LM, McEvoy JP, et al. A comparison of ten-year cardiac risk estimates in schizophrenia patients from the CATIE study and matched controls. Schizophr Res 2005;80(1):45–53.

[9] Brown S, Birtwistle J, Roe L, et al. The unhealthy lifestyle of people with schizophrenia. Psychol Med 1999;29(3):697–701.

[10] Bachrach LL. What we know about homelessness among mentally ill persons: an analytical review and commentary. Hosp Community Psychiatry 1992;43(5):453–64.

[11] Lublin H, Eberhard J, Levander S. Current therapy issues and unmet clinical needs in the treatment of schizophrenia: a review of the new generation antipsychotics. Int Clin Psychopharmacol 2005;20(4):183–98.

[12] Samele C, Patel M, Boydell J, et al. Physical illness and lifestyle risk factors in people with their first presentation of psychosis. Soc Psychiatry Psychiatr Epidemiol 2007;42(2):117–24.

[13] McCreadie RG. Diet, smoking and cardiovascular risk in people with schizophrenia: descriptive study. Br J Psychiatry 2003;183:534–9.

[14] Elman I, Borsook D, Lukas SE. Food intake and reward mechanisms in patients with schizophrenia: implications for metabolic disturbances and treatment with second-generation antipsychotic agents. Neuropsychopharmacology 2006;31(10):2091–120.

[15] Dixon L. Dual diagnosis of substance abuse in schizophrenia: prevalence and impact on outcomes. Schizophr Res 1999;35(Suppl):S93–S100.

[16] Dickey B, Normand SL, Weiss RD, et al. Medical morbidity, mental illness, and substance use disorders. Psychiatr Serv 2002;53(7):861–7.

[17] Vanina Y, Podolskaya A, Sedky K, et al. Body weight changes associated with psychopharmacology. Psychiatr Serv 2002;53(7):842–7.

[18] Kilbourne AM, McCarthy JF, Welsh D, et al. Recognition of co-occurring medical conditions among patients with serious mental illness. J Nerv Ment Dis 2006;194(8):598–602.

[19] Folsom DP, McCahill M, Bartels SJ, et al. Medical comorbidity and receipt of medical care by older homeless people with schizophrenia or depression. Psychiatr Serv 2002;53(11):1456–60.

[20] Muck-Jorgensen P, Mors O, Mortensen PB, et al. The schizophrenic patient in the somatic hospital. Acta Psychiatr Scand Suppl 2000;(407):96–9.

[21] Newcomer JW, Nasrallah HA, Loebel AD. The Atypical Antipsychotic Therapy and Metabolic Issues National Survey: practice patterns and knowledge of psychiatrists. J Clin Psychopharmacol 2004;24(5 Suppl 1):S1–6.

[22] Buckley PF, Miller DD, Singer B, et al. Clinicians' recognition of the metabolic adverse effects of antipsychotic medications. Schizophr Res 2005;79(2–3):281–8.

[23] Mackin P, Watkinson HM, Young AH. Prevalence of obesity, glucose homeostasis disorders and metabolic syndrome in psychiatric patients taking typical or atypical antipsychotic drugs: a cross-sectional study. Diabetologia 2005;48(2):215–21.

[24] Nasrallah HA, Meyer JM, Goff DC, et al. Low rates of treatment for hypertension, dyslipidemia and diabetes in schizophrenia: data from the CATIE schizophrenia trial sample at baseline. Schizophr Res 2006;86(1–3):15–22.

[25] Weissman EM, Zhu CW, Schooler NR, et al. Lipid monitoring in patients with schizophrenia prescribed second-generation antipsychotics. J Clin Psychiatry 2006;67(9): 1323–6.

[26] Himelhoch S, Lehman A, Kreyenbuhl J, et al. Prevalence of chronic obstructive pulmonary disease among those with serious mental illness. Am J Psychiatry 2004;161(12):2317–9.

[27] Kreyenbuhl J, Dickerson FB, Medoff DR, et al. Extent and management of cardiovascular risk factors in patients with type 2 diabetes and serious mental illness. J Nerv Ment Dis 2006;194(6):404–10.

[28] de Leon J, Dadvand M, Canuso C, et al. Schizophrenia and smoking: an epidemiological survey in a state hospital. Am J Psychiatry 1995;152(3):453–5.

[29] de Leon J, Diaz FJ. A meta-analysis of worldwide studies demonstrates an association between schizophrenia and tobacco smoking behaviors. Schizophr Res 2005;76(2–3): 135–57.

[30] Olincy A, Harris JG, Johnson LL, et al. Proof-of-concept trial of an {alpha}7 nicotinic agonist in schizophrenia. Arch Gen Psychiatry 2006;63(6):630–8.

[31] Harris EC, Barraclough B. Excess mortality of mental disorder. Br J Psychiatry 1998;173: 11–53.

[32] Joukamaa M, Heliovaara M, Knekt P, et al. Mental disorders and cause-specific mortality. Br J Psychiatry 2001;179:498–502.

[33] Filik R, Sipos A, Kehoe PG, et al. The cardiovascular and respiratory health of people with schizophrenia. Acta Psychiatr Scand 2006;113(4):298–305.

[34] Hole DJ, Watt GCM, Davey-Smith G, et al. Impaired lung function and mortality risk in men and women: findings from the Renfrew and Paisley prospective population study. BMJ 1996;313(7059):711–5.

[35] Shopland DR. Tobacco use and its contribution to early cancer mortality with a special emphasis on cigarette smoking. Environ Health Perspect 1995;103(Suppl 8):131–42.

[36] Grinshpoon A, Barchana M, Ponizovsky A, et al. Cancer in schizophrenia: is the risk higher or lower? Schizophr Res 2005;73(2–3):333–41.

[37] Sokal J, Messias E, Dickerson FB, et al. Comorbidity of medical illnesses among adults with serious mental illness who are receiving community psychiatric services. J Nerv Ment Dis 2004;192(6):421–7.

[38] Hunninghake DB. Cardiovascular disease in chronic obstructive pulmonary disease. Proc Am Thorac Soc 2005;2(1):44–9.

[39] Critchley JA, Capewell S. Mortality risk reduction associated with smoking cessation in patients with coronary heart disease: a systematic review. JAMA 2003;290(1):86–97.

[40] Hedley AA, Ogden CL, Johnson CL, et al. Prevalence of overweight and obesity among US children, adolescents, and adults, 1999–2002. JAMA 2004;291(23):2847–50.

[41] Pi-Sunyer FX. The obesity epidemic: pathophysiology and consequences of obesity. Obes Res 2002;10(Suppl 2):97S–104S.

[42] Lapidus L, Bengtsson C, Larsson B, et al. Distribution of adipose tissue and risk of cardiovascular disease and death: a 12 year follow up of participants in the population study of women in Gothenburg, Sweden. Br Med J (Clin Res Ed) 1984;289(6454):1257–61.

[43] Ohlson LO, Larsson B, Svardsudd K, et al. The influence of body fat distribution on the incidence of diabetes mellitus. 13.5 years of follow-up of the participants in the study of men born in 1913. Diabetes 1985;34(10):1055–8.

[44] Calle EE, Thun MJ, Petrelli JM, et al. Body-mass index and mortality in a prospective cohort of U.S. adults. N Engl J Med 1999;341(15):1097–105.

[45] Flegal KM, Carroll MD, Ogden CL, et al. Prevalence and trends in obesity among US adults, 1999–2000. JAMA 2002;288(14):1723–7.

[46] Homel P, Casey D, Allison DB. Changes in body mass index for individuals with and without schizophrenia, 1987–1996. Schizophr Res 2002;55(3):277–84.

[47] Wirshing DA. Schizophrenia and obesity: impact of antipsychotic medications. J Clin Psychiatry 2004;65(Suppl 18):13–26.

[48] DeLeon A, Patel NC, Crismon ML. Aripiprazole: a comprehensive review of its pharmacology, clinical efficacy, and tolerability. Clin Ther 2004;26(5):649–66.

[49] Nonogaki K, Strack AM, Dallman MF, et al. Leptin-independent hyperphagia and type 2 diabetes in mice with a mutated serotonin 5-HT2C receptor gene. Nat Med 1998;4(10): 1152–6.

[50] Wirshing DA, Wirshing WC, Kysar L, et al. Novel antipsychotics: comparison of weight gain liabilities. J Clin Psychiatry 1999;60(6):358–63.

[51] Kim SF, Huang AS, Snowman AM, et al. Antipsychotic drug-induced weight gain mediated by histamine H1 receptor-linked activation of hypothalamic AMP-kinase. Proc Natl Acad Sci USA 2007;104(9):3456–9.

[52] Kroeze WK, Hufeisen SJ, Popadak BA, et al. H1-histamine receptor affinity predicts short-term weight gain for typical and atypical antipsychotic drugs. Neuropsychopharmacology 2003;28(3):519–26.

[53] Baptista T, Lacruz A, Meza T, et al. Antipsychotic drugs and obesity: is prolactin involved? Can J Psychiatry 2001;46(9):829–34.

[54] Allison DB, Mentore JL, Heo M, et al. Antipsychotic-induced weight gain: a comprehensive research synthesis. Am J Psychiatry 1999;156(11):1686–96.

[55] Henderson DC, Cagliero E, Gray C, et al. Clozapine, diabetes mellitus, weight gain, and lipid abnormalities: a five-year naturalistic study. Am J Psychiatry 2000;157(6):975–81.

[56] Goff DC, Cather C, Evins AE, et al. Medical morbidity and mortality in schizophrenia: guidelines for psychiatrists. J Clin Psychiatry 2005;66(2):183–94 [quiz: 147, 273–4].

[57] Lieberman JA, Stroup TS, McEvoy JP, et al. Effectiveness of antipsychotic drugs in patients with chronic schizophrenia. N Engl J Med 2005;353(12):1209–23.

[58] Zipursky RB, Gu H, Green AI, et al. Course and predictors of weight gain in people with first-episode psychosis treated with olanzapine or haloperidol. Br J Psychiatry 2005;187:537–43.

[59] Martin A, L'Ecuyer S. Triglyceride, cholesterol and weight changes among risperidone-treated youths. A retrospective study. Eur Child Adolesc Psychiatry 2002;11(3):129–33.

[60] Kelly DL, Conley RR, Love RC, et al. Weight gain in adolescents treated with risperidone and conventional antipsychotics over six months. J Child Adolesc Psychopharmacol 1998;8(3):151–9.

[61] Shaw JA, Lewis JE, Pascal S, et al. A study of quetiapine: efficacy and tolerability in psychotic adolescents. J Child Adolesc Psychopharmacol 2001;11(4):415–24.

[62] Executive Summary of the Third Report of the National Cholesterol Education Program (NCEP) Expert Panel on Detection, Evaluation, and Treatment of High Blood Cholesterol in Adults (Adult Treatment Panel III). JAMA 2001;285(19):2486–97.

[63] Centers for Disease Control and Prevention. National diabetes fact sheet: general information and national estimates on diabetes in the United States, 2005. Atlanta (GA): U.S. Department of Health and Human Services, Centers for Disease Control and Prevention; 2005. Available at: http://www.cdc.gov/diabetes/pubs/pdf/ndfs_2005.pdf.

[64] Mayor S. Diabetes affects nearly 6% of the world's adults. BMJ 2006;333(7580):1191.

[65] Chan JM, Rimm EB, Colditz GA, et al. Obesity, fat distribution, and weight gain as risk factors for clinical diabetes in men. Diabetes Care 1994;17(9):961–9.

[66] Colditz GA, Willett WC, Rotnitzky A, et al. Weight gain as a risk factor for clinical diabetes mellitus in women. Ann Intern Med 1995;122(7):481–6.

[67] Sullivan PW, Morrato EH, Ghushchyan V, et al. Obesity, inactivity, and the prevalence of diabetes and diabetes-related cardiovascular comorbidities in the U.S., 2000–2002. Diabetes Care 2005;28(7):1599–603.

[68] Lamberti JS, Crilly JF, Maharaj K, et al. Prevalence of diabetes mellitus among outpatients with severe mental disorders receiving atypical antipsychotic drugs. J Clin Psychiatry 2004;65(5):702–6.

[69] Susce MT, Villanueva N, Diaz FJ, et al. Obesity and associated complications in patients with severe mental illnesses: a cross-sectional survey. J Clin Psychiatry 2005;66(2): 167–73.

[70] Dixon L, Weiden P, Delahanty J, et al. Prevalence and correlates of diabetes in national schizophrenia samples. Schizophr Bull 2000;26(4):903–12.

[71] Ryan MC, Collins P, Thakore JH. Impaired fasting glucose tolerance in first-episode, drug-naive patients with schizophrenia. Am J Psychiatry 2003;160(2):284–9.

[72] Henderson DC, Cagliero E, Copeland PM, et al. Glucose metabolism in patients with schizophrenia treated with atypical antipsychotic agents: a frequently sampled intravenous glucose tolerance test and minimal model analysis. Arch Gen Psychiatry 2005;62(1):19–28.

[73] Arranz B, Rosel P, Ramirez N, et al. Insulin resistance and increased leptin concentrations in noncompliant schizophrenia patients but not in antipsychotic-naive first-episode schizophrenia patients. J Clin Psychiatry 2004;65(10):1335–42.

[74] Ramaswamy K, Masand PS, Nasrallah HA. Do certain atypical antipsychotics increase the risk of diabetes? A critical review of 17 pharmacoepidemiologic studies. Ann Clin Psychiatry 2006;18(3):183–94.

[75] Gianfrancesco F, White R, Wang RH, et al. Antipsychotic-induced type 2 diabetes: evidence from a large health plan database. J Clin Psychopharmacol 2003;23(4): 328–35.

[76] Caro JJ, Ward A, Levinton C, et al. The risk of diabetes during olanzapine use compared with risperidone use: a retrospective database analysis. J Clin Psychiatry 2002;63(12): 1135–9.

[77] Lambert BL, Chou CH, Chang KY, et al. Antipsychotic exposure and type 2 diabetes among patients with schizophrenia: a matched case-control study of California Medicaid claims. Pharmacoepidemiol Drug Saf 2005;14(6):417–25.

[78] Lambert MT, Copeland LA, Sampson N, et al. New-onset type-2 diabetes associated with atypical antipsychotic medications. Prog Neuropsychopharmacol Biol Psychiatry 2006;30(5):919–23.

[79] Lambert BL, Cunningham FE, Miller DR, et al. Diabetes risk associated with use of olanzapine, quetiapine, and risperidone in Veterans Health Administration patients with schizophrenia. Am J Epidemiol 2006;164(7):672–81.

[80] Guo JJ, Keck PE Jr, Corey-Lisle PK, et al. Risk of diabetes mellitus associated with atypical antipsychotic use among Medicaid patients with bipolar disorder: a nested case-control study. Pharmacotherapy 2007;27(1):27–35.

[81] Sacchetti E, Turrina C, Parrinello G, et al. Incidence of diabetes in a general practice population: a database cohort study on the relationship with haloperidol, olanzapine, risperidone or quetiapine exposure. Int Clin Psychopharmacol 2005;20(1):33–7.

[82] Newcomer JW. Second-generation (atypical) antipsychotics and metabolic effects: a comprehensive literature review. CNS Drugs 2005;19(Suppl 1):1–93.

[83] Stamler J, Wentworth D, Neaton JD. Is relationship between serum cholesterol and risk of premature death from coronary heart disease continuous and graded? Findings in 356,222 primary screenees of the Multiple Risk Factor Intervention Trial (MRFIT). JAMA 1986;256(20):2823–8.

[84] Austin MA, Hokanson JE, Edwards KL. Hypertriglyceridemia as a cardiovascular risk factor. Am J Cardiol 1998;81(4A):7B–12B.

[85] Meyer JM, Koro CE. The effects of antipsychotic therapy on serum lipids: a comprehensive review. Schizophr Res 2004;70(1):1–17.

[86] Clark ML, Johnson PC. Amenorrhea and elevated level of serum cholesterol produced by a trifluoromethylated phenothiazine (SKF 5354-A). J Clin Endocrinol Metab 1960;20: 641–6.

[87] Clark ML, Ray TS, Paredes A, et al. Chlorpromazine in women with chronic schizophrenia: the effect on cholesterol levels and cholesterol-behavior relationships. Psychosom Med 1967;29(6):634–42.

[88] Mefferd RB Jr, Labrosse EH, Gawienowski AM, et al. Influence of chlorpromazine on certain biochemical variables of chronic male schizophrenics. J Nerv Ment Dis 1958;127(2): 167–79.

[89] Vaisanen K, Rimon R, Raisanen P, et al. A controlled double-blind study of haloperidol versus thioridazine in the treatment of restless mentally subnormal patients. Serum levels and clinical effects. Acta Psychiatr Belg 1979;79(6):673–85.

[90] Shafique M, Khan IA, Akhtar MH, et al. Serum lipids and lipoproteins in schizophrenic patients receiving major tranquilizers. J Pak Med Assoc 1988;38(10):259–61.

[91] Atmaca M, Kuloglu M, Tezcan E, et al. Weight gain, serum leptin and triglyceride levels in patients with schizophrenia on antipsychotic treatment with quetiapine, olanzapine and haloperidol. Schizophr Res 2003;60(1):99–100.

[92] Atmaca M, Kuloglu M, Tezcan E, et al. Serum leptin and triglyceride levels in patients on treatment with atypical antipsychotics. J Clin Psychiatry 2003;64(5):598–604.

[93] Meyer JM. A retrospective comparison of weight, lipid, and glucose changes between risperidone- and olanzapine-treated inpatients: metabolic outcomes after 1 year. J Clin Psychiatry 2002;63(5):425–33.

[94] Weiden PJ, Daniel DG, Simpson G, et al. Improvement in indices of health status in outpatients with schizophrenia switched to ziprasidone. J Clin Psychopharmacol 2003;23(6): 595–600.

[95] Kingsbury SJ, Fayek M, Trufasiu D, et al. The apparent effects of ziprasidone on plasma lipids and glucose. J Clin Psychiatry 2001;62(5):347–9.

[96] Olfson M, Marcus SC, Corey-Lisle P, et al. Hyperlipidemia following treatment with antipsychotic medications. Am J Psychiatry 2006;163(10):1821–5.

[97] Itoh T, Horie S, Takahashi K, et al. An evaluation of various indices of body weight change and their relationship with coronary risk factors. Int J Obes Relat Metab Disord 1996;20(12):1089–96.

[98] Baptista T, Lacruz A, Angeles F, et al. Endocrine and metabolic abnormalities involved in obesity associated with typical antipsychotic drug administration. Pharmacopsychiatry 2001;34(6):223–31.

[99] Meyer JM. Effects of atypical antipsychotics on weight and serum lipid levels. J Clin Psychiatry 2001;62(Suppl 27):27–34 [discussion: 40–1].

[100] Meyer JM. Novel antipsychotics and severe hyperlipidemia. J Clin Psychopharmacol 2001;21(4):369–74.

[101] Chobanian AV, Bakris GL, Black HR, et al. The seventh report of The Joint National Committee on Prevention, Detection, Evaluation, and Treatment of High Blood Pressure: the JNC 7 report. JAMA 2003;289(19):2560–72.

[102] Henderson DC, Daley TB, Kunkel L, et al. Clozapine and hypertension: a chart review of 82 patients. J Clin Psychiatry 2004;65(5):686–9.

[103] Reaven GM. Banting lecture 1988. Role of insulin resistance in human disease. Diabetes 1988;37(12):1595–607.

[104] Haffner SM, Valdez RA, Hazuda HP, et al. Prospective analysis of the insulin-resistance syndrome (syndrome X). Diabetes 1992;41(6):715–22.

[105] Isomaa B, Almgren P, Tuomi T, et al. Cardiovascular morbidity and mortality associated with the metabolic syndrome. Diabetes Care 2001;24(4):683–9.

[106] Trevisan M, Liu J, Bahsas FB, et al. Syndrome X and mortality: a population-based study. Risk Factor and Life Expectancy Research Group. Am J Epidemiol 1998;148(10):958–66.

[107] Grundy SM, Cleeman JI, Daniels SR, et al. Diagnosis and management of the metabolic syndrome: an American heart association/national heart, lung, and blood institute scientific statement. Circulation 2005;112(17):2735–52.

[108] Ford ES, Giles WH, Dietz WH. Prevalence of the metabolic syndrome among US adults: findings from the third National Health and Nutrition Examination Survey. JAMA 2002;287(3):356–9.

[109] Kato MM, Currier MB, Gomez CM, et al. Prevalence of metabolic syndrome in Hispanic and non-Hispanic patients with schizophrenia. Prim Care Companion J Clin Psychiatry 2004;6(2):74–7.

[110] Correll CU, Frederickson AM, Kane JM, et al. Metabolic syndrome and the risk of coronary heart disease in 367 patients treated with second-generation antipsychotic drugs. J Clin Psychiatry 2006;67(4):575–83.

[111] De Hert MA, van Winkel R, Van Eyck D, et al. Prevalence of the metabolic syndrome in patients with schizophrenia treated with antipsychotic medication. Schizophr Res 2006;83(1):87–93.

[112] Meyer J, Loh C, Leckband SG, et al. Prevalence of the metabolic syndrome in veterans with schizophrenia. J Psychiatr Pract 2006;12(1):5–10.

[113] McEvoy JP, Meyer JM, Goff DC, et al. Prevalence of the metabolic syndrome in patients with schizophrenia: baseline results from the Clinical Antipsychotic Trials of Intervention Effectiveness (CATIE) schizophrenia trial and comparison with national estimates from NHANES III. Schizophr Res 2005;80(1):19–32.

[114] Bobes J, Arango C, Aranda P, et al. Cardiovascular and metabolic risk in outpatients with schizophrenia treated with antipsychotics: results of the CLAMORS study. Schizophr Res 2007;90(1–3):162–73.

[115] Saari KM, Lindeman SM, Viilo KM, et al. A 4-fold risk of metabolic syndrome in patients with schizophrenia: the Northern Finland 1966 Birth Cohort study. J Clin Psychiatry 2005;66(5):559–63.

[116] Heiskanen T, Niskanen L, Lyytikainen R, et al. Metabolic syndrome in patients with schizophrenia. J Clin Psychiatry 2003;64(5):575–9.

[117] Newcomer JW. Metabolic considerations in the use of antipsychotic medications: a review of recent evidence. J Clin Psychiatry 2007;68(Suppl 1):20–7.

[118] Fiore MC, Hatsukami DK, Baker TB. Effective tobacco dependence treatment. JAMA 2002;288(14):1768–71.

[119] Dalack GW, Meador-Woodruff JH. Acute feasibility and safety of a smoking reduction strategy for smokers with schizophrenia. Nicotine Tob Res 1999;1(1):53–7.

[120] George TP, Ziedonis DM, Feingold A, et al. Nicotine transdermal patch and atypical antipsychotic medications for smoking cessation in schizophrenia. Am J Psychiatry 2000;157(11):1835–42.

[121] Tidey JW, O'Neill SC, Higgins ST. Contingent monetary reinforcement of smoking reductions, with and without transdermal nicotine, in outpatients with schizophrenia. Exp Clin Psychopharmacol 2002;10(3):241–7.

[122] Chou KR, Chen R, Lee JF, et al. The effectiveness of nicotine-patch therapy for smoking cessation in patients with schizophrenia. Int J Nurs Stud 2004;41(3):321–30.

[123] Hartman N, Leong GB, Glynn SM, et al. Transdermal nicotine and smoking behavior in psychiatric patients. Am J Psychiatry 1991;148(3):374–5.

[124] Addington J, el-Guebaly N, Campbell W, et al. Smoking cessation treatment for patients with schizophrenia. Am J Psychiatry 1998;155(7):974–6.

[125] Ziedonis DM, George TP. Schizophrenia and nicotine use: report of a pilot smoking cessation program and review of neurobiological and clinical issues. Schizophr Bull 1997;23(2):247–54.

[126] Evins AE, Cather C, Rigotti NA, et al. Two-year follow-up of a smoking cessation trial in patients with schizophrenia: increased rates of smoking cessation and reduction. J Clin Psychiatry 2004;65(3):307–11 [quiz: 452–3].

[127] George TP, Vessicchio JC, Termine A, et al. A placebo controlled trial of bupropion for smoking cessation in schizophrenia. Biol Psychiatry 2002;52(1):53–61.

[128] Evins AE, Cather C, Deckersbach T, et al. A double-blind placebo-controlled trial of bupropion sustained-release for smoking cessation in schizophrenia. J Clin Psychopharmacol 2005;25(3):218–25.

[129] Weiner E, Ball MP, Summerfelt A, et al. Effects of sustained-release bupropion and supportive group therapy on cigarette consumption in patients with schizophrenia. Am J Psychiatry 2001;158(4):635–7.

[130] Reus VI, Obach RS, Coe JW, et al. Varenicline: new treatment with efficacy in smoking cessation. Drugs Today (Barc) 2007;43(2):65–75.

[131] Nides M, Oncken C, Gonzales D, et al. Smoking cessation with varenicline, a selective {alpha}4beta2 nicotinic receptor partial agonist: results from a 7-week, randomized, placebo- and bupropion-controlled trial with 1-year follow-up. Arch Intern Med 2006;166(15):1561–8.

[132] Kroon LA. Drug interactions and smoking: raising awareness for acute and critical care providers. Crit Care Nurs Clin North Am 2006;18(1):53–62, xii.

[133] Loh C, Meyer JM, Leckband SG. A comprehensive review of behavioral interventions for weight management in schizophrenia. Ann Clin Psychiatry 2006;18(1): 23–31.

[134] Kwon JS, Choi JS, Bahk WM, et al. Weight management program for treatment-emergent weight gain in olanzapine-treated patients with schizophrenia or schizoaffective disorder: a 12-week randomized controlled clinical trial. J Clin Psychiatry 2006;67(4):547–53.

[135] Littrell KH, Hilligoss NM, Kirshner CD, et al. The effects of an educational intervention on antipsychotic-induced weight gain. J Nurs Scholarsh 2003;35(3):237–41.

[136] Brar JS, Ganguli R, Pandina G, et al. Effects of behavioral therapy on weight loss in overweight and obese patients with schizophrenia or schizoaffective disorder. J Clin Psychiatry 2005;66(2):205–12.

[137] Evans S, Newton R, Higgins S. Nutritional intervention to prevent weight gain in patients commenced on olanzapine: a randomized controlled trial. Aust N Z J Psychiatry 2005;39(6):479–86.

[138] Weber M, Wyne K. A cognitive/behavioral group intervention for weight loss in patients treated with atypical antipsychotics. Schizophr Res 2006;83(1):95–101.

[139] Daniel DG, Zimbroff DL, Potkin SG, et al. Ziprasidone 80 mg/day and 160 mg/day in the acute exacerbation of schizophrenia and schizoaffective disorder: a 6-week placebo-controlled trial. Ziprasidone Study Group. Neuropsychopharmacology 1999;20(5): 491–505.

[140] Keck P Jr, Buffenstein A, Ferguson J, et al. Ziprasidone 40 and 120 mg/day in the acute exacerbation of schizophrenia and schizoaffective disorder: a 4-week placebo-controlled trial. Psychopharmacology (Berl) 1998;140(2):173–84.

[141] Hirsch SR, Kissling W, Bauml J, et al. A 28-week comparison of ziprasidone and haloperidol in outpatients with stable schizophrenia. J Clin Psychiatry 2002;63(6):516–23.

[142] Gupta S, Masand PS, Virk S, et al. Weight decline in patients switching from olanzapine to quetiapine. Schizophr Res 2004;70(1):57–62.

[143] Meyer JM, Pandina G, Bossie CA, et al. Effects of switching from olanzapine to risperidone on the prevalence of the metabolic syndrome in overweight or obese patients with schizophrenia or schizoaffective disorder: analysis of a multicenter, rater-blinded, open-label study. Clin Ther 2005;27(12):1930–41.

[144] Essock SM, Covell NH, Davis SM, et al. Effectiveness of switching antipsychotic medications. Am J Psychiatry 2006;163(12):2090–5.

[145] Henderson DC, Copeland PM, Daley TB, et al. A double-blind, placebo-controlled trial of sibutramine for olanzapine-associated weight gain. Am J Psychiatry 2005;162(5): 954–62.

[146] Henderson DC, Fan X, Copeland PM, et al. A double-blind, placebo-controlled trial of sibutramine for clozapine-associated weight gain. Acta Psychiatr Scand 2007;115(2): 101–5.

[147] Kim JH, Yim SJ, Nam JH. A 12-week, randomized, open-label, parallel-group trial of top-iramate in limiting weight gain during olanzapine treatment in patients with schizophrenia. Schizophr Res 2006;82(1):115–7.

[148] Ko YH, Joe SH, Jung IK, et al. Topiramate as an adjuvant treatment with atypical antipsychotics in schizophrenic patients experiencing weight gain. Clin Neuropharmacol 2005;28(4):169–75.

[149] Poyurovsky M, Fuchs C, Pashinian A, et al. Attenuating effect of reboxetine on appetite and weight gain in olanzapine-treated schizophrenia patients: a double-blind placebo-controlled study. Psychopharmacology (Berl) 2007.

[150] Poyurovsky M, Isaacs I, Fuchs C, et al. Attenuating effect of reboxetine on appetitie and weight gain in olanzapine-treated schizophrenia patients: a double-blind, placebo-controlled study. Psychopharmacology 2007;192(3):441–8.

[151] Deberdt W, Winokur A, Cavazzoni PA, et al. Amantadine for weight gain associated with olanzapine treatment. Eur Neuropsychopharmacol 2005;15(1):13–21.

[152] Graham KA, Gu H, Lieberman JA, et al. Double-blind, placebo-controlled investigation of amantadine for weight loss in subjects who gained weight with olanzapine. Am J Psychiatry 2005;162(9):1744–6.

[153] Klein DJ, Cottingham EM, Sorter M, et al. A randomized, double-blind, placebo-controlled trial of metformin treatment of weight gain associated with initiation of atypical antipsychotic therapy in children and adolescents. Am J Psychiatry 2006;163(12):2072–9.

[154] Baptista T, Martinez J, Lacruz A, et al. Metformin for prevention of weight gain and insulin resistance with olanzapine: a double-blind placebo-controlled trial. Can J Psychiatry 2006;51(3):192–6.

[155] Cavazzoni P, Tanaka Y, Roychowdhury SM, et al. Nizatidine for prevention of weight gain with olanzapine: a double-blind placebo-controlled trial. Eur Neuropsychopharmacol 2003;13(2):81–5.

[156] Assuncao SS, Ruschel SI, Rosa Lde C, et al. Weight gain management in patients with schizophrenia during treatment with olanzapine in association with nizatidine. Rev Bras Psiquiatr 2006;28(4):270–6.

[157] Atmaca M, Kuloglu M, Tezcan E, et al. Nizatidine treatment and its relationship with leptin levels in patients with olanzapine-induced weight gain. Hum Psychopharmacol 2003;18(6):457–61.

[158] Atmaca M, Kuloglu M, Tezcan E, et al. Nizatidine for the treatment of patients with quetiapine-induced weight gain. Hum Psychopharmacol 2004;19(1):37–40.

[159] Poyurovsky M, Pashinian A, Gil-Ad I, et al. Olanzapine-induced weight gain in patients with first-episode schizophrenia: a double-blind, placebo-controlled study of fluoxetine addition. Am J Psychiatry 2002;159(6):1058–60.

[160] Bustillo JR, Lauriello J, Parker K, et al. Treatment of weight gain with fluoxetine in olanzapine-treated schizophrenic outpatients. Neuropsychopharmacology 2003;28(3):527–9.

[161] Poyurovsky M, Tal V, Maayan R, et al. The effect of famotidine addition on olanzapine-induced weight gain in first-episode schizophrenia patients: a double-blind placebo-controlled pilot study. Eur Neuropsychopharmacol 2004;14(4):332–6.

[162] Van Gaal LF, Rissanen AM, Scheen AJ, et al. Effects of the cannabinoid-1 receptor blocker rimonabant on weight reduction and cardiovascular risk factors in overweight patients: 1-year experience from the RIO-Europe study. Lancet 2005;365(9468):1389–97.

[163] Pi-Sunyer FX, Aronne LJ, Heshmati HM, et al. Effect of rimonabant, a cannabinoid-1 receptor blocker, on weight and cardiometabolic risk factors in overweight or obese patients: RIO-North America: a randomized controlled trial. JAMA 2006;295(7):761–75.

[164] Hill MN, Gorzalka BB. Is there a role for the endocannabinoid system in the etiology and treatment of melancholic depression? Behav Pharmacol 2005;16(5–6):333–52.

[165] Gadde KM, Allison DB. Cannabinoid-1 receptor antagonist, rimonabant, for management of obesity and related risks. Circulation 2006;114(9):974–84.

[166] Tuomilehto J, Lindstrom J, Eriksson JG, et al. Prevention of type 2 diabetes mellitus by changes in lifestyle among subjects with impaired glucose tolerance. N Engl J Med 2001;344(18):1343–50.

[167] Knowler WC, Barrett-Connor E, Fowler SE, et al. Reduction in the incidence of type 2 diabetes with lifestyle intervention or metformin. N Engl J Med 2002;346(6):393–403.

[168] Franz MJ, Bantle JP, Beebe CA, et al. Evidence-based nutrition principles and recommendations for the treatment and prevention of diabetes and related complications. Diabetes Care 2003;26(Suppl 1):S51–61.

[169] Standards of medical care for patients with diabetes mellitus. Diabetes Care 2003;26(90001):S33–50.

[170] Standards of medical care in diabetes. Diabetes Care 2005;28(Suppl 1):S4–S36.

[171] Effect of intensive blood-glucose control with metformin on complications in overweight patients with type 2 diabetes (UKPDS 34). UK Prospective Diabetes Study (UKPDS) Group. Lancet 1998;352(9131):854–65.

[172] Intensive blood-glucose control with sulphonylureas or insulin compared with conventional treatment and risk of complications in patients with type 2 diabetes (UKPDS 33). UK Prospective Diabetes Study (UKPDS) Group. Lancet 1998;352(9131):837–53.

[173] Costa J, Borges M, David C, et al. Efficacy of lipid lowering drug treatment for diabetic and non-diabetic patients: meta-analysis of randomised controlled trials. BMJ 2006;332(7550):1115–24.

[174] Tight blood pressure control and risk of macrovascular and microvascular complications in type 2 diabetes: UKPDS 38. UK Prospective Diabetes Study Group. BMJ 1998;317(7160):703–13.

[175] Melkersson K, Hulting A-L. Recovery from new-onset diabetes in a schizophrenic man after withdrawal of Olanzapine. Psychosomatics 2002;43(1):67–70.

[176] Rigalleau V, Gatta B, Bonnaud S, et al. Diabetes as a result of atypical anti-psychotic drugs—a report of three cases. Diabet Med 2000;17(6):484–6.

[177] Standards of medical care in diabetes-2007. Diabetes Care 2007;30(Suppl 1):S4–S41.

[178] Snow V, Aronson MD, Hornbake ER, et al. The Clinical Efficacy Assessment Subcommittee of the American College of Pysicians. lipid control in the management of type 2 diabetes mellitus: a clinical practice guideline from the American College of Physicians. Ann Intern Med 2004;140(8):644–9.

[179] Arauz-Pacheco C, Parrott MA, Raskin P. Hypertension management in adults with diabetes. Diabetes Care 2004;27(Suppl 1):S65–7.

[180] Hayward RA, Hofer TP, Vijan S. Narrative review: lack of evidence for recommended low-density lipoprotein treatment targets: a solvable problem. Ann Intern Med 2006;145(7):520–30.

[181] Caniato RN, Alvarenga ME, Garcia-Alcaraz MA. Effect of omega-3 fatty acids on the lipid profile of patients taking clozapine. Aust N Z J Psychiatry 2006;40(8):691–7.

[182] De Hert M, Kalnicka D, van Winkel R, et al. Treatment with rosuvastatin for severe dyslipidemia in patients with schizophrenia and schizoaffective disorder. J Clin Psychiatry 2006;67(12):1889–96.

[183] Hanssens L, De Hert M, Kalnicka D, et al. Pharmacological treatment of severe dyslipidaemia in patients with schizophrenia. Int Clin Psychopharmacol 2007;22(1):43–9.

[184] Appel LJ, Moore TJ, Obarzanek E, et al. A clinical trial of the effects of dietary patterns on blood pressure. DASH Collaborative Research Group. N Engl J Med 1997;336(16):1117–24.

[185] Chobanian AV, Bakris GL, Black HR, et al. Seventh report of the Joint National Committee on Prevention, Detection, Evaluation, and Treatment of High Blood Pressure. Hypertension 2003;42(6):1206–52.

[186] Barzilay JI, Davis BR, Cutler JA, et al. Fasting glucose levels and incident diabetes mellitus in older nondiabetic adults randomized to receive 3 different classes of antihypertensive

treatment: a report from the Antihypertensive and Lipid-Lowering Treatment to Prevent Heart Attack Trial (ALLHAT). Arch Intern Med 2006;166(20):2191–201.

[187] Baymiller SP, Ball P, McMahon RP, et al. Serum glucose and lipid changes during the course of clozapine treatment: the effect of concurrent beta-adrenergic antagonist treatment. Schizophr Res 2003;59(1):49–57.

[188] Lehman AF, Lieberman JA, Dixon LB, et al. Practice guideline for the treatment of patients with schizophrenia. 2nd edition. Am J Psychiatry 2004;161(2 Suppl):1–56.

[189] Consensus Development Conference on Antipsychotic Drugs and Obesity and Diabetes. Diabetes Care 2004;27(2):596–601.

[190] Marder SR, Essock SM, Miller AL, et al. Physical health monitoring of patients with schizophrenia. Am J Psychiatry 2004;161(8):1334–49.

[191] Schizophrenia and diabetes 2003: expert consensus meeting, Dublin, 3-4 October 2003: consensus summary. Br J Psychiatry Suppl 2004;47:S112–4.

[192] Woo V, Harris S, Houlden R. Canadian Diabetes Association position paper: antipsychotic medications and associated risks of weight gain and diabetes. Canadian Journal of Diabetes 2005;29(2):111–2.

[193] Lambert TJ, Chapman LH. Diabetes, psychotic disorders and antipsychotic therapy: a consensus statement. Med J Aust 2004;181(10):544–8.

[194] Cohn TA, Sernyak MJ. Metabolic monitoring for patients treated with antipsychotic medications. Can J Psychiatry 2006;51(8):492–501.

[195] van Winkel R, De Hert M, Van Eyck D, et al. Screening for diabetes and other metabolic abnormalities in patients with schizophrenia and schizoaffective disorder: evaluation of incidence and screening methods. J Clin Psychiatry 2006;67(10):1493–500.

[196] Citrome L, Yeomans D. Do guidelines for severe mental illness promote physical health and well-being? J Psychopharmacol 2005;19(6 Suppl):102–9.

[197] Leucht S, Fountoulakis K. Improvement of the physical health of people with mental illness. Curr Opin Psychiatry 2006;19(4):411–2.

[198] Druss BG, Rohrbaugh RM, Levinson CM, et al. Integrated medical care for patients with serious psychiatric illness: a randomized trial. Arch Gen Psychiatry 2001;58(9):861–8.

Understanding and Treating "First-Episode" Schizophrenia

Peter J. Weiden, MD[a],*, Peter F. Buckley, MD[b],
Michael Grody, MD[c]

[a]Department of Psychiatry, University of Illinois Medical Center, Chicago, IL
[b]Department of Psychiatry, Medical College of Georgia, Augusta, GA
[c]The Zucker Hillside Hospital, North Shore-Long Island Jewish Health System, Glen Oaks, NY

"First-episode schizophrenia" is a clinical and research term that often is used to emphasize the special issues that arise when working with this patient population. Although the incidence rate of first-episode schizophrenia makes this population a relatively small percentage of a usual clinical caseload, it is a critically important time for the future of the course of the illness. The hope is that proper management during this critical period can influence favorably the long-term trajectory of illness and outcome for the individual patient. A growing body of evidence suggests that certain approaches and interventions are more helpful than others. The notion that schizophrenia has an inexorable downhill course or is a deteriorating illness is being challenged by more sophisticated understanding of what happens before the initial episode and new understanding of the complex interactions between predisposing genetic or biologic vulnerabilities and exposure to specific environmental risk factors during adolescence and early adulthood. One premise of this review is that proper understanding and treatment interventions during the early phases of the illness can make an enormous difference in the eventual long-term outcome. But, the concepts and definitions regarding "first-episode" are often murky, and treatment services can easily miss some of the treatment opportunities discussed below.

WHAT IS MEANT BY FIRST-EPISODE SCHIZOPHRENIA?

"First-episode" is a clinical term referring to a patient who has only recently formally presented, been evaluated, and been treated for schizophrenia within the treatment services of mental health system. At some point during this initial treatment, the person has been evaluated and received a diagnosis of probable or definite schizophrenia. A related term, "first-episode psychosis" is sometimes used to identify a person recently identified as acutely psychotic but for whom a formal diagnosis has not yet been established. In this instance, the presumption

*Corresponding author. E-mail address: pweiden@psych.uic.edu (P.J. Weiden).

0193-953X/07/$ – see front matter
doi:10.1016/j.psc.2007.04.010
© 2007 Elsevier Inc. All rights reserved.
psych.theclinics.com

is that the individual probably will receive a diagnosis in which psychosis is a common presenting sign—affective disorder, schizophrenia, or substance abuse. This distinction is more than merely semantic, because the term "first-episode schizophrenia" pertains only to the subgroup of individuals who have psychotic symptoms at initial diagnosis and who eventually are diagnosed as having schizophrenia. Given that the clinical presentation of a first episode of acute psychosis eventually will include other diagnoses, the reader needs to keep in mind the difference and the retrospective nature of matching the course of illness before diagnosis with the eventual course and outcome once the diagnosis is made. To clarify these issues, some of the terms and concepts pertaining to first-episode schizophrenia are shown in Table 1.

This article focuses on the group of individuals who, after presenting with psychotic symptoms, go on to receive a probable or definite diagnosis of schizophrenia. Given that the diagnosis has been made, the article then retrospectively considers three broad phases of the illness trajectory for such a patient:

1. The period in adolescence or adulthood between the first signal of a possible problem and the time the person is first seen for acute treatment of what later is diagnosed as schizophrenia
2. The initial treatment episode when the person is first evaluated, almost always in the setting of a clinical crisis when there are prominent psychosis symptoms
3. The period after the diagnosis of "first-episode schizophrenia" is made, when the patient is embarking on an initial period of treatment after stabilization

These three phases may not have clear boundaries and may overlap. Nonetheless, they represent distinct theoretical and practical divisions in understanding and treating the first-episode schizophrenia patient.

These phases also are translatable into certain transitions that are part of the illness trajectory (Fig. 1):

The transition from no identifiable symptom to the retrospectively identified onset of some sign, symptom, or behavioral abnormality that later is viewed as the initial phases of schizophrenia (the start of the prodromal period)
The transition from nonpsychotic prodromal symptoms to retrospectively identified psychotic symptoms that fulfill the necessary diagnostic criteria for the diagnosis of schizophrenia
The transition from living in the community with disturbances that are not formally evaluated or treated within a mental health care system to having had an initial treatment episode and formal mental health evaluation
The transition from being treated for an acute psychotic episode to being stabilized and receiving a psychiatric diagnosis consistent with schizophrenia that includes discussion of vulnerability of recurrence and a recommendation of ongoing antipsychotic treatment

Although not every first-episode patient goes through these exact transitions, the person, at the very least, makes a transition from not having been formally treated in a mental health care system to being identified as a patient who has

Table 1
Terms commonly used in the literature discussing first-episode schizophrenia

Term	Definition	Comments and Issues
First-episode schizophrenia	No consensus definition, but most studies anchor the definition to treatment exposure, either by time since diagnosis was made or duration of antipsychotic treatment. Note that the anchoring of the time point is based on the time of clinical presentation that triggered a formal diagnostic evaluation.	Perhaps more accurate to consider as "first-presentation" because the definition is anchored to the relatively brief time since initial treatment (medication) exposure rather than other specific disease markers over and above standard diagnostic criteria for schizophrenia and related psychotic disorders
Precursor signs and symptoms	Signs and symptoms from a diagnostic cluster that are observed to precede the disorder but are not specific and do not predict future diagnosis with certainty	Most of the nonpsychotic signs and symptoms occurring during prodromal period are nonspecific and are common signs of other disorders such as depression or substance abuse
Prodrome (or "prodromal period")	Period before meeting the full-blown criteria of disorder (schizophrenia), when some signs and symptoms are nevertheless present	Can be defined only retrospectively, after a diagnosis of schizophrenia is made and confirmed. In other words, initial prodromal symptoms are not specific to an eventual schizophrenia diagnosis.
Duration of untreated psychosis (also known as "DUP")	Time from first discernable psychotic symptom to the first point of treatment for a possible diagnosis of schizophrenia	Psychotic symptoms usually occur only after other nonpsychotic symptoms have been present for some time. Also, there may be challenges in accurately dating onset of first psychotic symptom.

a psychotic disorder of probable or definite schizophrenia. This definition is in keeping with much of the literature addressing the epidemiologic risk factors, initial presentation, and initial course of treatment after the diagnosis of schizophrenia is established. This article therefore does not address evaluation or treatment issues pertaining to patients who are considered at high risk for schizophrenia but

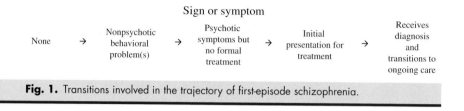

Sign or symptom

Fig. 1. Transitions involved in the trajectory of first-episode schizophrenia.

who do not meet diagnostic criteria for schizophrenia or to persons presenting with first-episode psychotic symptoms who receive another psychiatric diagnosis.

ENVIRONMENTAL RISK FACTORS DURING ADOLESCENCE AND YOUNG ADULTHOOD

The epidemiology of schizophrenia is reviewed elsewhere in this issue. In this article the focus is narrowed to recent developments in the understanding of emerging environmental risk factors that may be considered causal risk factors for the diagnosis of first-episode schizophrenia. There has been a major shift from the previously accepted concept that the risk of schizophrenia arises primarily from a neurodevelopmental disorder that is extant by the time of infancy, remains latent during childhood, and environmental influences during adolescence or young adulthood have little effect on the ultimate risk of schizophrenia. More recent epidemiologic studies have shown that social environment may be an important risk factor in determining transition from "at risk" to actual "first episode" diagnosis. In other words, given that more people are vulnerable to develop schizophrenia than eventually develop schizophrenia, what are some of the identifiable concurrent risk factors that may add to the overall risk of transitioning from never having schizophrenia to the onset of a first episode? Causal risk factors are neither necessary nor sufficient for the development schizophrenia, but their presence would mean that some people who otherwise would not develop schizophrenia are exposed to this causal risk factor and go on to develop the illness. Research suggests that in the general population low-grade psychotic experiences are a common but transitory developmental phenomenon [1]. In other words, many more people in the general population are vulnerable to schizophrenia than actually develop the full-blown disorder that is called "first-episode schizophrenia" by the clinicians who treat the unfortunate individuals who make this transition. Using two independent general population samples, investigators examined the hypothesis that common, nonclinical developmental expressions of psychosis may become abnormally persistent when synergistically combined with developmental exposures, such as cannabis use, trauma, or urbanicity [2], that may impact on behavioral and neurotransmitter sensitization, ultimately leading to a first episode of schizophrenia.

Adolescents and young adults exposed to the following environmental risk factors may be at increased risk for developing schizophrenia: (1) living in a densely populated urban environment ("urbanicity"), (2) specific types of social adversity related to discrimination, disconnection, or cultural isolation, and (3) exposure to cannabis by marijuana use in early adolescence or young adulthood before the onset of full schizophrenia symptoms. Remember that the term "causal risk factor" does not mean that these factors are necessary or sufficient; rather, they seem most relevant when a person is already at high risk for schizophrenia.

Urbanicity as a Risk Factor for Schizophrenia

There is a renewed interest in the social environment as a causal risk factor for the development of schizophrenia and other psychotic disorders. Estimates of the increased risk of urban environment as a causal risk factor for schizophrenia are as high as 30% of attributable risk within these high-risk populations. A Danish population registry study that took into account years spent living in urban environments found evidence for "a dose-response relationship between urbanicity during upbringing [at any time during childhood or adolescence] and schizophrenia risk" [3]. In a prospective study of risk factors in a cohort of 918 adolescents for future onset of psychotic disorder, baseline signs of psychotic types of experiences interacted with urban environment so that about 4 years later those exposed to both factors were more than twice as likely to develop a psychotic disorder than those who exposed to only one of these risk factors. These findings support the suggestion that the outcome of the developmental expression of psychosis is worse in urban environments. The environment may impact the risk for psychotic disorder by causing an abnormal persistence of developmentally common expressions of psychotic experiences [4]. "The excess incidence of [first-episode psychosis] in Southeast London compared with [less urban sites] of Nottingham or Bristol is consistent with a dose-response relationship with urbanicity demonstrated in several recent studies" [5].

Social Adversity as a Risk Factor for Schizophrenia

Although the association between minority ethnicity and risk of schizophrenia has been known for some time, the precise nature of this relationship has been a matter of debate. Recent prospective studies of new-incident cases of schizophrenia in three sites across the United Kingdom have shown a gradient effect of social adversity on the future risk of diagnosis of schizophrenia. The Etiology and Ethnicity in Schizophrenia and Other Psychoses study was "designed to better understand and disentangle the relationships between urbanicity, social class, ethnicity, immigration and other environmental factors that might contribute to the risk of schizophrenia and other psychotic disorders" [5]. This study evaluating the differential rates and risk factors for the higher incidence of cases of schizophrenia and other psychotic disorders among ethnic minorities and recent immigrants in the United Kingdom found that "black and minority ethnic" individuals had more than three times the risk of having an incident diagnosis of schizophrenia compared with "white British" (IRR, 3.6; 95% confidence interval

[CI], 2.7–4.9). This risk was not explained by urbanicity, which was itself an independent risk factor for new-onset psychosis, as discussed in the previous section. For example, although immigration is a risk factor for first-episode schizophrenia in United Kingdom, the percentage of others within the same immigrant group living in the local neighborhood also was found to be an independent risk factor. One ecologic study showed that minority adolescents growing up in neighborhoods that were less populated by the same minority had a higher risk of schizophrenia than minority adolescents living in neighborhoods that had greater minority representation [6]. Another cohort study also showed an interaction between baseline reporting of lifetime history of traumatic events and the subsequent emergence of psychotic symptoms on follow-up in a sample of community-dwelling adolescents [7].

Marijuana Exposure as a Causal Risk Factor

Substance and alcohol use is traditionally considered a precipitant but not a cause of schizophrenia. More recent studies challenge this attitude, especially for marijuana (cannabis). Findings in a series of studies suggest that exposure to marijuana may be a causal factor in some (but not all) episodes of new-onset schizophrenia among heavy marijuana users. The first major epidemiologic report suggesting some causal association came from a 15-year follow-up of 45,570 Swedish army recruits showing that those who had histories of moderate marijuana use (ie, used marijuana on more than 15 occasions) were six times more likely to develop schizophrenia than less-frequent users or nonusers [8,9]. Marijuana was the only substance associated with an increased risk for schizophrenia; exposure to other drugs of abuse or alcohol was not [10]. In a separate survey of non–mentally ill adolescents and young adults followed for 4 years after a baseline evaluation [11] (age range, 14–24 years; n = 2437), a report of cannabis use at the baseline evaluation increased the likelihood of reporting psychotic symptoms 4 years later (adjusted odds ratio, 1.67; 95% CI, 1.13–2.46). Consistent with a model of interaction with prior vulnerability, the effect of cannabis use was much stronger when the baseline evaluation also showed a predisposition for psychosis (23.8% adjusted difference in risk; 95% CI, 7.9–39.7%). Marijuana exposure is most detrimental to individuals who already are prone to psychosis before first marijuana use [12]. Marijuana seems to be a specific risk factor, and increased risk for schizophrenia does not generalize to other drugs or alcohol. Studies of drug use in non–mentally ill populations find a relationship between marijuana use, but not alcohol use, and tendencies toward psychosis [13]. A 3-year follow-up (1997–1999) is reported of a general population of 4045 psychosis-free persons and of 59 subjects in the Netherlands who had a baseline diagnosis of psychotic disorder. Substance use was assessed at baseline, at 1-year follow-up, and at 3-year follow-up. Baseline cannabis use predicted the presence at follow-up of any level of psychotic symptoms (adjusted odds ratio, 2.76; 95% CI, 1.18–6.47) as well as a severe level of psychotic symptoms (odds ratio, 24.17; 95% CI, 5.44–107.46). Results confirm previous suggestions that cannabis use increases the risk of both the incidence of psychosis in psychosis-free persons and a poor prognosis for those with an established vulnerability to psychotic disorder [14].

This information linking marijuana use and increased risk of schizophrenia may be of tremendous importance in educating siblings and other family members of individuals who have schizophrenia. Although still controversial, the quality and sophistication of the epidemiologic research challenge the primacy of genetic or in utero/postnatal predisposition and suggest that there may be some causal risk factors for development of incident cases of schizophrenia that can be modified from a public health perspective. These new findings have important implications for the management of first-episode patients as well as the families who are exposed to the same environmental factors [15].

TIME PERIOD BETWEEN INITIAL ONSET AND INITIAL CLINICAL PRESENTATION

When considered from the perspective of disease onset, the term "first-episode schizophrenia" is misleading. When clinicians first encounter such a patient, usually in crisis only recently, the illness can seem to have "come out of nowhere." Despite the overwhelming nature of the acute symptoms at time of clinical presentation, the underlying neurobiologic processes already have been present for considerable time. A person who soon will receive a diagnosis of first-episode schizophrenia is likely to have been very symptomatic for some time. When the patient's history is better understood, it becomes clear that things have not been not completely "right" for a long time, even if there were no obvious or flagrant psychotic symptoms. The threshold that finally is crossed, resulting in a treatment assessment or intervention, usually involves a symptom or behavior that has been present for a while but finally has become so bad that it elicits a response. In other words, once the diagnosis of schizophrenia is established, it is usual to find that the person has met diagnostic criteria for schizophrenia for a considerable period of time already. In fact, the only thing that is "first-episode" is that the clinicians now are aware that the case exists. It is more precise, therefore, to think of "first-episode" schizophrenia as "first-clinical-presentation" schizophrenia.

Course of "Prodromal" Symptoms: What Comes First?

Psychotic symptoms are most likely to be the most prominent symptoms at time of diagnosis. Psychotic symptoms, however, are usually a late sign of schizophrenia, and only 25% of patients who have schizophrenia report having experienced psychotic symptoms sometime in childhood. In most patients the onset of psychotic symptoms occurs in early adulthood, typically in the mid 20s for men and late 20s for women. Rather than psychotic symptoms, the earliest signs usually are an array of developmental disturbances that include neurologic soft signs, minor physical anomalies, and mild cognitive, sensory, and motor impairments (eg, inattention at school, poor scholastic performance, motor "clumsiness") [16,17]. Although this pattern has been well described in large, population-based studies, the signs are too subtle to be of any diagnostic value in individual patients. Current diagnostic criteria for schizophrenia do not include these early developmental signs, and generally they are not included in the retrospective category considered "prodromal" onset, as described in the next section.

Nature of "Prodromal" Symptoms Before the Onset of Psychosis

Social withdrawal, social anxiety, depression, and other interpersonal and functional problems often begin well before there is any signal of a more specific or more definitive psychotic disturbance. These behavioral changes usually cross a threshold into a noticeable and clinically significant problem well before the next threshold is crossed (the demonstration of psychotic symptoms or other criteria that permit a formal diagnosis of schizophrenia). From a developmental perspective, this experience supports the hypothesis that the initial neurochemical problems antecedent to schizophrenia probably are not caused by excess dopamine. In fact, this stage of prodrome is more consistent with hypotheses of dopamine hypoactivity in the frontal cortex.

Transition From Nonpsychotic "Prodromal" to Psychotic Symptoms

Because a diagnosis of schizophrenia requires persistent psychotic symptoms, it is inevitable that a person who later is diagnosed with first-episode schizophrenia will pass a threshold for psychosis and meet criteria for persistent psychotic symptoms. Although psychotic symptoms are part of the definition, the fact that they almost are always a later sign of the disorder is very important, both theoretically and clinically. The late arrival of psychotic symptoms is consistent with the hypothesis that psychosis is not a primary component of the disorder but is a secondary response to a perhaps more fundamental disturbance.

Unfortunately the onset of psychosis usually is not sufficient in its own right to trigger a prompt medical or psychiatric evaluation. Instead, the psychotic symptoms and all of the fallout from being psychotic usually fester for some time before receiving clinical attention or treatment. By the time the patient is initially seen for evaluation and help, there already is a good chance that significant psychosocial damage has resulted from the festering psychotic state. It is common for overt psychotic symptoms to have been present for a considerable period of time before the first treatment contact. Although there probably is a further delay between the onset of psychotic symptoms and their recognition as such by others, the delay often continues despite awareness of others that the person is seriously disturbed. Reasons for the further delay in getting treatment include stigma, inability to know how to respond, and, most common, lack of awareness on the part of the psychotic person himself or herself. In the first-episode literature, the time period between first established report of a psychotic symptom and initial treatment intervention for the acute psychotic episode is known as "duration of untreated psychosis," or DUP. A meta-analysis of DUP found that the average DUP was 9 months but may be as long as 2 years. The fact that a long DUP exists across a wide range of cultures and treatment services speaks to the strength of the resistance and barriers to initial care for persons who have psychotic symptoms. In the meantime, DUP is a measurable baseline component of the first-episode experience and has been the subject of considerable academic interest, especially regarding its role as a potentially modifiable prognostic indicator of future long-term outcome beyond the initial treatment episode.

Most studies of DUP and outcome have shown a correlation between the length of the DUP and treatment outcome, in that a longer DUP predicts poorer outcomes. What is more controversial is why this seems to be the case. One hypothesis is that the stigma that was a barrier to seeking help remains a barrier afterwards. Another hypothesis is that the DUP is of itself neurotoxic and somehow alters the central nervous system in a way that makes the patient less responsive to medication. If that supposition is true, patients who have a longer period of untreated psychosis may be unable to achieve the level of recovery that would have been possible if the psychosis had been treated sooner. The data supporting this hypothesis are, at present, mixed. The qualitative signs and symptoms of the actual "first-episode" of psychosis do not seem to be affected strongly by the DUP, but the DUP does seem to be one of the predictors of initial response to antipsychotic medication (a shorter DUP predicting a better likelihood of antipsychotic response). In a meta-analysis of 43 publications, Perkins and colleagues [18,19] showed a shorter DUP to be associated with a better response to antipsychotic medication "as measured by improvement or endpoint severity of global psychopathology (5 studies), positive symptom severity (13 studies), and negative symptom severity (14 studies)." In addition, at the time of first treatment, duration of previously untreated psychosis was found to be associated with severity of negative symptoms [19]. Because the presence of psychotic symptoms means the crossing of a threshold that is an unequivocal sign of a serious condition for which antipsychotic medication is indicated, shortening the DUP becomes a measurable outcome for efforts to shorten the time between a diagnosis of schizophrenia being made and treatment for psychotic symptoms. The potential advantage of recognizing the significance of the DUP is that it may reveal potential interventional treatment strategies that improve outcome. Shortening the DUP is theoretically important in understanding the potentially toxic effects of untreated psychotic symptoms on eventual treatment response. From a public health and interventional vantage point, it should be explored whether the DUP is influenced by factors connected with the fundamental pathology of schizophrenia, such as poor premorbid function, by factors unrelated to disease pathology, such as access to care and socioeconomic status, or perhaps by a combination of the two [18]. Nonetheless, other neurobiologic findings of first-episode schizophrenia show that even by the time the first psychotic symptoms manifest, other biologic processes have taken place that signify that onset of psychosis is not a primary threshold of illness progression.

NEUROBIOLOGY AT THE TIME OF PRESENTATION OF FIRST-EPISODE SCHIZOPHRENIA

The observation in the mid 1970s that patients who have chronic schizophrenia have demonstrable brain abnormalities on CT was a "wake-up call" for psychiatrists. The evolution of brain imaging studies has confirmed and extended these early findings. In particular, this work has shown conclusively that these changes are present (to a similar extent and magnitude) in patients who have first-episode schizophrenia [20–28]. Two recent sequential MRI studies [29,30] provided evidence of subtle abnormalities in the brains of patients genetically at high risk of developing schizophrenia and found preliminary evidence of reduction in temporal lobe structures in ultra–high-risk patients who converted from high-risk status to actual schizophrenia. Although these observations are provocative, they are not yet clinically useful. Therefore, an MRI scan in a first-episode patient probably would be read as normal by a neuroradiologist, even though the overall pattern of MRIs shows subtle differences when contrasted with appropriately matched comparison groups.

Although clinically they are too subtle to be useful, there nevertheless is ample evidence of an array of structural and neurochemical brain changes detectable even at the first episode of schizophrenia [31]. Current theories concerning the origins of schizophrenia account for these changes as evidence of a neurodevelopmental basis for schizophrenia arising from early noxious events (in utero and perhaps also in early childhood or adolescence) that either are genetic or environmental or involve some combination of the two types of events. Although this neurodevelopmental model has held ascendancy in conceptualizing the onset and cause(s) of schizophrenia, there also is evidence that progressive brain changes (neurodegenerative processes) occur in some patients who have schizophrenia within the first 2 years of the course of illness [23,32]. These results make it harder for clinicians to translate the neuroanatomic findings from this body of research into a cohesive message about future outlook and prognosis. There is ample evidence paralleling neurobiologic findings that the clinical symptoms of schizophrenia are as pronounced in a first episode as in more chronic stages of the illness. Negative symptoms are common, with one study reporting prominent primary negative symptoms (not attributed to either depression or extrapyramidal side effects [EPS]) in more than one quarter of first-episode patients [33,34]. Cognitive deficits, including memory, attention, and executive performance, are common across a broad array of functions. In the Calgary first-episode study, deficits across a range of cognitive measures were found in 111 first-episode patients that were comparable to deficits found in 76 patients who had chronic illness [35]. Other studies have reported a similar extent of pervasive cognitive impairment in first-episode patients [36,37]. Short-term (1- to 2-year follow-up) studies of neurocognitive functioning suggest some improvement in selective measures such as attention and visual learning but persistent disability in other core functions such as verbal memory [38,39]. This observation is important because cognitive impairment is considered a greater barrier than psychotic symptoms to achieving vocational rehabilitation [40]. Perhaps one way of describing these findings is to state that by the time of first clinical presentation of schizophrenia, the neurobiologic evidence indicates that significant changes to the brain have happened well before the immediate clinical crisis. This hard evidence goes along with the clinical evidence that the person probably has not been completely well for quite some time. Moving forward, the evidence suggests that further progression of illness, if it occurs, is not as severe as what has happened already. In other words, these data seem to be consistent with the possibility of recovery, analogous to rehabilitation after a nonprogressive central nervous system injury such as stroke.

CLINICAL PRESENTATION OF FIRST-EPISODE SCHIZOPHRENIA
Because social isolation and psychotic symptoms usually are present for some time before the initial contact with a mental health service, it is interesting to consider the sort of "tipping point" that marks the transition to receiving treatment. Most of the time, this transition is related to the degree of disturbance, disruption, or danger posed by the psychotic symptoms. Patients may present with either suicidal or violent behavior, perhaps because such triggering events finally lead to presentation to a treatment service [41]. The first presentation of psychosis is frightening and distressing. Patients are very perplexed, and family members are distraught. The patient's bizarre behavior and resistance to treatment make it all too easy to ignore how terrifying psychotic symptoms can be for the patient [42]. Therefore, by the time the clinician first sees the patient, the illness is further aggravated by a crisis that is the result of such behavior. The net result is that the initial contact with mental health services often happen in an atmosphere of extreme stress and social chaos.

To make matters worse, there is a lag time between the atmosphere of crisis and uncertainty and the eventual diagnosis and establishment of a clear treatment plan. It takes time to reconstruct what actually happened from history provided by the patient and family toward the end of the crisis, and after the treatment team has had a chance to complete a medical and psychiatric evaluation. As one might expect, pathways to care are many and diverse. Addington and colleagues [43] traced the presentation to services of 86 patients who had first-episode psychosis and found that most patients came into care through emergency services. The pernicious interaction between psychiatric symptoms and treatment delay is also shown by studies relating avoidance of health care to social isolation and impairments in social functioning [44]. Meanwhile, the mental health care system that is the initial point of entry generally is accustomed to caring for persistently ill, multiepisode patients and therefore is less likely to be attuned to the needs and emotional vulnerability of patients and families at this first stage of care. These systems barriers are even more challenging for first-episode patients who have multiple barriers to becoming engaged in the treatment process [45].

One of the most vexing and persistent problems in treating first-episode patients is "denial of illness" or "lack of insight," which for purposes of this article are considered the same. Although "lack of insight" sometimes is a state-related part of an acute psychotic episode [46,47], lack of insight often persists as psychotic symptoms resolve [48]. More than 50% of stabilized patients who have first-episode schizophrenia deny that they are ill after the acute episode is over [49,50]. A growing convergence in the literature shows that denial of illness or "lack of insight" is one of the strongest predictors of future nonadherence to antipsychotic medication [51–54].

To address the clinical need of first-episode patients better, and also to provide a foundation for clinical research in this area, there has been an international trend to develop specialty programs focused on the needs of the first-episode patient. A specialty service with mental health staff focused on the initial onset may help reduce some of the overwhelming nature of the experience of entering into mental health care treatment for the first time, especially because such programs provide a more distinct entry point to appropriate services [55]. Of course, these services are useful only when available, and they are not yet universally available in a way that is analogous to having surgical trauma centers strategically placed for ready access in urban areas. What these centers have demonstrated is that it is possible to study the pathways to care for first-episode patients within communities. Another assumption of specialty services is that because first-episode schizophrenia is the first opportunity for mental health services to begin treatment for those who develop schizophrenia, it is important that every effort be made to "get it right" from the very beginning of the treatment process.

IMMEDIATE TREATMENT OF A FIRST-EPISODE PSYCHOSIS PATIENT

Before a Formal Diagnosis of Schizophrenia is Established

It is important to remember that the diagnostic evaluation may take some time, and that only when it is apparent that the person has a probable or definite diagnosis of schizophrenia is it possible to consider the initial presentation as one of schizophrenia. Although a diagnosis of first-episode schizophrenia sometimes can be be made with some confidence within days to weeks of initial clinical contact, it often may require considerable time and effort to work through the differential diagnosis and to make such a diagnosis with a reasonable degree of clinical certainty.

As discussed, for individuals eventually diagnosed as having schizophrenia there usually is little question about the presence or absence of psychotic symptoms. The DUP literature shows that for patients who ultimately receive a diagnosis of schizophrenia or schizophreniform disorder, the threshold for meeting criteria for psychotic symptoms probably was crossed long before the immediate evaluation. Therefore, often the diagnostic challenge is focused on the differential diagnosis of acute psychosis. Although a review of this topic is beyond the scope of this article, the evaluation often is handicapped by the absence of a reliable and accurate history of symptoms. The patient often is unwilling or unable to disclose the full extent of symptoms, the family is too overwhelmed or shocked, and, almost by definition, medical records are un-available. Furthermore, stigma and fear may impede the patient's or family's willingness to report fully the severity or magnitude of the problem. Therefore, clinicians must keep in mind that the true nature of the course of illness will tend to unfold over time, and that the history reported during the first days and weeks often underrepresents the severity and the duration of the problem. Establishing the longitudinal course before onset is feasible but requires train-ing and consensus definitions [56,57]. Furthermore, the overlap between pri-mary affective illness and schizophrenia is well known and becomes a differential that sometimes cannot be answered with 100% certainty at the ini-tial evaluation. Once a diagnosis of schizophrenia (or schizophreniform disor-der) is made by experienced mental health clinicians, however, it is likely that the diagnosis of schizophrenia will remain stable and valid over time. Many pa-tients who have first-episode psychosis present with active substance abuse, which poses major diagnostic challenges, particularly in determining whether the drug abuse and schizophrenia are causally related [41].

Immediate Psychopharmacologic Intervention

Because psychotic symptoms are likely to be the primary focus of treatment, the primary pharmacologic question will be the choice of antipsychotic medica-tion. Because this treatment is the "default" mode, a few considerations con-cerning medication issues should be kept in mind before prescribing an antipsychotic agent. Many first-episode patients have never received psychiat-ric medications. Once an antipsychotic medication is prescribed, that changes forever. Therefore, clinicians need to be mindful of the importance of obtaining and recording the physical and mental status before starting medication and to consider whether delaying initiation of medication is appropriate. Table 2 lists the newer antipsychotics, and suggested starting doses and intervals for dose increases. The reader should note that these doses and dose titration schedule would be considered to be on the low end of the therapuetic range for more persistently ill patients. This illustrates the importance of being able to rapidly identify "first episode" patients and systems to be able to implement pharmaco-logic treatment plans that address the treatment needs of this patient population.

Although the clinician may use an antipsychotic medication before a primary diagnosis is established, this class of medication will not help clarify the primary diagnosis. That is, antipsychotic agents treat acute psychotic symptoms regard-less of whether the diagnosis ultimately turns out to be schizophrenia, bipolar disorder, or substance-induced psychosis. Perhaps a practical approach is to consider clinical situations when the use of antipsychotic agents should be de-layed or is contraindicated. Before starting treatment with a medication, some of the issues that might need to be considered include (1) possible pregnancy and whether knowledge of pregnancy would affect the use of a medication; (2) whether there is any possibility of behavioral or neurologic toxicity from recent exposure to antipsychotic medication; (3) whether there is a need for

Table 2
Initial dose and titration schedule for a first episode patient with no complicating conditions affecting dosing*

	Usual starting dose (mg/day) Avg (range)	Interval between dose increases	Usual dose increment	Usual initial target dose range (mg/day)	
				Low Avg (range)	High Avg (range)
Aripiprazole	10 (5–15)	1 week	5 (or 10 mg)	10 (5–15)	25 (20–30)
Olanzapine	10 (5–15)	1 week	5 mg	10 (7.5–12.5)	22.5 (20–30)
Quetiapine	150 (50–250)	3 days (but wide range)	150 mg (but wide range)	300 (wide range)	800 (600–1000)
Risperidone	1.5 (1–2)	1 week (but wide range)	1.5 mg (but wide range)	2 (1–3)	6 (5–8)
Ziprasidone	60 (40–100)	4 days	40 or 60 mg	100 (60–140)	200 (160–240)
Haloperidol	3 (1–4)	1 week	2–4 mg	5 (2–8)	10 (10–15)

*Mean doses and standard deviations from survey results converted to "real world" doses.

From Weiden PJ, Preskorn SH, Fahnestock, P, et al. A roadmap: translating the psychopharmacology of antipsychotics to individualized treatment for severe mental illness. J Clin Psych 2007;68(Supp X):1–48. Copyright © 2007, Comprehensive NeuroScience Inc., White Plains, NY; with permission.

a careful neurologic examination unaffected by the possible neurologic side effects of antipsychotic medication.

MANAGING DIAGNOSTIC UNCERTAINTY

As discussed, there is a period of time after the assessment has been done and before a tentative diagnosis is made. Because of the stress on the family and the patient, the work-up should be timely, and basic aspects of the evaluation (physical examination, neurologic assessment, laboratory and interview screening for drug and alcohol use) should be undertaken as soon as possible. Clinicians should know that there is a tendency for both patients and family to underreport the duration of symptoms before the initial presenting episode; therefore, initial reports should be considered tentative, and the history of duration of untreated symptoms (psychotic and nonpsychotic) should be reassessed later. A retrospective life chart should be developed with a focus on assessing the degree of social isolation that may have been one of the earliest signs of a developing illness. Social withdrawal is a particularly useful diagnostic sign: if it occurred before the manifestation of recognizable psychotic symptoms, it may be possible to rule out affective symptoms (patient is not lonely or sad during protracted periods of social isolation) and substance abuse (the patient was too socially withdrawn to be able to purchase or use illicit drugs). Once psychotic symptoms occur, it may be more difficult to disentangle concurrent mood symptoms from those psychotic symptoms more consistent with schizophrenia [58,59]. Diagnostic stability is better for men than women, and a diagnosis of schizophrenia tends to be more stable than a diagnosis of schizophreniform disorder. Regardless of the theoretical aspects of diagnostic stability, patients and families should be prepared to contend with changes in their formal psychiatric diagnosis whenever they change psychiatrists or treatment services.

CHOICE OF ANTIPSYCHOTIC AGENT

Clinicians should aim for excellent results when treating a first-episode patient because first-episode status is associated with a higher likelihood of achieving an excellent medication response. In one of the classic studies of first-episode schizophrenia, Robinson and colleagues [60] found that 87% of first-episode patients achieved an excellent response to antipsychotic medication, with a median time to response of 9 weeks. This favorable response was achieved using older antipsychotics, so the theoretical feasibility of achieving excellent therapeutic responses is not just a characteristic of the newer, atypical antipsychotic medications. There are, however, several other crucial considerations in medication selection that, taken together, strongly favor the use of one of the newer atypical antipsychotic agents rather than an older medication when initiating treatment with an antipsychotic agent. The relative advantages of the newer agents include the reduced neurologic burden relative to older conventional agents, their superior effectiveness at relapse prevention, and their relatively favorable effects on mood and cognition.

In terms of efficacy, safety, and tolerability, the issues pertaining to the specific choice of an antipsychotic medication for first-episode patients are similar, but not exactly the same, to those pertaining to the choice of antipsychotic for more persistently ill patients who have schizophrenia. We will discuss some of the specific aspects of differences between antipsychotics that may be particularly relevant in the treatment of the "first-episode patient.

When choosing medications for patients with established medication histories, clinicians can guide the selection in part on the person's past history of efficacy and tolerability. Most of the time, information will be available about the patients treatment system and any constraints. By definition this is not available for first episode patients. The lack of prior treatment trials means that the patient's pharmacologic history cannot be used as one of the factors guiding the choice of medication. There often will be uncertainties as to the final diagnosis and therefore about the recommendation for ongoing antipsychotic therapy after the acute episode resolves. Moreover, practical concerns such as location or access to ongoing treatment and medication are unknown at the time of the initial medication choice. These uncertainties may represent practical constraints on possible medication selection. While this may sound obvious, these practical matters are sometimes forgotten when medication are started in crisis settings. Advanced planning about these service and access needs of first episode patients is a crucial aspect of the initial medication selection process.

Given the stress and frequent opposition to treatment that are such common elements of the first-episode experience, any distressing or unexpected reaction to medication may result in long-term rejection of further treatment and may fuel a sense of distrust and alienation from mental health care services. Therefore, in choosing the medication the prescriber needs to be mindful of the need to minimize the risk of sudden, unexpected adverse events that would result in long-term avoidance of medications. Similarly, the prescriber of antipsychotic agent must be mindful that first-episode patients are more sensitive and more vulnerable than patients who have more chronic disease to common and distressing side effects of antipsychotics. This vulnerability may present in several ways, with more severe side effects, faster onset of side effects, and greater distress and discomfort caused by the same side effect.

There is nothing beneficial about having any side effect. Formerly it was believed that EPS might be a marker for the efficacy of antipsychotics. It now is clear that EPS actually are a marker of poor response and should be avoided whenever possible, regardless of the agent chosen. It also has been the lead author's experience that there often is a routine procedure in emergency rooms or inpatient units regarding the as-needed administration of antipsychotics that can best be described as "one size fits all." The combination of lack of insight and fear about what is happening in an adversarial situation often coincides with a standard policy of an as-needed intramuscular administration of the haloperidol/lorazepam combination for "agitation." Even though the initial pharmacologic treatment plan may have taken into account the sensitivity of the first-episode patient to low doses and used a dose titration strategy meant to minimize treatment-emergent side effects, this approach is obliterated by the automatic as-needed administration of haloperidol without regard to the needs of the first-episode patient. Once this medication is administered, it cannot be undone, and it may lead to persistent nonadherence or to irreversible neurologic effects [61]. Note that this case is different from the theoretical idea that it may be possible to use very low doses of conventional antipsychotics in a first episode of schizophrenia without necessarily inducing severe EPS [62].

The overall approach to medication choice has shifted overwhelmingly to the preferential use of the newer atypical antipsychotics instead of the older, first-generation antipsychotic medications. Although the short-term response rates of the newer and older antipsychotics are about equivalent, the newer medications have better long-term effectiveness for first-episode patients. One of the most compelling reasons to favor the newer agents is the lower likelihood of EPS, which translates to lower rates of sudden episodes of neurologic events that cause the patient to avoid long-term treatment and to lower coprescription of anticholinergic agents such as benztropine. Formerly, anticholinergic agents were overwhelmingly likely to be coprescribed with the antipsychotic agent, leading to distressing peripheral anticholinergic problems and exacerbating the cognitive dysfunction associated with the illness itself. Thus far, however, there is no consensus or clear evidence supporting use of one specific atypical antipsychotic over another, although the use of clozapine as a first-line agent does not seem to have clear-cut advantages [63]. Excellent reviews on medication treatment of first-episode schizophrenia have been published recently [62,64,65].

Although there is widespread agreement that the use of atypical antipsychotics for first-episode patients is preferred in theory, this use is not always followed in practice. In particular, a vexing problem is a "one size fits all" approach seen in many emergency psychiatric services. Often, clinicians working in these settings believe that the high-potency conventional antipsychotics such as haloperidol "work faster" than the newer medications or routinely prescribe intramuscular haloperidol to be used as needed in case of "agitation" or medication refusal. Unfortunately the net effect of this approach is that many first-episode patients are in fact exposed to older agents such as haloperidol under circumstances that are likely to pose significant neurologic risks as well as jeopardize the therapeutic engagement process that is fragile under the best of circumstances.

AFTER A DIAGNOSIS OF FIRST-EPISODE SCHIZOPHRENIA IS MADE

Once the clinician believes that the diagnosis is probable or definite schizophrenia, the issue of informing the patient and family becomes of critical importance. There is no debate that the patient and family need education and guidance about the nature of psychotic symptoms and the risk of possible recurrence. There is controversy in first-episode schizophrenia about the best way to convey this information. In particular, there is concern that using the word "schizophrenia" too soon, even if the diagnosis of schizophrenia is very likely, might alienate and stigmatize the patient in a way that could do more harm than good. Many first-episode services have developed their own approaches to patient and family education. It is important to be mindful of the issues involved. Whether one uses the diagnostic term "schizophrenia," uses a more tentative approach ("it may be schizophrenia"), or focuses on the psychotic symptoms without extensive discussion of the diagnosis should be considered and discussed with involved colleagues before the meeting with the patient or family when the diagnosis is discussed.

Psychosocial Interventions for First-Episode Patients

Helping patients and families acquire insight into a potentially lifelong and debilitating illness while preserving hope and supporting morale during a first episode of schizophrenia is a challenge for clinicians. The issues that arise in providing psychotherapy during a first episode are somewhat different from those that are a focus of psychotherapy at more advanced stages of the illness. A recent review of psychosocial interventions targeting first-episode patients was most noticeable for the paucity of focused intervention studies in this vital area [66]. Most of the literature on psychosocial intervention for first-episode patients pertains to what are described as "multimodal interventions," that is, a programmatic effort made possible by a specialty service focusing on the unique needs of this target population during this critical time period. Studies have evaluated comprehensive interventions, which include community outreach and early diagnosis with broad and specialized focus on pharmacologic and psychosocial services designed for this phase of illness. On the one hand, specific treatment interventions ("single-element interventions") were focused primarily on family interventions and individual cognitive behavior therapy (CBT) interventions. Readers should keep in mind that these interventions often occur in the milieu of a highly motivated and trained specialty staff. Incorporating such interventions into nonspecialty clinical services actually may result in larger improvements in care given to "first episode" patients entering treatment service systems that did not have ways to identify these individuals.

A study of the possible long-term benefits of an intensive short-term CBT intervention given during the first-episode of treatment did not show any enduring benefits of CBT on persistent symptoms or subsequent relapse [43]. Known as the Study of Cognitive Reality Alignment Therapy in Early Schizophrenia, it compared two "active" psychotherapies–CBT or supportive counseling–with a standard-of-care comparison group [55,67,68]. The long-term outcome showed no differences in persistent symptoms, nonadherence, relapse or rehospitalization. Although disappointing to those hoping to show specificity of CBT, this study is very informative in guiding the design of other CBT-based interventions for first-episode patients.

Support for relatives also is crucial at this early stage. Relatives need clear, comprehensible information on schizophrenia that covers symptoms, biology, course, and treatment. The National Alliance for the Mentally Ill (NAMI), founded in 1979, is a key source of information and support (available at NA-MI.org). Most NAMI chapters run a very well-received program for relatives called the "Family-to-Family" program [69]. Dixon [70] has confirmed the benefit of this program in allaying anxiety and providing valuable information. Studies have found that psychoeducational programs for families produce an impressive reduction in relapse rates among ill family members [71]. One way that family approaches may differ for first-episode schizophrenia is that the multifamily approach, in which several families (along with their ill relatives) meet together, may be effective in theory [72] but may be logistically too difficult to implement when focused primarily on first-episode patients and their families [73], The unpredictability and inconsistent attendance of first-episode patients makes this treatment approach feasible only in tertiary services for first-episode patients. Under most clinical circumstances, family psychoeducation should be done for each family separately and tailored to the specific health beliefs and concerns of the particular family environment.

Psychopharmacology After the Diagnosis is Established
Transitioning from acute to maintenance pharmacotherapy
A major practical effect of establishing a diagnosis of schizophrenia is that it establishes the need for ongoing antipsychotic therapy beyond the end of the acute psychotic episode. If a diagnosis of schizophrenia can be made with confidence, then long-term maintenance antipsychotics are indicated. This is often a point of confusion. Many schizophrenia patients can achieve full remission after their first episode is successfully treated. But, the degree of improvement does not change the need for ongoing antipsychotic medication. It is the primary diagnosis that drives the recommendation. This is, of course, one of the most important consequences of the diagnostic endeavor. (Other possibilities include a presumptive diagnosis of an affective disorder, for which maintenance treatment might be changed to a mood-stabilizing agent, or a primary diagnosis of substance abuse/dependence, for which referral to a psychosocial treatment program specializing in drug and alcohol problems would become the primary focus.) In some cases it may not be possible to achieve a sufficient degree of confidence to recommend maintenance antipsychotic therapy even though clinical intuition suggests that a diagnosis of schizophrenia is most likely. In this discussion it is assumed that the diagnosis of schizophrenia is established and that maintenance antipsychotic treatment is clearly indicated.

Assuming that the treatment response has been adequate and that the antipsychotic medication is reasonably well tolerated, the current antipsychotic usually remains the choice for ongoing treatment. The time course of response to the acute psychotic episode is such that patients remain quite sensitive to symptom recurrence soon after responding to medication and being stabilized to continue with ongoing medication treatment. Accordingly, in theory, the antipsychotic dose needed to achieve acute efficacy should be continued well into the maintenance treatment period (eg, 3–6 months into outpatient treatment) before any dose lowering is recommended. In practice this continuation of medication is easier said than done. First-episode patients typically are greatly relieved after the acute psychotic episode resolves, and are eager to put this experience behind them. The clinical import is that during the initial postacute treatment period (which often corresponds with the transition from inpatient to outpatient care), the patient attempts to put this experience behind them by ending treatment and stopping medication. Sometimes it is possible to work out a compromise so that the patient agrees to continue the medication but at a dose that is lower than before and lower than optimal for preventing relapse. In other words, the pharmacologic principle is that it is better for the patient to take some medication, even if it is not an optimal dose, if it is the only compromise that is acceptable. Likewise, the medication regimen needs to be tailored to what the patient is willing to take rather than to what has been prescribed. The medication regimen should be simplified even at the sacrifice of optimal efficacy. The overall approach here should be to prescribe the best pharmacologic regimen possible rather than the best possible pharmacologic regimen!

Changing antipsychotic medication

The time course of antipsychotic response is longer than the usual 4- to 6-week time period [74]. At the same time one should calibrate the response criteria to target a relatively complete control of positive and negative symptoms relative to what might be considered acceptable for a more persistently ill (chronic) patient. The initial goals of treatment should be aggressive and aim for resolution of positive symptoms and a return to premorbid (eg, before prodromal period) status. A detailed discussion of how to define a "good response" is beyond the scope of this article; it is important to note that full or almost full symptom remission is the goal of antipsychotic therapy. It is necessary to determine whether one antipsychotic agent works and to ensure that an appropriate dose of the antipsychotic was used before switching to another. Given the absence of fixed-dose studies of atypical antipsychotics in first-episode patients, dosing guidelines for using these agents in first-episode schizophrenia are generally extrapolated from available information on dosing in more chronic forms of schizophrenia. Typically, for first-episode patients, it is recommended that clinicians attempt to use the lower end of the therapeutic dosage range, at least during the initial phases of the first therapeutic treatment trial. Dosing recommendations for first-episode patients are derived from the *Expert Consensus Guidelines on Optimizing Pharmacologic Treatment of Psychotic Disorders* [75]. As in any other clinical situation, antipsychotic medications should be changed when the initial antipsychotic regimen does not have adequate efficacy or has unacceptable side effects. The caveat here is how the fact that the patient is early in the course of treatment may affect the operational criteria for "inadequate efficacy" or "intolerable side effects." The magnitude of weight gain and dyslipidemia from some of the newer agents is as large in first-episode cohorts as it is in chronically ill patients [76], however, and this weight gain is becoming recognized as a significant limitation of some of the newer antipsychotic medications.

Treatment of postpsychotic depression
In contrast to other chronic mental illnesses, such as depression or alcoholism, suicide is likely to occur earlier in the course of schizophrenia. This observation, however, is a generalization, and suicidal behavior may be a risk for patients at any stage of the illness. Demoralization and consequent depression in reaction to the magnitude of impending lifelong disability can occur early in the course of schizophrenia [44] and are considered major risk factors—along with other general and demographic characteristics—for suicide in patients who have schizophrenia. Birchwood and colleagues [77] have described the chronology and course of depression in patients following an acute episode of schizophrenia. Although not a first-episode sample, patients whose depressive symptoms persisted as a postpsychotic depression had a higher rate of suicidal behavior than patients who had depressive symptoms only during the acute episode of psychosis. In a Scandinavian follow-up study of a cohort of 321 patients with a first episode of psychosis, 26% of patients had a history of suicidal behavior, and 26% had suicidal thoughts within the week before their initial assessment. During the 1-year follow-up of these patients, 31 (11%) attempted suicide. The presence of hallucinations and a history of suicidal behavior were predictors of suicidal behavior in this population [78].

Adherence to the primary antipsychotic medication should be evaluated before initiating adjunctive antidepressant therapy. Usually the risk of precipitating a relapse from prescribing antidepressants when patients are "covered" with a parallel antipsychotic is too high, and other strategies (eg, hospitalization) might be considered.

Medication nonadherence: it is not a matter of "whether?" but "when?"
To prevent relapse, maintenance antipsychotic treatment is as important for first-episode patients as it is for multiepisode, or "revolving door," schizophrenic patients [64]. Therefore, at least from a theoretical perspective, a diagnosis of schizophrenia establishes the need for ongoing maintenance antipsychotic medication, and the clinician should not waiver from the commitment to promoting long-term adherence to ongoing antipsychotic therapy. Translating this evidence-based knowledge into a useful treatment plan is easier said than done. Despite clinicians' recommendations otherwise, the question usually is not so much whether the first-episode patient will stop antipsychotic medications too soon. The answer to that question is almost always "Yes." The correct question is "When will the medication be stopped?"

Given the problem of poor compliance in first-episode schizophrenia, one treatment option is to consider the use of a long-acting route of medication. Until recently only the older antipsychotics were available in long-acting preparations. Given the other advantages of the newer antipsychotics, the older medications generally were not recommended for patients in such early stages of the illness, not because of the need for injection per se but because of their side effect profile. The newer atypical antipsychotics now are the first-line treatment for schizophrenia [79,80]. Before long-acting risperidone became available, the major drawback of the first-line atypical agents was the lack of long-acting versions for continuous drug delivery. Clinicians had to struggle with the trade-off between recommending an oral atypical medication with superior efficacy and a reduced side burden or one of the older, less efficacious antipsychotic medications that can be given by long-acting injection [81,82]. This dilemma has changed with the availability of one of the atypical antipsychotics in a long-acting route of drug delivery [83–85]. Whether a long-acting route of medication delivery is more effective than oral administration within the class of newer atypical antipsychotics for first-episode patients is not known, but at least one randomized, prospective study has compared the long-term outcomes of first-episode patients treated with long-acting risperidone and those treated with an oral atypical antipsychotic agent. Preliminary findings show that most stabilized first-episode patients voluntarily accept a recommendation that they switch from an oral to a long-acting injection. The caveat here is that this acceptance is within the subset of first-episode patients who already had accepted a recommendation for outpatient follow-up, and that "acceptance" is defined as receiving one long-acting injection. Therefore, the impact of the long-acting route on first-episode outcome still is not known, but early results show that it is acceptable, and making the recommendation does not seem have any short-term detrimental effects on the therapeutic alliance or medication attitudes [82,86,87].

Choosing the maintenance antipsychotic medication for long-term treatment
Although the approach to choosing a maintenance antipsychotic is very similar to that used for choosing an antipsychotic before completing the final diagnostic evaluation for the "first-episode" patient during the acute psychotic episode, it is not the same. There is a general agreement within the expert community in the United States that, whenever possible, the first-line antipsychotic should be one of the first-line (nonclozapine) atypical antipsychotics. Provocative preclinical data and new neuroimaging data suggest that there may be differences in neuroprotective effects favoring the newer medications. Looked at another way, the older conventional antipsychotics may be more neurotoxic [88–90]. In a first-episode comparative treatment study, patients randomly assigned to either olanzapine or haloperidol received sequential neuroimaging assessments [88]. Over the course of 1 year, patients taking haloperidol showed a divergent pattern on MRI compared with patients treated with olanzapine. Patients treated with haloperidol showed a loss of gray and white cortical matter and enlarged ventricular volume. Because no comparable longitudinal MRI data exist for the other atypical antipsychotics, it is not known whether this finding is unique to olanzapine or is a class effect of the atypical agents relative to the older agents. Although the interpretation of MRI data is still speculative, it would parallel the clinical finding of lower rates of tardive dyskinesia from the newer medication [91]. Because tardive dyskinesia is a de facto marker

of central nervous system neurotoxicity, it is perhaps not a surprise that MRI studies show differential effects as well.

Beyond the general approach to favor one of the atypical antipsychotic, there is no consensus on the choice of the specific antipsychotic for long-term therapy. The issue of long-term safety is, of course, a very important consideration. The specific medication should take into account the patient's specific symptomatic profile, risk factors for adverse effects, and the adverse-effect profile of each antipsychotic agent under consideration. Of particular relevance in medication choice is minimizing the long-term medical risks of treatment, which include the neurologic risks of persistent EPS and tardive dyskinesia and the potential exacerbation of risk factors for diabetes mellitus and cardiovascular disease. Finally, medication adherence issues, if not already a central issue, are likely to be a major concern sometime within the first year of maintenance antipsychotic therapy.

The problem of poor adherence in first-episode schizophrenia
The treatment of a first-episode of schizophrenia is of critical importance in that it may establish—for better or worse—the acceptability of ongoing treatment in the years ahead. Despite responding relatively well, most will stop their medication within the first year of treatment. Naturalistic follow-up studies of ecologic samples find that only 25% of first-episode patients take antipsychotic medication consistently for the first year after starting treatment [92,93]. Many clinicians feel that being a "first episode" reduces the risk of relapse after medication discontinuation. Not so. The chances of relapsing from medication discontinuation are no different than chronically ill populations. In follow-up, nonadherence to medication is the greatest predictor of relapse [60,94]. Looked at another way, in terms of achieving improvements and recovery, continued medication adherence is by far and away the strongest clinical predictor of a patient's remaining stable and being able to achieve a sustained remission [95,96]. No pharmacologic or psychosocial treatment intervention studied so far has been able to prevent medication nonadherence among first-episode patients [97–99]. In a naturalistic follow-up study of a first-episode cohort treated in routine practice settings [92,93], less than one fifth of the first-episode cohort took antipsychotic medication consistently throughout the follow-up, and 65% had discontinued the antipsychotic medication for more than 2 weeks. The slope of the nonadherence curve shows that about one third of the cohort had a medication gap in the first 3 months after discharge. The slope then becomes more gradual, with another one third showing a first gap between 3 and 12 months. A first-episode patient has much to lose from stopping medication. The patient will probably suffer the pain and consequences of another acute psychotic episode much sooner rather than later. Today, nonadherence is a greater obstacle to the successful treatment of first-episode schizophrenia than any limitations in the efficacy of the newer medications.

Why do first-episode patients stop their medication? Many factors contribute to nonadherence, including efficacy problems, access barriers, and illness-related factors.

One of the basic elements of adherence, at least when it is self-directed, is to acknowledge that there is a problem that might need treatment. Therefore, failure to acknowledge or understand that there is a problem for which medications might be helpful becomes the primary motivational barrier to ongoing voluntary adherence. There is ample evidence that insight is impaired at the first onset of illness. Accordingly, it follows that for these patients adherence would be a substantial problem even when treatment for schizophrenia is first introduced. Novac [100] reported that medication noncompliance was best predicted by positive symptoms at admission and by lack of insight at discharge. In a similar study assessing compliance over the first 3 months of treatment among 59 Finnish first-episode patients, poor compliance was associated with side effects, male gender, lack of social activities, and global, but not positive, symptom severity [101,102]. First-episode patients are especially reluctant to accept a formal diagnosis of schizophrenia, or any other similar disorder with the associated stigma or a future of illness-based limitations and the need for ongoing treatment [103]. Refusal to accept such a diagnostic label may or may not extend to rejecting possible benefits from medication. This consideration is of particular importance for understanding nonadherence in immediate aftermath of a first episode of schizophrenia. The linking of medications to diagnosis is problematic for many first-episode patients who do not accept a diagnosis of mental illness but who otherwise might be willing to acknowledge that medications may be helpful for recovery.

Interventions for impending medication nonadherence in first-episode schizophrenia. One possible strategy to address the adherence problem in first-episode schizophrenia is to stop trying to fight against the overwhelming likelihood that a first-episode patient will stop antipsychotic medication too soon. Instead of trying to prevent nonadherence, perhaps it is better to focus on an overall strategy that reduces the harm from nonadherence. It might be more realistic to consider initial medication nonadherence as an expectable part of the recovery process. This expectation might change the therapeutic attitude from a pointless struggle to stop nonadherence and instead place a greater emphasis on maintaining the therapeutic alliance at all times regardless of the person's current adherence status. Such a long-term perspective may prevent the initial episodes of nonadherence after a first-episode from becoming entrenched in the years to come. From a research perspective, first-episode cohorts comprise an ideal population to study the potential impact of innovative therapeutic approaches. First-episode randomized pharmacologic studies comparing different antipsychotic agents show, at best, only marginal differences among medications in time until nonadherence [97,104]. These same studies show that nonpharmacologic factors such as the therapeutic alliance or insight are much more relevant predictors than are the side effects of the medication [99]. The authors' research group at SUNY Downstate Medical Center currently is conducting a prospective study evaluating the effectiveness of recommending a long-acting atypical antipsychotic (long-acting risperidone microspheres) shortly after an initial episode of schizophrenia has been treated and the patient has stabilized. Early findings show that the majority of first-episode patients who successfully engage in outpatient treatment during the first month after discharge are willing to accept a recommendation of trying a long-acting route of antipsychotic medication. Initial reluctance to try a long-acting injection is usually amenable to a tailored psychoeducation intervention focusing on matching the goals of antipsychotic therapy to the long-term goals of the patient and family [105]. Whether the acceptance of a long-acting atypical antipsychotic translates into better clinical outcomes in terms of better adherence, stability, and sustained recovery is still under investigation.

SUMMARY

The understanding and therapeutic focus in schizophrenia have shifted, in part from the recognition that neurobiologic damage occurs early and often in the course of the illness. First-episode schizophrenia therefore constitutes a window of opportunity for timely, comprehensive, and effective therapeutic interventions. The next phase of longitudinal studies evaluating treatment outcome in first-episode schizophrenia will provide information about whether improved care at the onset of illness can translate into a better long-term outcome. Simultaneously, studies in high-risk persons and prodromal studies will determine whether shifting the definition of onset to an earlier "incipient" stage and intervening assertively at that point can result in improved outcomes and perhaps even a reduction in the incidence of schizophrenia. Gathering information from these lines of inquiry will take some years, but if they converge it will be possible to offer a much more optimistic view of schizophrenia to patients and relatives when they present to mental health care services. In fact, the awareness of these research efforts and promotion of such work in the public domain is already a powerful source of encouragement for individuals who currently struggle with schizophrenia.

References

[1] van Os J, Hanssen M, Bijl RV, et al. Strauss (1969) revisited: a psychosis continuum in the general population? Schizophr Res 2000;45(1–2):11–20.

[2] Cougnard A, Marcelis M, Myin-Germeys I, et al. Does normal developmental expression of psychosis combine with environmental risk to cause persistence of psychosis? A psychosis proneness-persistence model. Psychol Med 2007;37(4):1–15.

[3] Pedersen CB, Mortensen PB. Evidence of a dose-response relationship between urbanicity during upbringing and schizophrenia risk. Arch Gen Psychiatry 2001;58(11):1039–46.

[4] Spauwen J, Krabbendam L, Lieb R, et al. Evidence that the outcome of developmental expression of psychosis is worse for adolescents growing up in an urban environment. Psychol Med 2006;36(3):407–15.

[5] Kirkbride JB, Fearon P, Morgan C, et al. Heterogeneity in incidence rates of schizophrenia and other psychotic syndromes: findings from the 3-center AeSOP study. Arch Gen Psychiatry 2006;63(3):250–8.

[6] Boydell J, van Os J, McKenzie K, et al. Incidence of schizophrenia in ethnic minorities in London: ecological study into interactions with environment. BMJ 2001;323(7325): 1336–8.

[7] Spauwen J, Krabbendam L, Lieb R, et al. Impact of psychological trauma on the development of psychotic symptoms: relationship with psychosis proneness. Br J Psychiatry 2006;188:527–33.

[8] Andreasson S, Allebeck P, Rydberg U. Schizophrenia in users and nonusers of cannabis. A longitudinal study in Stockholm County. Acta Psychiatr Scand 1989;79(5):505–10.

[9] Andreasson S, Allebeck P, Engstrom A, et al. Cannabis and schizophrenia. A longitudinal study of Swedish conscripts. Lancet 1987;2(8574):1483–6.

[10] Zammit S, Allebeck P, Andreasson S, et al. Self reported cannabis use as a risk factor for schizophrenia in Swedish conscripts of 1969: historical cohort study. BMJ 2002;325(7374):1199.

[11] Henquet C, Murray R, Linszen D, et al. The environment and schizophrenia: the role of cannabis use. Schizophr Bull 2005;31(3):608–12.

[12] Henquet C, Krabbendam L, Spauwen J, et al. Prospective cohort study of cannabis use, predisposition for psychosis, and psychotic symptoms in young people. BMJ 2005;330 (7481):11.

[13] Verdoux H, Sorbara F, Gindre C, et al. Cannabis use and dimensions of psychosis in a non-clinical population of female subjects. Schizophr Res 2003;59(1):77–84.

[14] van Os J, Bak M, Hanssen M, et al. Cannabis use and psychosis: a longitudinal population-based study. Am J Epidemiol 2002;156(4):319–27.

[15] McGrath JJ. The surprisingly rich contours of schizophrenia epidemiology. Arch Gen Psychiatry 2007;64(1):14–6.

[16] Cannon TD, Zorilla LE, Shtasel D, et al. Neuropsychological functioning in siblings discordant for schizophrenia and healthy volunteers. Arch Gen Psychiatry 1994;51:651–61.

[17] Verdoux H, van Os J. Psychotic symptoms in non-clinical populations and the continuum of psychosis. Schizophr Res 2002;54(1–2):59–65.

[18] Perkins DO. Review: longer duration of untreated psychosis is associated with worse outcome in people with first episode psychosis. Evid Based Ment Health 2006;9(2):36.

[19] Perkins DO, Gu H, Boteva K, et al. Relationship between duration of untreated psychosis and outcome in first-episode schizophrenia: a critical review and meta-analysis. Am J Psychiatry 2005;162(10):1785–804.

[20] Bagary MS, Symms MR, Barker GJ, et al. Gray and white matter brain abnormalities in first-episode schizophrenia inferred from magnetization transfer imaging. Arch Gen Psychiatry 2003;60(8):779–88.

[21] Price G, Cercignani M, Bagary MS, et al. A volumetric MRI and magnetization transfer imaging follow-up study of patients with first-episode schizophrenia. Schizophr Res 2006;87(1–3):100–8.

[22] Cahn W, Hulshoff Pol HE, Lems EB, et al. Brain volume changes in first-episode schizophrenia: a 1-year follow-up study. Arch Gen Psychiatry 2002;59(11):1002–10.

[23] Cahn W, van Haren NE, Hulshoff Pol HE, et al. Brain volume changes in the first year of illness and 5-year outcome of schizophrenia. Br J Psychiatry 2006;189:381–2.

[24] Sumich A, Chitnis XA, Fannon DG, et al. Unreality symptoms and volumetric measures of Heschl's gyrus and planum temporal in first-episode psychosis. Biol Psychiatry 2005;57(8):947–50.

[25] Keshavan MS, Rabinowitz J, DeSmedt G, et al. Correlates of insight in first episode psychosis. Schizophr Res 2004;70(2–3):187–94.

[26] Job DE, Whalley HC, McConnell S, et al. Voxel-based morphometry of grey matter densities in subjects at high risk of schizophrenia. Schizophr Res 2003;64(1):1–13.

[27] Kasai K, Shenton ME, Salisbury DF, et al. Progressive decrease of left superior temporal gyrus gray matter volume in patients with first-episode schizophrenia. Am J Psychiatry 2003;160(1):156–64.

[28] Kasai K, Shenton ME, Salisbury DF, et al. Progressive decrease of left Heschl gyrus and planum temporale gray matter volume in first-episode schizophrenia: a longitudinal magnetic resonance imaging study. Arch Gen Psychiatry 2003;60(8):766–75.

[29] Pantelis C, Lambert TJ. Managing patients with "treatment-resistant" schizophrenia. Med J Aust 2003;178(Suppl):S62–6.

[30] Pantelis C, Yucel M, Wood SJ, et al. Structural brain imaging evidence for multiple pathological processes at different stages of brain development in schizophrenia. Schizophr Bull 2005;31(3):672–96.

[31] Pantelis C, Velakoulis D, McGorry PD, et al. Neuroanatomical abnormalities before and after onset of psychosis: a cross-sectional and longitudinal MRI comparison. Lancet 2003;361(9354):281–8.

[32] Steen RG, Mull C, McClure R, et al. Brain volume in first-episode schizophrenia: systematic review and meta-analysis of magnetic resonance imaging studies. Br J Psychiatry 2006;188:510–8.

[33] Malla AK, Takhar JJ, Norman RM, et al. Negative symptoms in first episode non-affective psychosis. Acta Psychiatr Scand 2002;105(6):431–9.

[34] Malla AK, Norman RM, Manchanda R, et al. One year outcome in first episode psychosis: influence of DUP and other predictors. Schizophr Res 2002;54(3):231–42.

[35] Addington J, Brooks BL, Addington D. Cognitive functioning in first episode psychosis: initial presentation. Schizophr Res 2003;62(1–2):59–64.

[36] Amminger GP, Edwards J, Brewer WJ, et al. Duration of untreated psychosis and cognitive deterioration in first-episode schizophrenia. Schizophr Res 2002;54(3):223–30.

[37] Amminger GP, Edwards J, McGorry PD. Estimating cognitive deterioration in schizophrenia. Br J Psychiatry 2002;181:164, [author reply 165].

[38] Albus M, Hubmann W, Scherer J, et al. A prospective 2-year follow-up study of neurocognitive functioning in patients with first-episode schizophrenia. Eur Arch Psychiatry Clin Neurosci 2002;252(6):262–7.

[39] Albus M, Hubmann W, Mohr F, et al. Neurocognitive functioning in patients with first-episode schizophrenia: results of a prospective 5-year follow-up study. Eur Arch Psychiatry Clin Neurosci 2006;256(7):442–51.

[40] Velligan DI, Bow-Thomas CC, Mahurin RK, et al. Do specific neurocognitive deficits predict specific domains of community function in schizophrenia? J Nerv Ment Dis 2000;188(8):518–24.

[41] Green AI, Canuso CM, Brenner MJ, et al. Detection and management of comorbidity in patients with schizophrenia. Psychiatr Clin North Am 2003;26(1):115–39.

[42] Weiden PJ, Havens LL. Psychotherapeutic management techniques in the treatment of outpatients with schizophrenia. Hosp Community Psychiatry 1994;45:549–55.

[43] Addington J, Van Mastrigt S, Hutchinson J, et al. Pathways to care: help seeking behaviour in first episode psychosis. Acta Psychiatr Scand 2002;106(5):358–64.

[44] Drake RJ, Haley CJ, Akhtar S, et al. Causes and consequences of duration of untreated psychosis in schizophrenia. Br J Psychiatry 2000;177:511–5.

[45] Tait L, Birchwood M, Trower P. Predicting engagement with services for psychosis: insight, symptoms and recovery style. Br J Psychiatry 2003;182:123–8.

[46] Weiler MA, Fleisher MH, McArthur-Campbell D. Insight and symptom change in schizophrenia and other disorders. Schizophr Res 2000;45(1–2):29–36.

[47] Rossell SL, Coakes J, Shaleske J, et al. Insight: its relationship with cognitive function, brain volume and symptoms in schizophrenia. Psychol Med 2003;33:111–9.

[48] Carroll A, Fattah S, Clyde Z, et al. Correlates of insight and insight change in schizophrenia. Schizophr Res 1999;35(3):247–53.

[49] Amador XF, Flaum MM, Andreasen NC, et al. Awareness of illness in schizophrenia and schizoaffective and mood disorders. Arch Gen Psychiatry 1994;51:826–36.

[50] Amador XF, Strauss DH, Yale SA, et al. Awareness of illness in schizophrenia. Schizophr Bull 1991;17(1):113–32.

[51] Appelbaum PS, Gutheil TG. Drug refusal: a study of psychiatric inpatients. Am J Psychiatry 1980;137:3.

[52] Hoge SK, Appelbaum PS, Lawlor T, et al. A prospective, multicenter study of patients' refusal of antipsychotic medication. Arch Gen Psychiatry 1990;47:949–56.

[53] McEvoy JP, Appelbaum PS, Apperson LJ, et al. Why must some schizophrenic patients be involuntarily committed? The role of insight. Compr Psychiatry 1989;30:13–7.

[54] Weiden P, Dixon L, Frances A, et al. Neuroleptic noncompliance in Schizophrenia. In: Tamminga C, Schulz C, editors. Advances in neuropsychiatry and psychopharmacology, schizophrenia research, vol. 1. New York: Raven Press; 1991. p. 285–96.

[55] Lewis S, Tarrier N, Haddock G, et al. Randomised controlled trial of cognitive-behavioural therapy in early schizophrenia: acute-phase outcomes. Br J Psychiatry Suppl 2002;43: s91–7.

[56] Perkins DO, Leserman J, Jarskog LF, et al. Characterizing and dating the onset of symptoms in psychotic illness: the Symptom Onset in Schizophrenia (SOS) inventory. Schizophr Res 2000;44(1):1–10.

[57] Miller TJ, McGlashan TH, Rosen JL, et al. Prodromal assessment with the structured interview for prodromal syndromes and the scale of prodromal symptoms: predictive validity, interrater reliability, and training to reliability. Schizophr Bull 2003;29(4): 703–15.

[58] Chaves AC, Addington J, Seeman M, et al. One-year stability of diagnosis in first-episode nonaffective psychosis: influence of sex. Can J Psychiatry 2006;51(11):711–4.

[59] Addington J, Chaves A, Addington D. Diagnostic stability over one year in first-episode psychosis. Schizophr Res 2006;86(1–3):71–5.

[60] Robinson D, Woerner MG, Alvir J, et al. Predictors of response from a first-episode of schizophrenia or schizoaffective disorder. Am J Psychiatry 1999;156:544–9.

[61] Mujica R, Weiden PJ. NMS associated with IM haloperidol administration in a patient maintained on olanzapine. Am J Psychiatry 2001;158(4):650–1.

[62] Kelly DL, Conley RR, Carpenter WT. First-episode schizophrenia: a focus on pharmacological treatment and safety considerations. Drugs 2005;65(8):1113–38.

[63] Woerner MG, Robinson DG, Alvir JM, et al. Clozapine as a first treatment for schizophrenia. Am J Psychiatry 2003;160(8):1514–6.

[64] Robinson DG, Woerner MG, Delman HM, et al. Pharmacological treatments for first-episode schizophrenia. Schizophr Bull 2005;31(3):705–22.

[65] Bradford DW, Perkins DO, Lieberman JA. Pharmacological management of first-episode schizophrenia and related nonaffective psychoses. Drugs 2003;63(21):2265–83.

[66] Penn DL, Waldheter EJ, Perkins DO, et al. Psychosocial treatment for first-episode psychosis: a research update. Am J Psychiatry 2005;162(12):2220–32.

[67] Tarrier N, Lewis S, Haddock G, et al. Cognitive-behavioural therapy in first-episode and early schizophrenia. 18-month follow-up of a randomised controlled trial. Br J Psychiatry 2004;184:231–9.

[68] Tarrier N, Haddock G, Barrowclough C, et al. Are all psychological treatments for psychosis equal? The need for CBT in the treatment of psychosis and not for psychodynamic psychotherapy. Psychol Psychother 2002;75(Pt 4):365–74, [discussion: 375–9].

[69] Weiden P. A clinician's guide to the NAMI Family-to-Family education program. J Pract Psychiatry Behav Health 1999;6:353–6.

[70] Dixon L. Providing services to families of persons with schizophrenia: present and future. J Ment Health Policy Econ 1999;2(1):3–8.

[71] McFarlane WR, Dixon L, Lukens E, et al. Family psychoeducation and schizophrenia: a review of the literature. J Marital Fam Ther 2003;29(2):223–45.

[72] Schooler NR, Keith S, Severe J, et al. Relapse and rehospitalization during maintenance treatment of schizophrenia: the effects of dose reduction and family treatment. Arch Gen Psychiatry 1997;54:453–63.

[73] Fjell A, Bloch Thorsen GR, Friis S, et al. Innovations: psychoeducation: multifamily group treatment in a program for patients with first-episode psychosis: experiences from the TIPS Project. Psychiatr Serv 2007;58(2):171–3.

[74] Emsley R, Rabinowitz J, Medori R. Time course for antipsychotic treatment response in first-episode schizophrenia. Am J Psychiatry 2006;163(4):743–5.

[75] Kane JM, Leucht S, Carpenter D, et al. The expert consensus guideline series. Optimizing pharmacologic treatment of psychotic disorders. Introduction: methods, commentary, and summary. J Clin Psychiatry 2003;64(Suppl 12):5–19.

[76] Zipursky RB, Gu H, Green AI, et al. Course and predictors of weight gain in people with first-episode psychosis treated with olanzapine or haloperidol. Br J Psychiatry 2005;187: 537–43.

[77] Birchwood M, Iqbal Z, Chadwick P, et al. Cognitive approach to depression and suicidal thinking in psychosis. 1. Ontogeny of post-psychotic depression. Br J Psychiatry 2000;177: 516–21.

[78] Nordentoft M, Laursen TM, Agerbo E, et al. Change in suicide rates for patients with schizophrenia in Denmark, 1981-97: nested case-control study. BMJ 2004;329(7460): 261.

[79] Kane JM, Leucht S, Carpenter D, et al. The expert consensus guideline series: optimizing pharmacologic treatment of psychotic disorders. J Clin Psychiatry 2003;64(Suppl 12): 1–100.

[80] Leucht S, Barnes TRE, Kissling W, et al. Relapse prevention in schizophrenia with new-generation antipsychotics: a systematic review and exploratory meta-analysis of randomized, controlled trials. Am J Psychiatry 2003;160(7):1209–22.

[81] Weiden P, Glazer W. Assessment and treatment selection for "revolving door" inpatients with schizophrenia. Psychiatr Q 1997;68(4):377–92.

[82] Weiden PJ. Understanding depot therapy in schizophrenia. J Pract Psychiatry Behav Health 1995;1:182–4.

[83] Turner M, Eerdekens M, Jacko M, et al. Long-acting injectable risperidone: safety and efficacy in stable patients switched from conventional depot antipsychotics. Presented at the 43rd Annual Meeting of the New Clinical Drug Evaluation Unit (NCDEU). Boca Raton (FL); May 27–30, 2003.

[84] Kane JM, Eerdekens M, Keith SJ, et al. Efficacy and safety of a novel long-acting risperidone microspheres formulation. Am J Psychiatry 2003;60:1125–32.

[85] Rasmussen M, Eardekeus M, Lowenthal R, et al. Kinetics and safety of a novel depot formulation. Presented at the XI World Congress of Psychiatry. Hamburg (Germany), 1999.

[86] Weiden PJ. Using depot therapy. J Pract Psychiatry Behav Health 1995;1:247–50.

[87] Weiden PJ, Rapkin B, Zygmunt A, et al. Postdischarge medication compliance of inpatients converted from an oral to a depot regimen. Psychiatr Serv 1995;46(10):1049–54.

[88] Lieberman JA, Tollefson GD, Charles C, et al. Antipsychotic drug effects on brain morphology in first-episode psychosis. Arch Gen Psychiatry 2005;62(4):361–70.

[89] Ho BC, Alicata D, Ward J, et al. Untreated initial psychosis: relation to cognitive deficits and brain morphology in first-episode schizophrenia. Am J Psychiatry 2003;160(1): 142–8.

[90] Wakade CG, Mahadik SP, Waller JL, et al. Atypical neuroleptics stimulate neurogenesis in adult rat brain. J Neurosci Res 2002;69(1):72–9.

[91] Tarsy D, Baldessarini RJ. Epidemiology of tardive dyskinesia: is risk declining with modern antipsychotics? Mov Disord 2006;21(5):589–98.

[92] Mojtabai R, Lavelle J, Gibson PJ, et al. Atypical antipsychotics in first admission schizophrenia: Medication continuation and outcomes. Schizophr Bull 2003;29(3):519–30.

[93] Mojtabai R, Lavelle J, Gibson PJ, et al. Gaps in use of antipsychotics after discharge by first-admission patients with schizophrenia, 1989–1996. Psychiatr Serv 2002;53(3): 337–9.

[94] Robinson D, Woerner MG, Alvir J, et al. Predictors of relapse following response from a first-episode of schizophrenia or schizoaffective disorder. Arch Gen Psychiatry 1999;56:241–7.

[95] Robinson DG, Woerner MG, McMeniman M, et al. Symptomatic and functional recovery from a first episode of schizophrenia or schizoaffective disorder. Am J Psychiatry 2004;161(3):473–9.

[96] Robinson D, Woerner MG, Alvir J, et al. Predictors of medication discontinuation by patients with first-episode schizophrenia and schizoaffective disorder. Schizophr Res 2002;57:209–19.

[97] Perkins DO, Johnson JL, Hamer RM, et al. Predictors of antipsychotic medication adherence in patients recovering from a first psychotic episode. Schizophr Res 2006;83(1): 53–63.

[98] Weiden P, Mott T, Curcio N. Recognition and management of neuroleptic noncompliance in schizophrenia. In: Shriqui C, Nasrallah H, editors. Contemporary issues in the treatment of schizophrenia. Washington, DC: APA Press; 1995. p. 411–34.

[99] McEvoy JP, Johnson J, Perkins D, et al. Insight in first-episode psychosis. Psychol Med 2006;36(10):1–9.

[100] Novak-Grubic V, Tavcar R. Predictors of noncompliance in males with first-episode schizophrenia, schizophreniform and schizoaffective disorder. Eur Psychiatry 2002;17(3): 148–54.

[101] Kampman O, Illi A, Poutanen P, et al. Four-year outcome in non-compliant schizophrenia patients treated with or without home-based ambulatory outpatient care. Eur Psychiatry 2003;18(1):1–5.

[102] Kampman O, Laippala P, Vaananen J, et al. Indicators of medication compliance in first-episode psychosis. Psychiatry Res 2002;110(1):39–48.

[103] Bebbington P. The content and context of compliance. Int Clin Psychopharmacol 1995;9(Suppl 5):41–50.

[104] McEvoy JP, Lieberman JA, Stroup TS, et al. Effectiveness of clozapine versus olanzapine, quetiapine, and risperidone in patients with chronic schizophrenia who did not respond to prior atypical antipsychotic treatment. Am J Psychiatry 2006;163(4):600–10.

[105] Weiden PJ, Schooler NR, Goldfinger S, et al. Acceptance of maintenance antipsychotic recommendation for patients with "first-episode" schizophrenia: preliminary results from an effectiveness study of oral vs. long-acting atypical antipsychotic. Psychiatric Services Annual Meeting. New York; October 4, 2006.

Psychiatr Clin N Am 30 (2007) 511–533

PSYCHIATRIC CLINICS
OF NORTH AMERICA

ELSEVIER
SAUNDERS

Treatment-Resistant Schizophrenia

Helio Elkis, MD, PhD

Department and Institute of Psychiatry, University of Sao Paulo Medical School (FMUSP),
Rua Ovidio Pires de Campos 785, 05403-010-São Paulo-SP-Brazil, Brazil

I n the history of psychiatry, the introduction of antipsychotics undoubtedly represented a major milestone. The discovery of chlorpromazine, the first of the first-generation antipsychotics (FGAs) in the 1950s brought high hopes for treating schizophrenia, allowing both psychotic symptoms and hospital stays to be reduced and enabling patients to return to a social setting. From the outset of chlorpromazine use, however, it was clear that a specific group of patients remained symptomatic and therefore were considered refractory or resistant to phenothiazine [1].

Indeed, the definition of treatment-resistant schizophrenia (TRS) proves problematic to this day, in that schizophrenia is, by definition, a chronic disease, and long-term studies have shown that 80% to 90% of patients develop some kind of social or occupational dysfunction [2]. Chronicity frequently is taken as a synonym of refractoriness, and some authors use parameters such as the number of patient hospitalizations [3] or chronic hospitalizations [4] to define TRS. Regarding this latter item, Conley and Kelly [4] pointed out that factors such as poor compliance, weak social support programs, or a history of violence can keep patients chronically hospitalized without their having TRS.

Indeed in medicine there is a clear distinction between chronicity and refractoriness, because there are various chronic diseases, for example diabetes and hypertension, that, despite their chronicity, do in fact respond to treatment, with patients remaining stable with the same doses of hypoglycemic agents or antihypertensives throughout their lives.

Sometimes the term "TRS" or "refractory schizophrenia" is mistakenly thought to result from a lack of compliance, and some authors argue that it suggests "nothing can be done," embedding the notion that the patient is resisting the treatment, rather than the illness itself is resistant to treatment. Therefore it has been suggested that the term for "incomplete recovery" be used instead of "treatment refractory" [5]. In addition to distinguishing the concepts of chronicity and refractoriness, it is necessary to define what is meant by response to treatment, a concept that distinguishes remission from recovery. "Response to treatment" is a reduction in the severity of symptoms, as assessed by

E-mail address: helkis@usp.br

0193-953X/07/$ – see front matter
doi:10.1016/j.psc.2007.04.001
© 2007 Elsevier Inc. All rights reserved.

some sort of scale. "Remission" means an almost total absence of symptomatology for a certain period of time, whereas "recovery" is the absence of the disease for a long period. For instance, "remission" in rheumatoid arthritis is considered as absence of fatigue, minimal morning stiffness, absence of pain and swelling in joints, and normal hemo-sedimentation. When used analogously for schizophrenia, "remission" currently is defined as a minimum period of 6 months during which psychotic symptoms, symptoms of disorganization, and negative symptoms have low levels of clinical severity [6] corresponding to levels of three or less for the respective symptoms on the Brief Psychiatric Rating Scale (BPRS) [7] or the Positive and Negative Syndrome Scale (PANSS) scales [8].

The concept of TRS sometimes is associated with remission, which would imply an almost complete absence of symptoms, but also is related to response (ie, reduction in symptoms as compared with a previously established baseline level of severity).

PREVALENCE AND CLINICAL CHARACTERISTICS OF TREATMENT-RESISTANT SCHIZOPHRENIA

In a meta-analysis of the outcome literature of the treatment of schizophrenia encompassing the twentieth century, Hegarty and colleagues [9] observed that, after the introduction of neuroleptic therapy, only 48% of patients who had chronic schizophrenia had a favorable outcome, and approximately 20% of first-episode patients did not respond to conventional antipsychotic treatment after 1 year of treatment [10]. Generally it is assumed that 20% to 30% of patients who have schizophrenia do not respond to treatment with conventional antipsychotics [11,12], but some authors have mentioned higher rates (up to 60%) [13].

Meltzer and colleagues [14] observed a mean difference of 2 years of age at disease onset, together with predominance in the male gender in patients with TRS as compared with non-TRS patients. Similarly, Henna and Elkis [3] observed that patients who had TRS were predominantly male and experienced a higher number of hospitalizations than those who responded to treatment. The age of onset for patients who had TRS was around 17 years, compared with around 20 years for patients who responded to treatment. Other correlates are the number of episodes of illness, history of obstetric complications, long duration of untreated psychosis, and history of substance abuse [15].

In terms of the psychopathology, some authors assessed homogeneous populations of patients who had TRS using well-known rating scales to detect symptom clusters in an attempt to elicit a distinctive psychopathologic profile of TRS. Thus Lindenmayer and colleagues [16] used the PANSS [8] to evaluate 157 patients who had TRS and found a factor structure similar to their original factor-analysis study in TRS patients who were responsive to treatment [17], that is, positive, negative, excitement, cognitive, and depressive factors.

Using the BPRS [7] to evaluate 1074 patients who had schizophrenia that did not respond to antipsychotic agents and 197 patients who met the definition of

TRS, McMahon and colleagues [18] observed through confirmatory factor analysis that 13 of the 18 items of the BPRS loaded into four factors: reality distortion (grandiosity, suspiciousness, hallucinatory behavior, unusual thought content), disorganization (conceptual disorganization, mannerism and posturing, disorientation), negative symptoms (emotional withdrawal, motor retardation, blunted affect), and anxiety/depression (anxiety, guilty feelings, depression). The authors proposed that such factors should be used in analyzing the data from clinical trials involving patients who have TRS.

In the program investigating schizophrenia at the Institute of Psychiatry of the University of São Paulo Medical School, the author and colleagues analyzed data from an homogenous population of 96 patients [19] narrowly defined as having TRS based on Kane and colleagues' [11] criteria, for which the details are given later, and assessed by an anchored version of the BPRS [20,21]. Using factor analysis these investigators found that 16 of the 18 items of the scale clustered into four dimensions: negative/disorganization (emotional withdrawal, disorientation, blunted affect, mannerisms and posturing, conceptual disorganization), excitement (excitement, hostility, tension, grandiosity, uncooperativeness), positive factors (unusual thought content, suspiciousness, hallucinatory behavior), and depression (depression, guilt feelings, motor retardation), which are quite similar to some of the factors found by McMahon and colleagues [18] (ie, depressive and positive factors) but are dissimilar regarding negative and excitement factors. The inability to segregate negative and disorganization factors may result from the smaller sample size of the study.

Some authors argue that altered cognition and higher rates of suicide should be included among the clinical characteristics of TRS [13]. Altered cognition now is considered one of the best predictors of outcome in schizophrenia [22].

OPERATIONAL DEFINITIONS OF TREATMENT-RESISTANT SCHIZOPHRENIA

As discussed in the previous section, the psychopathology of TRS seems not to differ essentially from nonresistant schizophrenia, except that, by most current definitions, TRS implies the persistence of psychotic symptoms despite a certain number of adequate treatments [4,5,23–25]. Others authors propose that other symptom dimensions, such as negative and cognitive symptoms and the ability to return to the best premorbid level of functioning, should be included in the definition [2,13,26].

Therefore the definition of TRS is necessarily multidimensional, and a simple dichotomous definition is inadequate. Some authors have tried to construct operational definitions based on only one dimension, such as symptom reduction. For example, Csernansky and colleagues [27] developed a 10-item scale for chart review assessing the severity of symptoms such as delusions, hallucinations, and bizarre behavior with degrees of severity ranging from zero (absence) to four (marked). May and colleagues [28] constructed a bi-dimensional scale with six levels of resistance evaluated by the severity of symptoms and by social adaptation.

Brenner and colleagues [29] conceived of TRS as a continuum from resistance to refractoriness and developed a scale [30] comprising two dimensions: psychopathology, as assessed by the BPRS [7] and skills ability, as measured by the Living Skills Survey [31]. According to Brenner and Merlo [30], other authors such as Wilson and Keefe also developed operational criteria for TRS based on changes on the BPRS and the Clinical Global Impression (CGI) scale. These criteria are summarized in Table 1.

The operational criteria most widely used for the definition of TRS in clinical studies are those of Kane and colleagues [11] which enabled the selection of patients who had TRS for the study that introduced clozapine to the therapeutic armamentarium for schizophrenia, thereby paving the way for the emergence

Table 1
Early operational criteria for treatment-resistant schizophrenia

Author, Year	Criteria	Instrument (s)
Csernansky et al, 1983 [27]	Past response to antipsychotics based on reduction of items of the scale	10-item chart-review scale
May et al, 1988 [28]	Response based on a scale developed by the author	6-item scale of remission or recovery ranging from excellent (1) to refractory (6). Each item has two dimensions: clinical and social
Wilson, 1989 [30]	Psychotic symptoms persisting for more than 2.5 years after treatment with three neuroleptics of different classes (1000 mg chlorpromazine dosage equivalent) for 8 weeks within the last 5 years	BPRS $\geq$ 45 (with severity in items such as hallucinations, delusions, thought disorders as or more severe as other items)
Brenner et al, 1990 [29]	Criteria based on a scale developed by the author distinguishing three different concepts: remission, resistance, and refractoriness	Levels 1 and 2: remission Levels 3, 4, and 5: slight to severe resistance Levels 6 and 7: refractoriness Each level is evaluated by the BPRS, the CGI, and the Living Skills Survey
Keefe, 1991 [30]	No sufficient improvement after neuroleptic treatment (40 mg haloperidol/d) during 6 weeks	BPRS change < 20%; CGI level change < 2

Abbreviations: BPRS, Brief Psychiatric Rating Scale; CGI, Clinical Global Impression scale; PANNS, Positive and Negative Syndrome Scale.

of second-generation antipsychotic agents (SGAS). Kane's criteria are three dimensional, meaning that to be considered refractory, the patient must fulfill the following criteria or dimensions:

1. Historic: The patient must have a history of total or partial lack of response to previous treatment using two antipsychotics at adequate doses and periods.
2. Actual (severity of symptoms): The patient must present a certain level of psychopathologic severity as assessed by the BPRS and the GCI [32].
3. Prospective (confirmatory): Following treatment with haloperidol, the patient must present a reduction in BPRS and CGI symptomatology compared with values obtained at baseline.

Details of these criteria are shown in Table 2.

ALGORITHM DEFINITIONS OF TREATMENT-RESISTANT SCHIZOPHRENIA

To simplify clinical decision making, a number of treatment guidelines, such as the American Psychiatric Association [33] guidelines and the Schizophrenia Patient Outcomes Research Team [34] guidelines, or algorithms, such as the Texas Medication Algorithm Project [35], state that a patient who has not responded to two or three treatments using atypical antipsychotics for a duration of at least 4 to 6 weeks can be considered as having TRS and is eligible for treatment with clozapine.

The most recent algorithm, the Schizophrenia Algorithm of the International Pharmacological Algorithm Project (www.ipap.org) states that a patient

Table 2
Original criteria for treatment-resistant schizophrenia used in the clozapine trial

Dimensions	Criteria
Historical	At least three treatments with antipsychotics of at least two different chemical classes with doses equivalent to 1000 mg/d of chlorpromazine for a period of 6 weeks, without significant relief
	No period of good function within the preceding 5 years
Actual	A score of at least 45 in the BPRS (1–7 degrees of severity) with scores of at least 4 in two of the following items: conceptual disorganization, suspiciousness, hallucinatory behavior, or unusual thought content
	CGI ≥ 4 (moderately ill)
Prospective	No improvement after 6 weeks of treatment with haloperidol (up to 60 mg/d or higher); improvement is defined as A 20% reduction of the BPRS as compared with the level of severity defined by the actual criteria and/or
	A posttreatment CGI of ≤ 3 or a BPRS ≤ 35

Abbreviations: BPRS, Brief Psychiatric Rating Scale; CGI, Clinical Global Impression scale.
Data from Kane J, Hognifeld G, Singer J, et al. Clozapine for the treatment-resistant schizophrenic. A double-blind comparison with chlorpromazine. Arch Gen Psychiatry 1988;45:789–96.

who has not responded to two trials of 4 to 6 weeks' duration using mono-therapy with two different SGAs (or two trials with an FGA, if SGAs are not available) is considered to have TRS and is eligible for treatment with clo-zapine, for a six month trial with doses up to 900 mg/d (Fig. 1).

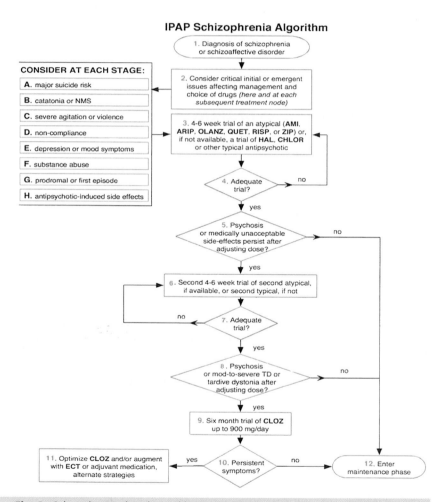

Fig. 1. Schizophrenia algorithm. (*Abbreviations:* Atypicals – AMI, amisulpride; ARIP, aripra-zole; CLOZ, clozapine; OLANZ, olanzapine; QUET, quetiapine; RISP, risperidone; ZIP, ziprasi-done; Typicals – CHLOR, chlorpromazine; FLU, fluphenazine; HAL, haloperidol; THIO, thiothixene; Other – AD, antidepressant; BZD, benzodiazepine; ECT, electroconvulsive therapy; IM, intramuscular; MS, mood stabilizer; TD, tardrive dyskinesia; NMS, Neuroleptic Malignant Syndrome. Updated 2004-06-17 interactive version at: www.ipap.org/schiz. *Courtesy of* The International Pharmacological Algorithm Project (IPAP). Copyright © 2006, IPAP. Available at: www.ipap.org; used with permission.)

CLINICAL AND BIOLOGIC CORRELATES OF TREATMENT RESPONSE

As previously described, a modern definition of TRS is the failure to respond to at least to two adequate trials of one SGA or FGA in monotherapy. The definition of an "adequate" trial implies the control of at least two variables: adequate doses and periods of treatment. "Apparent treatment resistance" or "incomplete recovery" should not be confused with TRS and may be caused by a variety of conditions that must be ruled before a diagnosis of TRS is established [5,36]. Factors that can lead to apparent treatment resistance or incomplete recovery include

- Poor compliance
- Lack of family support
- Substance abuse
- Physical comorbidity
- Intolerable side effects
- Incorrect dose schedule
- Poor therapeutic alliance

In terms of adequacy of dosage, a recent evidence-based review by Kinon and colleagues [37] recommends the following oral doses for an SGA for treatment-responsive schizophrenia and eventually in some cases of TRS:

- Risperidone: 4 to 6 mg/d
- Olanzapine: 10 to 20 mg/d
- Quetiapine: 300 to 600 mg/d
- Ziprasidone: 80 to 160 mg/d
- Aripiprazole: 15 to 30 mg/d

Clozapine is discussed later in this article.

In terms of an adequate period of trial, the majority of guidelines and/or algorithms recommend an antipsychotic agent be used for a minimum of 4 weeks before considering switching to another antipsychotic medication [33–35].

NEUROIMAGING CORRELATES OF TREATMENT-RESISTANT SCHIZOPHRENIA

Sheitman and Lieberman [26] propose that there may be two forms of treatment resistance: one that is present at the onset of the illness and thereafter and another that evolves as the illness progress. The latter form would be related to chronicity and the natural history of schizophrenia [26].

Combining neurodevelopmental and neurodegenerative aspects of the evolution of schizophrenia, these authors proposed that TRS develops according to three stages: (1) cortical pathology and deficient neuromodulatory capacity resulting from genetic/epigenetic etiologic factors occurring during childhood; (2) neurochemical sensitization leading to dopamine release and development of psychotic episodes occurring during adolescence; and (3) neurotoxicity with consequent development of structural neuronal changes in adulthood. Therefore it is conceivable that brain abnormalities may underlie the development of resistance to treatment in schizophrenia [26].

In fact, the relationship between structural brain abnormalities and response to conventional antipsychotic treatment in patients who have schizophrenia was the subject of pioneer studies that used methods such as pneumoencephalography [38] or CT [39] and demonstrated an inverse relationship between the degree of ventricular enlargement and treatment response.

Subsequent studies confirmed these findings, but Friedman and colleagues [40], in a meta-analysis of CT studies published between 1980 and 1989 that investigated the relationship between treatment response to antipsychotic agents and ventricular enlargement, found that such brain abnormality was not predictive of treatment response. A critical review of the literature on the same subject, published subsequently, arrived at the same conclusion [41]. In an 18-month follow-up study, however, Lieberman and colleagues [42] observed an increase in ventricular dimensions among patients classified as non-remitters when compared with controls or remitters.

Studies that relate brain abnormalities to treatment response can be classified in two main categories, according to their design [43]: (1) retrospective or cohort studies, which typically relate brain abnormalities to outcome measures, and (2) prospective or case- control studies, which relate treatment response to brain abnormalities. Reviews of retrospective studies suggest that ventricular enlargement is related to poor outcome [44], but in prospective studies ventricular enlargement is associated with response to conventional antipsychotics, and cortical atrophy mediates the effects of atypical neuroleptics [43].

Only a few case-controlled studies used a clear definition of treatment response to antipsychotic agents in schizophrenia, but such studies found a weak relationship between response to antipsychotic medications and brain abnormalities as measured by morphometric methods [45,46]. Moreover, to date, all the structural neuroimaging studies that investigated the relationship between treatment response and brain abnormalities have used relatively large-sized region-of-interest methods for measuring selected brain structures [43].

OTHER PSYCHOBIOLOGIC CORRELATES OF TREATMENT-RESISTANT SCHIZOPHRENIA

There are a few other neurobiologic correlates of TRS, such as plasma homovanillic acid which is seen in higher levels in first-episode patients who respond to treatment [42], altered T-cell functions, and alterations of the inflammatory process mediated by interleukins [47]. Response to treatment is highly mediated by genetic considerations, which are summarized later.

TREATMENT OPTIONS FOR TREATMENT-RESISTANT SCHIZOPHRENIA: REVIEW OF THE EVIDENCE

Pharmacologic Treatments

Beginning in the late 1970s and during the 1980s therapeutic attempts were made to treat TRS by using endorphins [48], prostaglandins [49], lithium [50], and FGAs [51], but none of these treatments proved effective.

With the advent of advent of clozapine in 1988 [11], which became the standard for the treatment of TRS, other SGAs (mainly risperidone, olanzapine, quetiapine, and ziprasidone) were tested as treatments for TRS in various clinical trials. The scope of this article does allow a discussion of these studies. The reader is referred to excellent reviews examining these clinical trials in detail that have appeared in the literature in recent years [4,13,15,22,24,52].

Instead, the author considers these clinical trials from the perspective of evidence-based medicine, because it is well established that systematic reviews and meta-analyses are the most important methods of research synthesis and take precedence over evidence obtained from single double-blind trials, open trials, cohort studies, case series, case reports, and expert opinions [53].

Systematic Reviews and Meta-Analysis of Controlled Trials of Second-Generation Antipsychotics versus First-Generation Antipsychotics or Second-Generation Antipsychotics in Patients Who Have Treatment-Resistant Schizophrenia

Meta-analyses of controlled trials involving patients who had TRS [54–57] and a systematic review [58] showed that clozapine is as effective or is more effective than other SGAs for treating TRS. Wahlbeck and colleagues' [54] meta-analysis included 30 trials of clozapine versus an FGA. Chakos and colleagues [55] meta-analysis reviewed trials of SGAs versus FGAs and also reviewed trials of SGAs versus other SGAs. Taylor and Duncan-McConnell [58] systematically reviewed controlled trials of an SGA versus an FGA. One of these studies [56], which compared clozapine with an FGA, challenged these results, criticizing methodologic bias (eg, the heterogeneity and duration of the studies, the initial psychopathology of patients, the year of publication, and sponsorship) in the clinical trials but still found a 0.44 effect in favor of clozapine. The meta-analysis of the Cochrane Center included only eight studies comparing clozapine with an SGA. This meta-analysis found a trend for clozapine to be more effective in improving positive symptoms but not negative symptoms; no differences were seen in other outcome variables, such relapse rates or global improvement. There was a trend for an SGA to be more effective in improving cognition; an update of this meta-analysis was released recently and is available at the Cochrane Website, wwww.cochrane.org. Details of these studies are provided in Table 3.

Two famous meta-analyses showed opposite results in terms of the efficacy of SGAs over FGAs. In one of these studies Geddes and colleagues [59] found that the superiority of an FGA is related to the dosage of the comparator (ie, when the dose of haloperidol was 12 mg or more, the SGA had no superiority over the FGA in efficacy or tolerability). Some of the studies in this meta-analysis involved controlled trials in which patients who had TRS were treated with clozapine, but no specific conclusions about clozapine treatment were reported. Davis and colleagues [60] challenged these results with another meta-analysis showing that clozapine had almost twice the effect size (0.49) of some other SGAs (0.29 for amisulpride; 0.25 for risperidone; 0.21 for

Table 3
Meta-analysis/systematic reviews of controlled trials of the effectiveness of second-generation antipsychotics versus first-generation antipsychotics or second-generation antipsychotics in patients who have treatment-resistant schizophrenia

Author, Year	Type of Review	Controlled Trials	Number of Subjects	Results/Conclusions
Wahlbeck et al, 1999 [54]	Meta-analysis	Clozapine versus FGA: 30 studies 12 versus chlorpromazine 13 versus haloperidol 1 versus trifluoperazine 1 versus thioridazine 1 versus clopenthixol 2 various	2530	Patients treated with clozapine showed more clinical improvement (NNT= 3) and less relapses (NNT=6) in long-term than in short-term studies (NNT = 20).
Taylor and Duncan-McConnell, 2000 [58]	Systematic review	Clozapine: 8 studies 3 versus chlorpromazine 1 versus fluphenazine 3 versus haloperidol 1 versus zotepine Risperidone: 4 studies 2 versus haloperidol 2 versus clozapine Olanzapine: 2 studies 1 versus chlorpromazine 1 versus haloperidol	1664	Clozapine is effective in TRS. Data on others SGAs are inconclusive.

Chakos et al, 2001 [55]	Meta-analysis	Clozapine versus FGA: 7 studies 1 versus standard care 2 versus chlorpromazine 4 versus haloperidol Olanzapine versus FGA: 2 studies 1 versus chlorpromazine 1 versus haloperidol Clozapine versus risperidone: 2 studies Risperidone versus haloperidol: 1 study	1916	Effect sizes: Clozapine versus FGA: 0.14 to 0.81 Olanzapine versus FGA: 0.18 to 0.29 Clozapine versus risperidone: 0.27 to 0.35 Risperidone versus Haloperidol: 0.14
Moncrieff, 2003 [56]	Systematic review and meta-analysis	Clozapine versus FGA: 9 studies 1 versus usual care 3 versus chlorpromazine 5 versus haloperidol	1199	High heterogeneity of studies. Meta-analysis using ITT showed a range of 0.38 (FEM) to 0.44 SDs (REM) favoring clozapine. Meta-regression: larger differences in short-term studies and in those sponsored by pharmaceutical companies.
Tuunainen et al, 2002/2006 [57]	Systematic review and meta-analysis	Clozapine versus SGA: 8 studies 2 versus olanzapine 1 versus remoxipride/ risperidone/zotepine 1 versus remoxipride 4 versus risperidone	795	Almost no differences between groups in terms of global improvement and relapses. Clozapine showed a trend for being more effective for positive symptoms. SGAs showed a trend for being more effective in cognitive functions.

Abbreviations: FGA, first-generation antipsychotic; FEM, fixed effect model; ITT, intention to treat; NNT, number needed to treat; REM, random effect model; SGA, second-generation antipsychotic; TRS, treatment-resistant schizophrenia.

olanzapine). The effect size for clozapine was obtained from studies involving populations of patients who had TRS, but the authors of this meta-analysis have not acknowledged this issue.

Pragmatic Trials

Unlike randomized, controlled trials, pragmatic or practical trials are designed to measure effectiveness in a real-world setting and population to provide more complete information for the physician in clinical practice [61].

Two recent important pragmatic trials support the effectiveness of clozapine over SGAs for the treatment of schizophrenia. Evoy and colleagues [62], in a phase II trial in the Clinical Antipsychotic Trials of Intervention Effectiveness study [63] (which involved about 1400 patients), studied 99 patients who had not responded to atypical antipsychotics in previous phases of the trial because of lack of efficacy [64]. Patients were assigned randomly to open-label clozapine (n = 49) or to blinded treatment with another SGA (olanzapine, n = 19; quetiapine n = 15; or risperidone n =16). When compared with other SGAs, clozapine had the greatest reductions in the PANSS total score and the lowest discontinuation rates; that is, the use of clozapine proved to be more effective than switching to another SGA in patients who previously had not responded to another SGA.

In another pragmatic trial Lewis and colleagues [65] studied 136 patients who had schizophrenia and who had showed a poor response to two or more antipsychotic medications. The patients were assigned randomly to receive clozapine (n = 67) or an SGA (risperidone, olanzapine, quetiapine, amisulpride) (n = 69). At the end of 1 year patients who received clozapine showed a reduction in psychopathology (PANSS score) and improved quality of life. The authors state that patients who have schizophrenia and who have had a previous poor response to two or more antipsychotic drugs should receive clozapine instead of another SGA.

Suicide

Because suicide is an important outcome dimension of TRS, it is important to mention the results of the 2-year International Suicide Prevention Trial [66] in which 980 patients who had schizophrenia (about 260 of whom had TRS), recruited from 67 medical centers in 11 countries, were assigned randomly to treatment with either clozapine or olanzapine. The rates of suicidal behavior or suicide attempts were significantly lower in patients taking clozapine than in those taking olanzapine, although the rates of deaths from suicide were not statistically different between groups. A number-needed-to-treat of 13 was obtained; that is, 1 less patient will have a suicidal event for every 13 high-risk patients treated with clozapine rather than olanzapine.

Predictors of Clozapine Response

Because of the importance of clozapine in treating TRS, the author and colleagues reviewed its main predictors of response. Chung and Remington [67] also have published an excellent review on this subject.

Clinical Predictors of response to clozapine
A number of authors have investigated the factors associated with response to clozapine in cohort studies and have found that high psychopathologic levels, female gender, early onset of the disorder, and years of schooling are predictors of good response [68–70]. Other authors however, have obtained opposite results in cohort studies and have found the best clozapine responders to be those who at baseline displayed lower levels of psychopathologic severity and less severe negative and extrapyramidal symptoms [71].

Dose response for clozapine
Doses of clozapine of 300 to 600 mg/d correlate with the plasma threshold for response [37,67].

Plasma levels
Although studies are not unanimous, plasmatic levels equal to or greater than 350 ng/mL and reaching 500 ng/mL tend to be associated with a good response when these levels are not influenced by the use of nicotine [67,72]. Miller and colleagues [73] and Potkin and colleagues [74], however, observed that around 30% of non-responders achieved plasma levels above the supposed adequate threshold.

Genetic factors in response to clozapine
It has been well established that genetic factors influence response to medication. Genetic variants caused by polymorphisms of the dopaminergic receptors D2, D3, and D4 and genetic variants of the serotoninergic receptors 5 HT2a, 5HT2c, and 5HT6 have been shown to influence the response to clozapine [75]. Glutamate and norepinephrine receptors were investigated also [67], and recently the metabolic activity of the prefrontal cortex of patients responsive to clozapine has been shown to be associated with alleles of the D1 receptor [76]. As reviewed by Chung and Remington [67], however, the available data on the genetic predictors of treatment response to clozapine presently are inconsistent.

Neuroimaging Factors for Response to Clozapine
Structural factors
The prefrontal region has an important role in the mediation of treatment response to atypical antipsychotics. Three CT studies consistently found that an increased prefrontal sulcal prominence was associated with a lesser response to clozapine [77–79]. An MRI study found that larger right prefrontal gray matter volumes were associated with better treatment response in patients taking clozapine, as compared with those treated with haloperidol [80]. One CT study [81] and one MRI study [82], however, found no relationship between prefrontal atrophy and treatment response to clozapine.

One of the most consistent findings observed in three studies was the reduction of the caudate in patients taking clozapine when compared with patients who received an FGA [83–86]; only one study reported negative results [80].

Functional factors

Studies using single photon emission tomography [87,88] and positron emission tomography [89] have observed an association between a reduction of metabolic activity in the prefrontal regions and clozapine response. A study by Chen and colleagues [90], however, showed opposite results (ie, increase prefrontal activity associated with clozapine response). Studies using positron emission tomography, which is a more precise technique, found reduced metabolic rates in the frontal lobes and increased metabolism in the striatum [91]. As previously mentioned, a later study by the same authors found an association between reduced metabolism in various brain areas and response to clozapine in patients who were homozygotes for the *2.2 DRD1* gene, whereas no such reduction was found in nonresponders who were homozygotes for *1.2 DRD1* [76].

Reviewing this evidence, Chung and Remington [67] suggested that as yet there are no predictors of treatment response to clozapine; rather, there are markers. The reduction in frontal cortex metabolism seen with positron emission tomography, the reduction of the caudate volume seen with MRI, the baseline severity of psychopathology, and clozapine plasma levels cannot be considered predictors of response because of the inconsistency of the data.

Polypharmacy

The use of polypharmacy in schizophrenia is widespread [92–95], although there is no evidence that this empiric therapeutic habit is superior to monotherapy. Some believe that combinations of SGAs are well tolerated and may be effective in the treatment of TRS [96]; others authors remain more cautious because of the lack of well-controlled studies [97] or possible evidence of harm (eg, increased mortality) [98]. In a naturalistic study in seven psychiatric hospitals, Janssen and colleagues [99] found that patients discharged with more than one antipsychotic medication had significantly poorer outcomes in both mental state and social functioning. Suzuki and colleagues [93] observed an improvement when patients treated with antipsychotic polytherapy were switched to monotherapy.

It is estimated, however, that approximately 30% of patients treated with clozapine do not respond adequately, remaining with persistent psychotic symptomatology despite having received adequate treatment for sufficient periods. Such patients are called "partial responders to clozapine," "clozapine resistant," or even "super-refractory" and represent a challenge for the treatment of TRS as well as a great economic burden [100].

The treatment of these patients is problematic, and pharmacologic and non-pharmacologic augmentation strategies remain the only options for this population, despite the lack of adequate evidence for their efficacy [12,100]. Many reviews have described such strategies in detail and are subsequently summarized [96,97,100–104].

Clozapine polypharmacy and other augmentation strategies

A narrow definition of partial or incomplete response to clozapine is the persistence of psychotic symptoms despite a trial of clozapine with adequate doses (ie, 300–900 mg/d) for a minimum of 8 weeks and for up to 6 months with plasma levels reaching 350 ng/mL [72]. Thus the improvement of psychotic symptoms is considered the main treatment target, and, as an apparent logical consequence, the addition of high-potency antipsychotic medications to clozapine has been proposed for the treatment of these symptoms.

Various antipsychotic agents have been used, supposedly to augment the antipsychotic properties of clozapine: amisulpride [105,106], aripiprazole [107], haloperidol [108], loxapine [109], olanzapine [110], pimozide [111], and ziprasidone [112]. The benefit of these augmentation strategies remains inconclusive because they were tested in case series or case reports, which have a low strength of evidence as compared with controlled trials [103,104].

More robust evidence is derived from four placebo-controlled trials, one with sulpiride [113] and three with risperidone [114–116] . Because of their importance, these trials are summarized here.

The study by Shiloh and colleagues [113] showed a significant improvement in positive and negative symptoms in the group that received clozapine plus sulpiride when compared with placebo group. It was suggested that this effect could be explained by the selective enhancement of D2 blockage by sulpiride.

It is well known that risperidone has a strong affinity for D2 receptors, but the hypothesis that the blocking these receptors would improve persistent positive symptoms in patients resistant to clozapine was supported only by the study by Josiassen and colleagues [114]. The studies by Yagcioglu [115] and by Honer [116] found no differences between the risperidone and placebo groups.

Therefore these studies did not support the hypothesis that adding a more potent antipsychotic to enhance or optimize D2 affinity would improve psychotic symptoms in persons who respond poorly to clozapine . In the study by Yagcioglu and colleagues [115], the placebo group showed a greater reduction in PANSS positive scores than the risperidone group, and the neuropsychologic evaluation of the same sample published in a subsequent study showed no benefit of risperidone in terms of cognitive functions [117].

Finally, when clozapine augmentation with antipsychotics fails, switching to another antipsychotic has been proposed. This strategy is considered to have a weak level of evidence [12]. Olanzapine was the antipsychotic most tested in four open trials [118–121].

Other medications were tested in controlled trials for augmenting clozapine efficacy in ameliorating negative or cognitive symptoms (eg, serine [122], cycloserine [123], glycine [124,125], ampakine), depression (fluoxetine [126], mirtazapine [127]), and mood (lithium [128], lamotrigine [129]). Other compounds such as allopurinol [130], valproic acid [131], carbamazepine [132], topiramate [133], and benzodiazepines [103] also were tested in clinical trials.

Nonpharmacologic augmentation strategies
Electroconvulsive therapy and transcranial magnetic stimulation. Although various guidelines [33] and algorithms [35] (www.ipap.org) recommend electroconvulsive therapy as an augmentation strategy for clozapine nonresponders, only

two studies provide evidence of efficacy for this intervention. Tang and Un-gvari [134], compared a group 15 patients who had TRS (some of whom were resistant to clozapine) with 15 controls (who had refused clozapine or had switched to another antipsychotic medication). After a certain number of sessions, the investigators observed improvement in the whole group in some outcome measures such as CGI score but not in psychopathologic mea-sures such as the BPRS. The authors did not provide a separate analysis of the clozapine-resistant subgroup to verify the effectiveness electroconvulsive ther-apy for these patients.

In an open-label study electroconvulsive therapy was administered to 11 clo-zapine nonresponders who showed improvement in positive and negative symptoms and in global score on the PANSS. The eight who responded were followed up for a mean period of 16 weeks; and the authors observed that four of them relapsed [135].

Although transcranial magnetic stimulation (TMS) has been used in con-trolled studies to treat medication-resistant auditory hallucinations [136–139], there is only one open-label trial in which TMS was administered to seven pa-tients being treated with clozapine. These patients showed improvement in the severity of their persistent hallucinations [140]. At the time this article is being written, the first controlled study of the use of TMS to treat persistent hallucina-tions in clozapine nonresponders (active TMS = 6 patients; "sham" treatment = 5 patients) by Rosa and colleagues [141] has been submitted for publication. The authors show that TMS can be administered safely to patients taking clozapine, but no significant differences between groups were seen because of lack of power.

Psychosocial strategies
Cognitive behavioral therapy has been used extensively in patients who are re-fractory to antipsychotic medications [142–144] but only two studies included patients resistant to clozapine [145,146] showing that this technique can help them control their symptoms, specially hallucinations. The authors have pre-sented preliminary data showing that cognitive behavioral therapy in patients who have severe symptoms and also are resistant to clozapine can improve general psychopathology and quality of life [147].

SUMMARY

TRS continues to be challenge for clinicians despite considerable progress in the therapeutics of schizophrenia with the advent of SGAs. The neurobiologic mechanisms underlying TRS are still unclear, and progress will come through better-designed studies and adequately powered randomized, controlled trials. The pharmacogenetic studies seem to be the most promising approach, spe-cially when they are integrated with clinical and neuroimaging findings.

SGAs should be used as the first two steps for treatment of psychotic epi-sodes of schizophrenia. The presently available evidence from randomized, controlled trials, practical trials, meta-analyses, guidelines, and algorithms indicates that clozapine is necessarily the third step. Ignoring this evidence is not justified unless patients develop intolerance or severe side effects with clozapine.

Special attention should be given to patients who do not respond to clozapine. Current augmentation strategies are essentially empiric and are based on case reports or open-label trials; therefore there currently is not enough evidence to recommend any of those treatments. There is an urgent need for intense research, particularly well-designed, randomized, controlled trials, in this population.

References

[1] Itil T, Keskiner A, Fink M. Therapeutic studies in therapy resistant schizophrenic patients. Compr Psychiatry 1966;7:488–93.

[2] Meltzer HY. Commentary: defining treatment refractoriness in schizophrenia. Schizophr Bull 1990;16:563–5.

[3] Henna J, Elkis H. Predictors of response and outcome in treatment resistant versus non treatment resistant schizophrenics patients. Schizophr Res 1999;36:281–2.

[4] Conley R, Kelly D. Management of treatment resistant schizophrenia. Biol Psychiatry 2001;50:898–911.

[5] Pantelis C, Lambert T. Managing patients with "treatment resistant" schizophrenia. Med J Aust 2003;5:s62–6.

[6] Andreasen N, Carpenter W, Kane J, et al. Remission in schizophrenia: proposed criteria and rationale for consensus. Am J Psychiatry 2005;162:441–9.

[7] Overall J, Gorham D. The Brief Psychiatric Rating Scale. Psychol Rep 1962;10:799–812.

[8] Kay SR, Fiszbein A, Opler LA. The Positive and Negative Syndrome Scale (PANSS) for schizophrenia. Schizophr Bull 1987;13(2):261–76.

[9] Hegarty JD, Baldessarini RJ, Tohen M, et al. One hundred years of schizophrenia: a meta-analysis of the outcome literature. Am J Psychiatry 1994;151(10):1409–16.

[10] Lieberman JA. Prediction of outcome in first-episode schizophrenia. J Clin Psychiatry 1993;54(Suppl):13–7.

[11] Kane J, Hognifeld G, Singer J, et al. Clozapine for the treatment-resistant schizophrenic. A double-blind comparison with chlorpromazine. Arch Gen Psychiatry 1988;45:789–96.

[12] Miller A, McEvoy J, Jeste D, et al. Treatment of chronic schizophrenia. In: Lieberman J, Stroup TS, Perkins D, editors. Textbook of schizophrenia. Washington, DC: The American Psychiatric Publishing; 2006. p. 365–81.

[13] Meltzer H, Kostacoglu A. Treatment-resistant schizophrenia. In: Lieberman J, Murray R, editors. Comprehensive care of schizophrenia: a textbook of clinical management. London (UK): Martin Dunitz; 2001. p. 181–203.

[14] Meltzer HY, Rabinowitz J, Lee MA, et al. Age at onset and gender of schizophrenic patients in relation to neuroleptic resistance. Am J Psychiatry 1997;154(4):475–82.

[15] Lindenmayer J. Treatment refractory schizophrenia. Psychiatr Q 2000;71:373–84.

[16] Lindenmayer JP, Czobor P, Volavka J, et al. Effects of atypical antipsychotics on the syndromal profile in treatment-resistant schizophrenia. J Clin Psychiatry 2004;65(4):551–6.

[17] Lindenmayer J, Bernstein-Hyman R, Grochowski S. The psychopathology of schizophrenia: initial validation of a five factor model. Psychopathology 1995;28:22–31.

[18] McMahon R, Kelly D, Kreyenbuhl J, et al. Novel factor-based symptom scores in treatment resistant schizophrenia: implications for clinical trials. Neuropsychopharmacology 2002;26:537–45.

[19] Alves T, Pereira JR, Elkis H. The psychopathological factors of refractory schizophrenia. J Bras Psiquiatr 2005;27:108–12.

[20] Woerner MG, Mannuzza S, Kane JM. Anchoring the BPRS: an aid to improved reliability. Psychopharmacol Bull 1988;24(1):112–7.

[21] Elkis H, Alves TM, Eizenman IB. Reliability of the Brazilian version of the BPRS Anchored. Schizophr Res 1999;36:7–8.

[22] Buckley P, Shendakar N. Treatment-refractory schizophrenia. Curr Opin Psychiatry 2005;18:165–73.

[23] Peuskens J. The evolving definition of treatment resistance. J Clin Psychiatry 1999; 60(suppl 12):4–8.

[24] Citrome L, Bilder R, Volavka J. Managing treatment resistant schizophrenia: evidence from randomized controlled trials. J Psychiatr Pract 2002;8:205–15.

[25] Siegfried S, Fleischhaker W, Lieberman J. Pharmacological treatment of schizophrenia. In: Lieberman J, Murray R, editors. Comprehensive care of schizophrenia: a textbook of clinical management. London (UK): Martin Dunitz; 2001. p. 59–94.

[26] Sheitman B, Lieberman J. The natural history and pathophysiology of treatment resistant schizophrenia. J Psychiatr Res 1988;32:143–50.

[27] Csernansky JG, Yesavage JA, Maloney W, et al. The treatment response scale: a retrospective method of assessing response to neuroleptics. Am J Psychiatry 1983;140(9): 1210–3.

[28] May PRA, Dencker SJ, Hubbard JW. A systematic approach to treatment resistance in schizophrenic disorders. In: Dencker SJ, Kulhanek F, editors. Treatment resistance in schizophrenia. Braunschweig (Germany): Viewag Verlag; 1988. p. 22–3.

[29] Brenner HD, Dencker SJ, Goldstein MJ, et al. Defining treatment refractoriness in schizophrenia. Schizophr Bull 1990;16(4):551–61.

[30] Brenner HD, Merlo MCG. Definition of therapy-resistant schizophrenia and its assessment. Eur Psychiatry 1995;10(suppl 1):11s–7s.

[31] Wallace C. Functional assessment in rehabilitation. Schizophr Bull 1986;24:112–7.

[32] Guy W. ECDEU Assessment Manual of Psychopharmacology, Publication No. ADM-76-36US. Rockville (MD): Department of Health, Education and Welfare; 1976.

[33] Lehman AF, Lieberman JA, Dixon LB, et al. Practice guideline for the treatment of patients with schizophrenia, second edition. Am J Psychiatry 2004;161(2 Suppl):1–56.

[34] Lehman AF, Kreyenbuhl J, Buchanan RW, et al. The Schizophrenia Patient Outcomes Research Team (PORT): updated treatment recommendations 2003. Schizophr Bull 2004;30(2):193–217.

[35] Miller AL, Hall CS, Buchanan RW, et al. The Texas Medication Algorithm Project antipsychotic algorithm for schizophrenia: 2003 update. J Clin Psychiatry 2004;65(4): 500–8.

[36] Morrison D. Management of refractory schizophrenia. Br J Psychiatry 1996;169(Suppl 31):15–20.

[37] Kinon BJ, Ahl J, Stauffer VL, et al. Dose response and atypical antipsychotics in schizophrenia. CNS Drugs 2004;18(9):597–616.

[38] Cazzullo CL. Biological and clinical studies on schizophrenia related to pharmacological treatment. Recent Adv Biol Psychiatry 1963;5:114–43.

[39] Weinberger DR, Bigelow LB, Kleinman JE, et al. Cerebral ventricular enlargement in chronic schizophrenia. An association with poor response to treatment. Arch Gen Psychiatry 1980;37:11–3.

[40] Friedman L, Lys C, Schulz SC. The relationship of structural brain imaging parameters to antipsychotic treatment response: a review. J Psychiatry Neurosci 1992;17(2): 42–54.

[41] Sharma T, Kerwin R. Biological determinants of difficult to treat patients with schizophrenia. Br J Psychiatry 1996;169(supp 31):5–9.

[42] Lieberman J, Alvir J, Koreen A, et al. Psychobiological correlates of treatment response in schizophrenia. Neurpsychopharmacology 1996;14(3S):13S–21S.

[43] Crosthwaite CG, Reveley MA. Structural imaging and treatment response in schizophrenia. In: Reveley MA, William Deakin JF, editors. The psychopharmacology of schizophrenia. London (UK): Arnold; 2000. p. 89–108.

[44] Staal WG, Hulshoff Pol HE, Schnack HG, et al. Structural brain abnormalities in chronic schizophrenia at the extremes of the outcome spectrum. Am J Psychiatry 2001;158(7): 1140–2.

[45] Lawrie SM, Ingle GT, Santosh CG, et al. Magnetic resonance imaging and single photon emission tomography in treatment-responsive and treatment-resistant schizophrenia. Br J Psychiatry 1995;167(2):202–10.

[46] Lawrie SM, Abukmeil SS, Chiswick A, et al. Qualitative cerebral morphology in schizophrenia: a magnetic imaging study and systematic literature review. Schizophr Res 1997;25:155–66.

[47] Altamura AC, Bassetti R, Cattaneo E, et al. Some biological correlates of drug resistance in schizophrenia: a multidimensional approach. World J Biol Psychiatry 2005;2(6 Suppl): 23–30.

[48] Verhoeven WM, van Praag HM, van Ree JM, et al. Improvement of schizophrenic patients treated with [des-Tyr1]-gamma-endorphin (DTgammaE). Arch Gen Psychiatry 1979; 36(3):294–8.

[49] Vaddadi KS, Gilleard CJ, Mindham RH, et al. A controlled trial of prostaglandin E1 precursor in chronic neuroleptic resistant schizophrenic patients. Psychopharmacology (Berl) 1986;88(3):362–7.

[50] Lerner Y, Mintzer Y, Schestatzky M. Lithium combined with haloperidol in schizophrenic patients. Br J Psychiatry 1988;153:359–62.

[51] Huang CC, Gerhardstein RP, Kim DY, et al. Treatment-resistant schizophrenia: controlled study of moderate- and high-dose thiothixene. Int Clin Psychopharmacol 1987;2(1):69–75.

[52] Emsley R. Role of the newer antipsychotics in the management of treatment-resistant schizophrenia. CNS Drugs 2001;13:409–20.

[53] Gray G. Evidence based psychiatry. Washington, DC: American Psychiatric Publishing; 2004.

[54] Wahlbeck K, Cheine M, Essali A, et al. Evidence of clozapine's effectiveness in schizophrenia: a systematic review and meta-analysis of randomized trials. Am J Psychiatry 1999;156(7):990–9.

[55] Chakos M, Lieberman J, Hoffman E, et al. Effectiveness of second-generation antipsychotics in patients with treatment-resistant schizophrenia: a review and meta-analysis of randomized trials. Am J Psychiatry 2001;158(4):518–26.

[56] Moncrieff J, Clozapine V. Conventional antipsychotic drugs for treatment-resistant schizophrenia: a re-examination. Br J Psychiatry 2003;183:161–6.

[57] Tuunainen A, Wahlbeck K, Gilbody S. Newer atypical antipsychotic medication in comparison to clozapine: a systematic review of randomized trials. Schizophr Res 2002;56(1–2):1–10.

[58] Taylor DM, Duncan-McConnell D. Refractory schizophrenia and atypical antipsychotics. J Psychopharmacol 2000;14(4):409–18.

[59] Geddes J, Freemantle N, Harrison P, et al. Atypical antipsychotics in the treatment of schizophrenia: systematic overview and meta-regression analysis. BMJ 2000; 321(7273):1371–6.

[60] Davis JM, Chen N, Glick ID. A meta-analysis of the efficacy of second-generation antipsychotics. Arch Gen Psychiatry 2003;60(6):553–64.

[61] Perkins DO. Clinical trials in schizophrenia with results for the real world. CNS Spectr 2006;11(7 Suppl 7):9–13.

[62] McEvoy JP, Lieberman JA, Stroup TS, et al. Effectiveness of clozapine versus olanzapine, quetiapine, and risperidone in patients with chronic schizophrenia who did not respond to prior atypical antipsychotic treatment. Am J Psychiatry 2006;163(4): 600–10.

[63] Stroup TS, McEvoy JP, Swartz MS, et al. The National Institute of Mental Health Clinical Antipsychotic Trials of Intervention Effectiveness (CATIE) project: schizophrenia trial design and protocol development. Schizophr Bull 2003;29(1):15–31.

[64] Lieberman JA, Stroup TS, McEvoy JP, et al. Effectiveness of antipsychotic drugs in patients with chronic schizophrenia. N Engl J Med 2005;353(12):1209–23.

[65] Lewis SW, Barnes TR, Davies L, et al. Randomized controlled trial of effect of prescription of clozapine versus other second-generation antipsychotic drugs in resistant schizophrenia. Schizophr Bull 2006;32(4):715–23.

[66] Meltzer HY, Alphs L, Green AI, et al. Clozapine treatment for suicidality in schizophrenia: International Suicide Prevention Trial (InterSePT). Arch Gen Psychiatry 2003;60(1): 82–91.

[67] Chung C, Remington G. Predictors and markers of clozapine response. Psychopharmacology (Berl) 2005;179(2):317–35.

[68] Ciapparelli A, Dell'Osso L, Pini S, et al. Clozapine for treatment-refractory schizophrenia, schizoaffective disorder, and psychotic bipolar disorder: a 24-month naturalistic study. J Clin Psychiatry 2000;61(5):329–34.

[69] Ciapparelli A, Dell'Osso L, Bandettini di Poggio A, et al. Clozapine in treatment-resistant patients with schizophrenia, schizoaffective disorder, or psychotic bipolar disorder: a naturalistic 48-month follow-up study. J Clin Psychiatry 2003;64(4):451–8.

[70] Ciapparelli A, Ducci F, Carmassi C, et al. Predictors of response in a sample of treatment-resistant psychotic patients on clozapine. Eur Arch Psychiatry Clin Neurosci 2004;254(5): 343–6.

[71] Umbricht DS, Wirshing WC, Wirshing DA, et al. Clinical predictors of response to clozapine treatment in ambulatory patients with schizophrenia. J Clin Psychiatry 2002;63(5): 420–4.

[72] Schulte P. What is an adequate trial with clozapine?: therapeutic drug monitoring and time to response in treatment-refractory schizophrenia. Clin Pharmacokinet 2003;42:607–18.

[73] Miller DD, Fleming F, Holman TL, et al. Plasma clozapine concentrations as a predictor of clinical response: a follow-up study. J Clin Psychiatry 1994;55(Suppl B):117–21.

[74] Potkin SG, Bera R, Gulasekaram B, et al. Plasma clozapine concentrations predict clinical response in treatment-resistant schizophrenia. J Clin Psychiatry 1994;55(Suppl B):133–6.

[75] Mancama D, Arranz MJ, Kerwin RW. Genetic predictors of therapeutic response to clozapine: current status of research. CNS Drugs 2002;16(5):317–24.

[76] Potkin SG, Basile VS, Jin Y, et al. D1 receptor alleles predict PET metabolic correlates of clinical response to clozapine. Mol Psychiatry 2003;8(1):109–13.

[77] Friedman L, Knutson L, Shurell M, et al. Prefrontal sulcal prominence is inversely related to response to clozapine in schizophrenia. Biol Psychiatry 1991;29(9):865–77.

[78] Honer WG, Smith GN, Lapointe JS, et al. Regional cortical anatomy and clozapine response in refractory schizophrenia. Neuropsychopharmacology 1995;13(1):85–7.

[79] Konicki PE, Kwon KY, Steele V, et al. Prefrontal cortical sulcal widening associated with poor treatment response to clozapine. Schizophr Res 2001;48(2–3):173–6.

[80] Arango C, Breier A, McMahon R, et al. The relationship of clozapine and haloperidol treatment response to prefrontal, hippocampal, and caudate brain volumes. Am J Psychiatry 2003;160(8):1421–7.

[81] Bilder RM, Wu H, Chakos MH, et al. Cerebral morphometry and clozapine treatment in schizophrenia. J Clin Psychiatry 1994;55(Suppl B):53–6.

[82] Lauriello J, Mathalon DH, Rosenbloom M, et al. Association between regional brain volumes and clozapine response in schizophrenia. Biol Psychiatry 1998;43(12): 879–86.

[83] Chakos MH, Lieberman JA, Alvir J, et al. Caudate nuclei volumes in schizophrenic patients treated with typical antipsychotics or clozapine. Lancet 1995;345(8947):456–7.

[84] Frazier JA, Giedd JN, Kaysen D, et al. Childhood-onset schizophrenia: brain MRI rescan after 2 years of clozapine maintenance treatment. Am J Psychiatry 1996;153(4):564–6.

[85] Scheepers FE, de Wied CC, Hulshoff Pol HE, et al. The effect of clozapine on caudate nucleus volume in schizophrenic patients previously treated with typical antipsychotics. Neuropsychopharmacology 2001;24(1):47–54.

[86] Scheepers FE, Gispen de Wied CC, Hulshoff Pol HE, et al. Effect of clozapine on caudate nucleus volume in relation to symptoms of schizophrenia. Am J Psychiatry 2001;158(4): 644–6.

[87] Rodriguez VM, Andree RM, Castejon MJ, et al. Fronto-striato-thalamic perfusion and clozapine response in treatment-refractory schizophrenic patients. A 99mTc-HMPAO study. Psychiatry Res 1997;76(1):51–61.

[88] Molina Rodriguez V, Montz Andree R, Perez Castejon MJ, et al. SPECT study of regional cerebral perfusion in neuroleptic-resistant schizophrenic patients who responded or did not respond to clozapine. Am J Psychiatry 1996;153(10):1343–6.

[89] Molina V, Reig S, Sarramea F, et al. Anatomical and functional brain variables associated with clozapine response in treatment-resistant schizophrenia. Psychiatry Res 2003; 124(3):153–61.

[90] Chen RY, Chen E, Ho WY. A five-year longitudinal study of the regional cerebral metabolic changes of a schizophrenic patient from the first episode using Tc-99m HMPAO SPECT. Eur Arch Psychiatry Clin Neurosci 2000;250(2):69–72.

[91] Potkin SG, Buchsbaum MS, Jin Y, et al. Clozapine effects on glucose metabolic rate in striatum and frontal cortex. J Clin Psychiatry 1994;55(Suppl B):63–6.

[92] McCue RE, Waheed R, Urcuyo L. Polypharmacy in patients with schizophrenia. J Clin Psychiatry 2003;64(9):984–9.

[93] Suzuki T, Uchida H, Tanaka KF, et al. Revising polypharmacy to a single antipsychotic regimen for patients with chronic schizophrenia. Int J Neuropsychopharmacol 2004;7(2): 133–42.

[94] Ananth J. Long term antipsychotic polypharmacy is common among Medicaid recipients with schizophrenia. Evid Based Ment Health 2005;8(2):55.

[95] Barbui C, Nose M, Mazzi MA, et al. Persistence with polypharmacy and excessive dosing in patients with schizophrenia treated in four European countries. Int Clin Psychopharmacol 2006;21(6):355–62.

[96] Lerner V, Libov I, Kotler M, et al. Combination of "atypical" antipsychotic medication in the management of treatment-resistant schizophrenia and schizoaffective disorder. Prog Neuropsychopharmacol Biol Psychiatry 2004;28(1):89–98 [Write to the Help Desk NCBI | NLM | NIH Department of Health & Human Services Privacy Statement | Freedom of Information Act | Disclaimer Dec 18 2006 06:34:27.].

[97] Freudenreich O, Goff D. Antipsychotic combination therapy in schizophrenia. A review of efficacy and risks of current medications. Acta Psychiatr Scand 2002;106:323–30.

[98] Waddington JL, Youssef HA, Kinsella A. Mortality in schizophrenia. Antipsychotic polypharmacy and absence of adjunctive anticholinergics over the course of a 10-year prospective study. Br J Psychiatry 1998;173:325–9.

[99] Janssen B, Weinmann S, Berger M, et al. Validation of polypharmacy process measures in inpatient schizophrenia care. Schizophr Bull 2004;30(4):1023–33.

[100] Buckley P, Miller A, Olsen J, et al. When symptoms persist: clozapine augmentation strategies. Schizophr Bull 2001;27(4):615–28.

[101] Barnes TR, McEvedy CJ, Nelson HE. Management of treatment resistant schizophrenia unresponsive to clozapine. Br J Psychiatry Suppl 1996;31:31–40.

[102] Williams L, Newton G, Roberts K, et al. Clozapine-resistant schizophrenia: a positive approach. Br J Psychiatry 2002;181:184–7.

[103] Remington G, Saha A, Chong SA, et al. Augmentation strategies in clozapine-resistant schizophrenia. CNS Drugs 2005;19(10):843–72.

[104] Mouaffak F, Tranulis C, Gourevitch R, et al. Augmentation strategies of clozapine with antipsychotics in the treatment of ultraresistant schizophrenia. Clin Neuropharmacol 2006;29(1):28–33.

[105] Munro J, Matthiasson P, Osborne S, et al. Amisulpride augmentation of clozapine: an open non-randomized study in patients with schizophrenia partially responsive to clozapine. Acta Psychiatr Scand 2004;110(4):292–8.

[106] Agelink MW, Kavuk I, Ak I. Clozapine with amisulpride for refractory schizophrenia. Am J Psychiatry 2004;161(5):924–5.

[107] Henderson DC, Kunkel L, Nguyen DD, et al. An exploratory open-label trial of aripiprazole as an adjuvant to clozapine therapy in chronic schizophrenia. Acta Psychiatr Scand 2006;113(2):142–7.

[108] Rajarethinam R, Gilani S, Tancer M, et al. Augmentation of clozapine partial responders with conventional antipsychotics. Schizophr Res 2003;60(1):97–8.

[109] Mowerman S, Siris SG. Adjunctive loxapine in a clozapine-resistant cohort of schizophrenic patients. Ann Clin Psychiatry 1996;8(4):193–7.

[110] Gupta S, Sonnenberg SJ, Frank B. Olanzapine augmentation of clozapine. Ann Clin Psychiatry 1998;10(3):113–5.

[111] Friedman J, Ault K, Powchik P. Pimozide augmentation for the treatment of schizophrenic patients who are partial responders to clozapine. Biol Psychiatry 1997;42(6):522–3.

[112] Kaye NS. Ziprasidone augmentation of clozapine in 11 patients. J Clin Psychiatry 2003;64(2):215–6.

[113] Shiloh R, Zemishlany Z, Aizenberg D, et al. Sulpiride augmentation in people with schizophrenia partially responsive to clozapine. A double-blind, placebo-controlled study. Br J Psychiatry 1997;171:569–73.

[114] Josiassen RC, Joseph A, Kohegyi E, et al. Clozapine augmented with risperidone in the treatment of schizophrenia: a randomized, double-blind, placebo-controlled trial. Am J Psychiatry 2005;162(1):130–6.

[115] Anil Yagcioglu AE, Kivircik Akdede BB, Turgut TI, et al. A double-blind controlled study of adjunctive treatment with risperidone in schizophrenic patients partially responsive to clozapine: efficacy and safety. J Clin Psychiatry 2005;66(1):63–72.

[116] Honer WG, Thornton AE, Chen EY, et al. Clozapine alone versus clozapine and risperidone with refractory schizophrenia. N Engl J Med 2006;354(5):472–82.

[117] Akdede BB, Anil Yagcioglu AE, Alptekin K, et al. A double-blind study of combination of clozapine with risperidone in patients with schizophrenia: effects on cognition. J Clin Psychiatry 2006;67(12):1912–9.

[118] Henderson DC, Nasrallah RA, Goff DC. Switching from clozapine to olanzapine in treatment-refractory schizophrenia: safety, clinical efficacy, and predictors of response. J Clin Psychiatry 1998;59(11):585–8.

[119] Dossenbach MRK, Beuzen JN, Avnon M, et al. The effectiveness of olanzapine in treatment-refractory schizophrenia when patients are nonresponsive to or unable to tolerate clozapine. Clin Ther 2000;22(9):1021–34.

[120] Littrell KH, Johnson CG, Hilligoss NM, et al. Switching clozapine responders to olanzapine. J Clin Psychiatry 2000;61(12):912–5.

[121] Lindenmayer JP, Czobor P, Volavka J, et al. Olanzapine in refractory schizophrenia after failure of typical or atypical antipsychotic treatment: an open-label switch study. J Clin Psychiatry 2002;63(10):931–5.

[122] Tsai GE, Yang P, Chung LC, et al. D-serine added to clozapine for the treatment of schizophrenia. Am J Psychiatry 1999;156(11):1822–5.

[123] Goff DC, Tsai G, Manoach DS, et al. D-cycloserine added to clozapine for patients with schizophrenia. Am J Psychiatry 1996;153(12):1628–30.

[124] Potkin SG, Jin Y, Bunney BG, et al. Effect of clozapine and adjunctive high-dose glycine in treatment-resistant schizophrenia. Am J Psychiatry 1999;156(1):145–7.

[125] Evins AE, Fitzgerald SM, Wine L, et al. Placebo-controlled trial of glycine added to clozapine in schizophrenia. Am J Psychiatry 2000;157(5):826–8.

[126] Buchanan RW, Kirkpatrick B, Bryant N, et al. Fluoxetine augmentation of clozapine treatment in patients with schizophrenia. Am J Psychiatry 1996;153(12):1625–7.

[127] Zoccali R, Muscatello MR, Cedro C, et al. The effect of mirtazapine augmentation of clozapine in the treatment of negative symptoms of schizophrenia: a double-blind, placebo-controlled study. Int Clin Psychopharmacol 2004;19(2):71–6.

[128] Small JG, Klapper MH, Malloy FW, et al. Tolerability and efficacy of clozapine combined with lithium in schizophrenia and schizoaffective disorder. J Clin Psychopharmacol 2003;23(3):223–8.

[129] Tiihonen J, Hallikainen T, Ryynanen OP, et al. Lamotrigine in treatment-resistant schizophrenia: a randomized placebo-controlled crossover trial. Biol Psychiatry 2003;54(11): 1241–8.

[130] Lara DR, Brunstein MG, Ghisolfi ES, et al. Allopurinol augmentation for poorly responsive schizophrenia. Int Clin Psychopharmacol 2001;16(4):235–7.

[131] Kando JC, Tohen M, Castillo J, et al. Concurrent use of clozapine and valproate in affective and psychotic disorders. J Clin Psychiatry 1994;55(6):255–7.

[132] Simhandl C, Meszaros K, Denk E, et al. Adjunctive carbamazepine or lithium carbonate in therapy-resistant chronic schizophrenia. Can J Psychiatry 1996;41(5):317.

[133] Tiihonen J, Halonen P, Wahlbeck K, et al. Topiramate add-on in treatment-resistant schizophrenia: a randomized, double-blind, placebo-controlled, crossover trial. J Clin Psychiatry 2005;66(8):1012–5.

[134] Tang WK, Ungvari GS. Efficacy of electroconvulsive therapy in treatment-resistant schizophrenia: a prospective open trial. Prog Neuropsychopharmacol Biol Psychiatry 2003;27(3):373–9.

[135] Kho KH, Blansjaar BA, de Vries S, et al. Electroconvulsive therapy for the treatment of clozapine nonresponders suffering from schizophrenia—an open label study. Eur Arch Psychiatry Clin Neurosci 2004;254(6):372–9.

[136] Hoffman RE, Hawkins KA, Gueorguieva R, et al. Transcranial magnetic stimulation of left temporoparietal cortex and medication-resistant auditory hallucinations. Arch Gen Psychiatry 2003;60(1):49–56.

[137] McIntosh AM, Semple D, Tasker K, et al. Transcranial magnetic stimulation for auditory hallucinations in schizophrenia. Psychiatry Res 2004;127(1–2):9–17.

[138] Hoffman RE, Gueorguieva R, Hawkins KA, et al. Temporoparietal transcranial magnetic stimulation for auditory hallucinations: safety, efficacy and moderators in a fifty patient sample. Biol Psychiatry 2005;58(2):97–104.

[139] Lee SH, Kim W, Chung YC, et al. A double blind study showing that two weeks of daily repetitive TMS over the left or right temporoparietal cortex reduces symptoms in patients with schizophrenia who are having treatment-refractory auditory hallucinations. Neurosci Lett 2005;376(3):177–81.

[140] d'Alfonso AA, Aleman A, Kessels RP, et al. Transcranial magnetic stimulation of left auditory cortex in patients with schizophrenia: effects on hallucinations and neurocognition. J Neuropsychiatry Clin Neurosci 2002;14(1):77–9.

[141] Rosa M, Gattaz W, Rosa M, et al. Effects of repetitive transcranial magnetic stimulation on auditory hallucinations refractory to clozapine. J Clin Psychiatry, in press.

[142] Sensky T, Turkington D, Kingdon D, et al. A randomized controlled trial of cognitive-behavioral therapy for persistent symptoms in schizophrenia resistant to medication. Arch Gen Psychiatry 2000;57(2):165–72.

[143] Dickerson FB. Cognitive behavioral psychotherapy for schizophrenia: a review of recent empirical studies. Schizophr Res 2000;43(2–3):71–90.

[144] Turkington D, Kingdon D, Weiden PJ. Cognitive behavior therapy for schizophrenia. Am J Psychiatry 2006;163(3):365–73.

[145] Pinto A, La Pia S, Mennella R, et al. Cognitive-behavioral therapy and clozapine for clients with treatment-refractory schizophrenia. Psychiatr Serv 1999;50(7):901–4.

[146] Valmaggia LR, van der Gaag M, Tarrier N, et al. Cognitive-behavioural therapy for refractory psychotic symptoms of schizophrenia resistant to atypical antipsychotic medication. Randomised controlled trial. Br J Psychiatry 2005;186:324–30.

[147] Barretto E, Avrichir B, Camargo M, et al. Randomized controlled trial of cognitive behavioral therapy for partial response to clozapine. Schizophr Res 2006;81(Suppl S):101.

Rehabilitation and Recovery in Schizophrenia

Dawn I. Velligan, PhD[a,*], Jodi M. Gonzalez, PhD[b]

[a]Department of Psychiatry, Division of Schizophrenia and Related Disorders-MSC 7792, University of Texas Health Science Center at San Antonio, 7703 Floyd Curl, San Antonio, TX 78229–3900, USA
[b]Department of Psychiatry, Division of Mood & Anxiety Disorders, University of Texas Health Science Center at San Antonio, University Plaza, 7526 Louis Pasteur, San Antonio, TX 78229–3900, USA

Schizophrenia is a severe and persistent mental illness characterized by a constellation of signs and symptoms including positive symptoms (hallucinations, delusions, disordered speech and behavior), negative symptoms (amotivation, asociality, poverty of speech and movement), and cognitive deficits (impaired information-processing speed, attention, memory, and executive functions [1,2]. Moreover, multiple domains of functional outcome, including performance of independent living skills, social functioning, and occupational/educational performance and attainment, are impaired for individuals who have schizophrenia [1,3]. Schizophrenia remains one of the top 10 leading causes of disability worldwide in young adults.

The focus of psychiatric rehabilitation is the management of persistent symptoms and the reduction of the long-term disability often associated with schizophrenia [4]. Medication management forms a foundation for the process of recovery which seeks to help each individual maximize his or her potential and outcomes [5,6]. The recovery model focuses on instilling hope for the future, setting individual goals, capitalizing on strengths, and building skills to allow the individual to grow and to achieve meaningful work, supportive social relationships, and a better quality of life [7]. Psychiatric remediation and rehabilitation techniques to promote recovery include a comprehensive and coordinated range of services addressing many domains of outcome.

The advent of novel medications for schizophrenia in the past decade has been paralleled by the development of a number of innovative, evidence-based rehabilitation strategies designed to improve specific areas of functional outcome [6]. This article describes a variety of psychosocial interventions targeting

This work is supported by National Institute of Mental Health grant R01 MH074047–01A1 to Dr. Velligan.

*Corresponding author. E-mail address: velligand@uthscsa.edu (D.I. Velligan).

0193-953X/07/$ – see front matter   © 2007 Elsevier Inc. All rights reserved.
doi:10.1016/j.psc.2007.05.001   psych.theclinics.com

improvements in psychiatric symptoms, cognition, and a broad range of functional outcomes and discusses the evidence base regarding the impact of these interventions on the recovery process for individuals who have schizophrenia.

COGNITIVE BEHAVIOR THERAPY

Cognitive Behavior Therapy (CBT) for schizophrenia is a treatment designed to address positive symptoms that remain after medication treatment has been optimized. Although available antipsychotic medications reduce positive symptoms, many patients continue to struggle with hallucinations or delusions that impact adjustment and quality of life. CBT is focused on helping individuals develop alternative explanations for the symptoms of their illness and reduce the impact of these symptoms on their behavior [8,9]. CBT is based partly on the evidence that emotional processes, information-processing deficits, and reasoning and appraisal biases contribute to the formation and maintenance of delusions and hallucinations and that these processes can be changed through cognitive intervention [10,11].

During the process of CBT, in the context of a strong therapeutic alliance, the client and therapist discuss and evaluate the specific content of delusions and hallucinations. The therapist works first to understand thoroughly the patient's perspective as to how the hallucinations and beliefs described have developed (eg, "The Secret Service started tapping my phone after I broke up with my girlfriend."), later raising questions about the sources of the problem (eg, "Could it be any agency other than the Secret Service"? "Did you know that when people have a relationship breakup they are under a great deal of stress?"), and eventually helping the individual conduct behavioral experiments to test explanations (eg, asking trusted family members whether they hear the clicks on the telephone line) and suggesting alternative explanations for events [8]. This process slowly allows clients to evaluate their own explanatory model for their experiences and to consider other possible explanations and interpretations of events.

A series of prospective, randomized, controlled clinical trials has demonstrated the efficacy of CBT for the treatment of persistent positive symptoms in patients who have schizophrenia [9,12–15]. The average effect sizes for CBT versus control treatments for reducing symptomatology are in the moderate range [9,16]. CBT is considered standard of care in the United Kingdom, and interest in this method of treatment continues to grow in the United States. [8,17]. Although researchers have worked to extend CBT into group settings, results have failed to demonstrate the efficacy of group CBT for decreasing symptoms [18]. Group CBT, however, has been found to lead to more positive evaluations of oneself and the future [18]. Research on CBT suggests it is a promising approach to addressing persistent symptoms in schizophrenia.

CBT approaches have also been applied to individuals who do not comply with medication because of poor insight into having a mental disorder [19–22]. The CBT approach provides more freedom to attempt to frame the issue of adherence in a way that is most acceptable to the patient's own perspective of the problem and the treatment options. Previous treatment failures, contradictory information, and disappointments in attaining goals are discussed. The clinician withholds comments and interventions regarding adherence until the client's perspective is fully understood. Over time the therapist helps clients make the connection between their own goals for recovery, the barriers to reaching those goals, and how medication may be able to assist in this process. Evidence supporting CBT-based compliance therapies has been mixed [21,23,24], but more methodologically rigorous trials of CBT for medication adherence are needed [25].

INTERVENTIONS TARGETING COGNITIVE IMPAIRMENTS
In the context of a generalized intellectual deficit, specific cognitive impairments are present in schizophrenia in the areas of information processing speed, attention, memory, and executive functions [1,26]. These cognitive impairments are believed to underlie much of the functional role impairment observed in schizophrenia [1,3]. Moreover, impairments in cognitive functioning have been found to interfere with skill acquisition in rehabilitation programs. The increasing recognition of the importance of addressing cognitive impairment has led to the development of several cognitive rehabilitation strategies for individuals who have schizophrenia. Some of these techniques seek to improve or restore cognitive abilities directly; others are considered compensatory in nature and attempt to bypass impairments in cognitive functioning to improve community outcomes [27].

Cognitive Remediation
Cognitive Remediation (CR) seeks to improve and/or restore cognitive functions directly using a variety of pen-and-paper or computerized tests requiring cognitive skills such as attention, planning, problem solving, and/or memory [27–32]. CR approaches are based on theories of cognitive development and approaches adapted from the treatment of brain-injured populations. A basic tenet of CR is that the brain's neuroplastic reserve can be enriched by cognitive experiences provided through training [33]. Improvements in cognitive and functional outcomes may be accomplished through a combination of drill and practice exercises and group or individual training sessions focusing on higher-level abstraction of social, work-related, or problem-solving themes [27]. Many successful CR programs are embedded in comprehensive rehabilitation programs where cognitive exercises work synergistically with psychosocial groups or other treatment modalities.

Many independent CR programs have been developed. The neuropsychologic educational approach to rehabilitation program created by Alice Medalia [31,32] is based on teaching techniques developed within educational psychology that promote intrinsic motivation and task engagement. The conceptual model favors a top-down approach that emphasizes higher-order, strategy-based methods of learning over drill and practice exercises that focus on learning of elementary cognitive skills (a bottom-up approach). Training involves participation in computer-based cognitive exercises (eg, computer games such as "Where in the World is Carmen San Diego?") that are designed to be engaging, enjoyable, and intrinsically motivating and require the recruitment of several cognitive skills within a contextualized format.

The Neurocognitive Enhancement Therapy program developed by Bell and colleagues [34,35] focuses on CR in the context of work rehabilitation. This program uses computerized software programs targeting attention, memory, and executive functions. Training begins with relatively simple exercises and proceeds to more complex ones. As an individual masters a task at a prespecified level, the parameters of the task are changed to allow mastery of increasingly difficult material. This approach is designed to keep motivation at optimum levels. In addition to computerized exercises, participants attend a weekly social-processing group where they are given feedback on work performance and suggestions for improvement are discussed.

Cognitive Remediation Therapy developed by Til Wykes [30] focuses on teaching patients to develop their own individualized set of problem-solving strategies. The individually delivered training program targets deficits in executive processes including cognitive flexibility, working memory, and planning. This program uses paper-and-pencil exercises for training, begins with simpler tasks and proceeds to more difficult ones, and emphasizes teaching through procedural learning, scaffolding, and errorless learning [36].

Cognitive Enhancement Therapy developed by the late Gerald Hogarty [33] is a comprehensive rehabilitation program designed to enhance abstraction of social themes and alter cognitive schemas for individuals who have recent-onset schizophrenia. Cognitive Enhancement Therapy is based on a neurodevelopmental model of schizophrenia that suggests that disturbances in neurodevelopment result in delays in social cognition. Social cognitive milestones such as perspective taking are therefore the focus of treatment. Computer-based cognitive exercises focus on attention, memory, and problem-solving abilities. In addition, participants attend a social-cognition training group. Social interaction is emphasized throughout treatment, and even the computer sessions are conducted in pairs of patients who assist one another by suggesting strategies and offering encouragement.

Reviews of the CR literature generally have been positive and have concluded that CR improves multiple domains of cognitive functioning not limited to the tasks used in the cognitive training [27,37–39]. Moreover, studies have established that improvements for individuals who have schizophrenia and who participate in CR programs are not limited to cognitive improvements. Depending on the type of CR program, improvements have been found in a range of outcomes, including independent living skills, obtaining employment, job tenure, hours worked, and money earned in vocational rehabilitation, improved social problem-solving skills, and social adjustment [27,28,30–34,40]. Effect sizes for improvements in specific training exercises generally have been large, with more moderate effect sizes for other cognitive outcomes and improvements in community functioning [40]. Although there is no consensus regarding which approach to CR is best for particular patients, the importance of an adequate amount of treatment, proper training of therapists conducting CR and motivational factors within the participant are mentioned as important factors for maximizing outcomes [27,40,41].

Compensatory or Adaptive Strategies to Bypass Cognitive Impairment
Rather than attempting to alter neurocognitive function per se, adaptive strategies attempt to bypass cognitive deficits by establishing supports or prosthetic devices in the environment to improve functioning. These techniques have been used for years in the rehabilitation of individuals who have head injuries or mental retardation. More recently, cognitive adaptation training (CAT) has applied these strategies to individuals with schizophrenia [42–44].

CAT is a psychosocial treatment that uses environmental supports such as alarms, signs, checklists, and the reorganization of belongings to cue and sequence adaptive behavior in the home environment. CAT treatment focuses on impairments in adaptive functioning in areas such as medication and appointment adherence, grooming and hygiene, care of living space, and leisure and social activities. Treatment strategies are based on a comprehensive assessment of cognitive functioning, behavior, and environment. CAT is based on the idea that impairments in executive functioning lead to problems in initiating and/or inhibiting appropriate behaviors. Using behavioral principles such as antecedent control, environments are set up to cue appropriate behaviors, discourage distraction, and maintain goal-directed activity. In addition, adaptations are customized for specific cognitive strengths or limitations in attention, memory, and fine motor control (eg, changing the color of signs frequently to capture attention, using Velcro closures instead of buttons for someone who has fine-motor problems). Examples of CAT interventions include signs asking "Did I take my medication?" placed on the back of the front door, medication containers with alarms to cue taking medication at specific times, reorganization of closets to prevent soiled or inappropriate clothing from being worn, money management or job-hunting notebooks, and checklists reminding the individual to perform specific grooming or leisure tasks.

CAT has been shown to improve adherence to medication, community functioning, and rates of relapse for individuals who have schizophrenia [42–44]. Large effect sizes (Cohen's D > 1.0) have been found for improvements in functioning and medication adherence with CAT relative to control and treatment-as-usual conditions [43–45]. Larger randomized trials are underway currently to examine issues regarding the length and durability of treatment effects and factors mediating treatment outcomes. Recent evidence suggests that environmental adaptations are highly likely to be used in a comprehensive program such as CAT in which supports are individualized and set up in the patient's home environment. Supports are far less likely to be used when they are generic and given to patients in the clinic rather than on home visits [45].

Adaptive supports for specific problems such as medication adherence also are available. One example is the Med-eMonitor (Informedix, Rockville, MD) device, which stores up to a month's supply of five different medications, cues the taking of medication at specific times with an alarm, asks the patient whether the medication has been taken, and downloads adherence data to a secure Website for retrieval by a case manager. Preliminary data suggest that such devices improve adherence to medication in schizophrenia [22]. Given the advances in the development of new technologies, it is likely that the use of electronic environmental supports will continue to increase in the treatment of schizophrenia.

Fig. 1 illustrates the two primary approaches to cognitive rehabilitation: restorative/enhancing versus compensatory. The ultimate goal of both strategies is to improve community functioning in individuals who have schizophrenia.

SOCIAL SKILLS TRAINING

Social skills deficits are common among individuals who have schizophrenia. Based on a neurodevelopmental model for schizophrenia, individuals who go on to develop schizophrenia have cognitive deficits that may have prevented or interfered with the acquisition of adequate social skills during development [46]. Many of these individuals may not have mastered the skills necessary to maintain adult relationships and to function successfully in their social roles. Social skills training teaches specific skills that lead to effective behavior in social interactions. Specific skills may include nonverbal behavior, such as appropriate eye contact and voice volume, conversational skills such as introducing

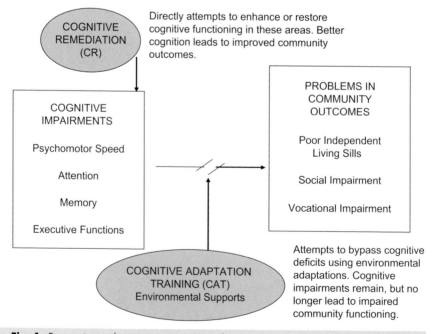

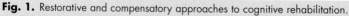

Fig. 1. Restorative and compensatory approaches to cognitive rehabilitation.

oneself to a new person and taking the perspective of another person, and problem-solving skills such as expressing dissatisfaction and generating solutions to interpersonal problems [46].

Although there are different models of social skills training, many interventions attempt to reduce cognitive demands by using visual aids and by modeling desired behaviors [47]. Most break complex social behaviors down into components that can be addressed through specific teaching techniques. Participants may be taught in a didactic manner the steps to perform a behavior, watch the behavior of a model, and then practice the behavior while receiving coaching and corrective feedback from the group [46,48]. When skills are improved, patients' interactions with others may become more successful and rewarding, leading to increased social participation.

Social skills training has been found to increase specific behaviors necessary to communicate effectively [46–49]. In addition, research indicates that social skills training decreases rates of relapse, reduces symptomatology, and improves social functioning [50–52]. Maintenance of gains in learning lasting as long as 2 years after training have been found [53]. It is difficult, however, to determine the extent to which these new social skills are generalized to the individual's environment outside the training context. Specific mechanisms to generalize training to the natural environment may be necessary to ensure transfer of skills to everyday life [53].

INTEGRATED TREATMENTS FOR COMORBID SUBSTANCE ABUSE IN SCHIZOPHRENIA

Between 20% and 75% of individuals who have schizophrenia have comorbid substance abuse disorders [54,55]. Comorbid substance abuse increases the likelihood of poor adherence to medication and is associated with more severe positive symptoms, more frequent hospitalizations, and poorer prognosis [55,56]. Moreover, individuals who have co-occurring substance abuse and schizophrenia are more likely than those who have schizophrenia alone to exhibit poor occupational and role functioning, to demonstrate higher levels of depression and anxiety, and to have unstable housing, poor access to health care, and more involvement with the legal system [55,57,58].

Although traditional 12-Step programs such as Alcoholics Anonymous or Narcotics Anonymous may be helpful for some patients, available data suggest that outcomes for patients are better in programs that integrate mental health and substance abuse treatments [59–65]. Integrated treatment has been found to decrease costs associated with the hospitalization and contact with the criminal justice system [55,66].

Integrated treatments for dual-diagnosis patients make use of many different treatment modalities including intensive case management, motivational interviewing, 12-Step programs focused on dual diagnosis, CBT, social skills training, contingency management, and family psychoeducation [66]. Many successful programs do not have abstinence from substance use as a goal but instead use a harm-reduction model that focuses on reducing the harmful consequences of substance abuse for the patient and society. One example of integrated treatment using a harm-reduction model is called "behavioral treatment for substance abuse in schizophrenia" [63]. The treatment involves motivational interviewing to develop treatment goals, urinalysis with social and small monetary reinforcements for "clean" urine, social skills training aimed at providing the patient with the skills necessary to refuse drugs when offered and to develop friendships with those who do not use drugs, education regarding how drugs affect the brain and medications for psychiatric illness, and teaching ways to cope with high-risk situations. This treatment has been found to decrease drug use and increase the frequency of "clean" urine drug screens [63]. More than 54% of individuals in integrated treatment had at least one 4-week period of clean urine test results compared with just over 16% of those in supportive group treatment. Multimodal treatments for substance abuse and schizophrenia are important to provide to assist individuals who have a dual diagnosis with the process of recovery.

VOCATIONAL REHABILITATION AND SUPPORTED EMPLOYMENT

Gainful employment is an important goal for many individuals who have schizophrenia. Gainful employment can enhance economic independence, self-esteem, and community adaptation [67,68]. Although most individuals who have schizophrenia state they want to work, employment rates range from only about 10% to 20% [69]. Train-and-place models of vocational rehabilitation that focus on prevocational training to prepare individuals for the job market have not been found to be particularly successful in helping individuals who have schizophrenia secure jobs in the competitive market place and have fallen out of favor [70]. In contrast, supported employment programs, including the individual placement and support model, emphasize rapid placement in a competitive job tailored to the individual's interests and strengths, the job training specific to the duties of the position, and ongoing support from a collaborative team [67,71,72]. Supported employment programs follow a place-then-train philosophy in which training takes place in the job setting with a job coach. This approach eliminates the need for generalization of behaviors to new settings.

Numerous randomized, controlled trials have found that individuals participating in these specialized vocational programs are more likely to obtain employment and to earn more money than those in comparison rehabilitation services [67,68,71–73]. More than 50% of individuals in supported employment programs have been found to work competitively versus less than 20% in comparison groups. This difference translates into an effect size close to 80 [68]. Retention of employment and achieving the full benefits of supported employment for a wider range of individuals remain obstacles that must be addressed. Factors that influence retention and success include negative symptoms of schizophrenia, recent hospitalization, cognitive deficits, and persistent psychotic symptoms [69,74]. Recent efforts that combine cognitive remediation and supported employment have demonstrated beneficial effects on both cognitive skills and employment outcomes [34,69]. Continued enhancements of the supported employment model are likely to extend positive outcomes to a broader range of individuals who have schizophrenia.

FAMILY PSYCHOEDUCATION

Research has consistently indicated that high levels of criticism and overinvolvement by family members can increase the risk of relapse for a person who has schizophrenia [7,75]. Moreover, being the primary caregiver for an individual who has schizophrenia can cause a significant amount of distress. Family psychoeducation offers information and support for family members who care for their relatives who have schizophrenia.

Although there are a number of different family treatment strategies, common elements include providing education about mental illness, helping members develop realistic expectations that take the illness into account, and providing training in communication and problem-solving skills. Family treatment can be provided for individual families or in group settings where members can learn information and effective coping skills and gain perspective from one another.

Decades of research indicate that family treatment results in lower rates of relapse in comparison to standard care or control treatments [76]. On average, the rate of relapse for individuals whose families participate in psychoeducation treatment is 24% compared with a rate of 64% for those receiving treatment as usual [75,77]. Treatments lasting 9 months or more have been found to produce more favorable outcomes than those of shorter duration [7]. Family intervention has been found to decrease the family's experience of burden and to increase members' ability to cope with the illness [78]. Moreover, there is evidence that participation in family treatment decreases health care costs resulting from the illness [7].

SUMMARY

A number of promising interventions have demonstrated efficacy for various aspects of schizophrenia. Much of the efficacy is domain specific. Interventions to address vocational needs or social skills do not necessarily improve symptomatology. Interventions designed to improve symptomatology and distress do not result in improved occupational functioning or social skills [75]. This experience suggests that an integrated approach to treatment involving multiple strategies may enhance the process of recovery and maximize a range of outcomes for individuals.

Implementation of Evidence-Based Psychosocial Rehabilitation Techniques into Community Practice

Although ways to treat many aspects of schizophrenia successfully have been identified, the illness remains one of the top 10 disabling conditions worldwide for young adults. Evidence-based treatments often are unavailable to large numbers of individuals who need or could benefit from them [79,80]. Issues of cost and reimbursement, the availability of trained service-delivery personnel, and overburdened health care systems remain significant obstacles.

The Website of the National Mental Health Information Center of the Substance Abuse and Mental Health Services Administration (http://mentalhealth. samhsa.gov/cmhs/communitysupport/toolkits/default.asp). provides tool kits designed to assist public mental health authorities in implementation of best practices such as supported employment and family psychoeducation. Information for consumers, families, and treatment providers is available. Recommendations include assembling a group of stakeholders to include consumers, families, and provider agencies to work on implementation of a specific practice, ensuring that all stakeholders have information about the efficacy, core principals, and resources necessary to deliver the intervention, identifying and overcoming practical and financial barriers to implementation and ensuring that performance outcome measures and financial incentives be put in place for service-delivery personnel. The use of a demonstration project is recommended to establish the effectiveness of the intervention for the stakeholders and to overcome financial and organizational barriers to implementation. By addressing these issues as they arise in a small demonstration project, implementation of the intervention on a larger-scale becomes possible. Consideration should be given to shifting resources from less successful programs to evidence-based practices. This strategy may improve the services delivered and outcomes for consumers while minimizing the financial burden for the agency. It also is important to establish mechanisms for ongoing training and supervision of staff at all levels and to continue to assess the fidelity with which the intervention is being applied. Research on implementation strategies for applying evidence-based practices in community settings continues to be important. A great deal of knowledge regarding what works has been gained. Putting in place the mechanisms to provide what works remains a significant challenge that must be addressed.

References

[1] Green MF. What are the functional consequences of neurocognitive deficits in schizophrenia? Am J Psychiatry 1996;153(3):321–30.

[2] Andreasen NC, Arndt S, Alliger R, et al. Symptoms of schizophrenia methods, meanings, and mechanisms. Arch Gen Psychiatry 1995;52:341–51.

[3] Velligan DI, Mahurin RK, Eckert SL, et al. Relationship between specific types of communication deviance and attentional performance in patients with schizophrenia. Psychiatry Res 1997;70:9–20.

[4] Liberman RP, Kopelowicz A, Smith TE. Psychiatric rehabilitation. In: Sadock BJ, Sadock V, editors. Kaplan and Sadock's comprehensive textbook of psychiatry. 7th edition. Baltimore (MD): Lippincott Williams & Wilkins; 1999. p. 3218–45.

[5] Bellack AS. Scientific and consumer models of recovery in schizophrenia: concordance, contrasts, and implications. Schizophr Bull 2006;32(3):432–42.

[6] Corrigan PW. Recovery from schizophrenia and the role of evidence-based psychosocial interventions. Expert Rev Neurother 2006;6(7):993–1004.

[7] Glynn SM, Cohen AN, Dixon LB, et al. The potential impact of the recovery movement on family interventions for schizophrenia: opportunities and obstacles. Schizophr Bull 2006;32(3):451–63.

[8] Turkington D, Kingdon D, Weiden PJ. Cognitive behavior therapy for schizophrenia. Am J Psychiatry 2006;163:365–73.

[9] Tarrier N, Wykes T. Is there evidence that cognitive behaviour therapy is an effective treatment for schizophrenia? a cautious or cautionary tale? Behav Res Ther 2004;42: 1377–401.

[10] Kuipers E, Garety P, Fowler D, et al. Cognitive, emotional, and social processes in psychosis: refining cognitive behavioral therapy for persistent positive symptoms. Schizophr Bull 2006;32(Suppl 1):S24–31.

[11] van der Gaag M. A neuropsychiatric model of biological and psychological processes in the remission of delusions and auditory hallucinations. Schizophr Bull 2006;32(Suppl 1): S113–22.

[12] Turkington D, Dudley R, Warman DM, et al. Cognitive-behavioral therapy for schizophrenia: a review. J Psychiatr Pract 2004;10(1):5–16.

[13] Rector N, Beck AT. Cognitive behavioural therapy for schizophrenia: an empirical review. J Nerv Ment Dis 2001;189:278–87.

[14] Lewis S, Tarrier N, Haddock G, et al. Randomised controlled trial of cognitive-behavioural therapy in early schizophrenia: acute-phase outcomes. Br J Psychiatry 2002;43(Suppl): S91–7.

[15] Tarrier N, Yusupoff L, Kinney C, et al. Randomised controlled trial of intensive cognitive behaviour therapy for patients with chronic schizophrenia. BMJ 1998;317:303–7.

[16] Zimmerman G, Favrod J, Trieu V, et al. The effect of cognitive behavioral treatment on the positive symptoms of schizophrenia spectrum disorders: a meta-analysis. Schizophr Res 2005;77:1–9.

[17] Keith SJ. Are we still talking to our patients with schizophrenia? Am J Psychiatry 2006;163(3):362–4.

[18] Barrowclough C, Haddock G, Lobban F, et al. Group cognitive-behavioural therapy for schizophrenia. Br J Psychiatry 2006;189:527–32.

[19] Kemp R, David A, Hayward P. Compliance therapy: an intervention targeting insight and treatment adherence in psychotic patients. Behavioural and Cognitive Psychotherapy 1996;24(4):331–50.

[20] Hayward P, Chan N, Kemp R, et al. Medication self-management: a preliminary report on an intervention to improve medication compliance. J Ment Health 1995;4(5):511–7.

[21] Kemp R, Kirov G, Everitt B, et al. Randomised controlled trial of compliance therapy. 18-month follow-up. Br J Psychiatry 1998;172:413–9.

[22] Velligan DI, Weiden PJ. Interventions to improve adherence to antipsychotic medications. Psychiatric Times 2006;23(9):50–3.

[23] Byerly MJ, Fisher R, Carmody T, et al. A trial of compliance therapy in outpatients with schizophrenia or schizoaffective disorder. J Clin Psychiatry 2005;66(8):997–1001.

[24] O'Donnell C, Donohoe G, Sharkey L, et al. Compliance therapy: a randomised controlled trial in schizophrenia. BMJ 2003;327(7419):834.

[25] McIntosh A, Conlon L, Lawrie SM, et al. A compliance therapy for schizophrenia. Cochrane Database Syst Rev 2006;3.

[26] Gold JM, Harvey PD. Cognitive deficits in schizophrenia. Psychiatr Clin of North Am 1993;16(2):295–312.

[27] Velligan DI, Kern RS, Gold JM. Cognitive rehabilitation for schizophrenia and the putative role of motivation and expectancies. Schizophr Bull 2006;32(3):474–85.

[28] Bell M, Bryson G, Greig T, et al. Neurocognitive enhancement therapy with work therapy: effects on neuropsychological test performance. Arch Gen Psychiatry 2001;58(8):763–8.

[29] Spaulding W, Reed D, Storzbach D, et al. The effects of a remediational approach to cognitive therapy for schizophrenia. In: Wykes T, Tarrier N, Lewis S, editors. Outcome and

innovation in psychological treatment of schizophrenia. West Sussex (UK): John Wiley & Sons, Ltd.; 1998. p. 145–60.

[30] Wykes T, Reeder C, Williams C, et al. Are the effects of cognitive remediation therapy (CRT) durable? Results from an exploratory trial in schizophrenia. Schizophr Bull 2003;61: 163–74.

[31] Medalia A, Revheim N, Casey M. The remediation of problem-solving skills in schizophrenia. Schizophr Bull 2001;27(2):259–67.

[32] Medalia A, Revheim N, Casey M. Remediation of problem-solving skills in schizophrenia: evidence of a persistent effect. Schizophr Res 2002;57(2–3):165–71.

[33] Hogarty GE, Flesher S, Ulrich R, et al. Cognitive enhancement therapy for schizophrenia: effects of a 2-year randomized trial on cognition and behavior. Arch Gen Psychiatry 2004;61(9):866–76.

[34] Wexler B, Bell M. Cognitive remediation and vocational rehabilitation for schizophrenia. Schizophr Bull 2005;31(4):931–41.

[35] Bell MD, Fiszdon J, Bryson G, et al. Effects of neurocognitive enhancement therapy in schizophrenia: normalisation of memory performance. Cognit Neuropsychiatry 2004;9(3):199–211.

[36] Wykes T, Reeder C. Cognitive remediation therapy for schizophrenia: an introduction. New York: Brunner-Routledge; 2005.

[37] Kurtz MM, Moberg PJ, Gur RC, et al. Approaches to cognitive remediation of neuropsychological deficits in schizophrenia: a review and meta-analysis. Neuropsychol Rev 2001;11(4):197–210.

[38] Twamley EW, Jeste DV, Bellack AS. A review of cognitive training in schizophrenia. Schizophr Bull 2003;29(2):359–82.

[39] Wykes T, van der Gaag M. Is it time to develop a new cognitive therapy for psychosis—cognitive remediation therapy (CRT)? Clin Psychol Rev 2001;21(8):1227–56.

[40] Medalia A, Richardson R. What predicts a good response to cognitive remediation interventions? Schizophr Bull 2005;31(4):942–53.

[41] Silverstein SM, Wilkniss SM. At issue: the future of cognitive rehabilitation of schizophrenia. Schizophr Bull 2004;30(4):679–92.

[42] Velligan DI, Bow-Thomas CC. Two case studies of cognitive adaptation training for outpatients with schizophrenia. Psychiatr Serv 2000;51(1):25–9.

[43] Velligan DI, Prihoda TJ, Ritch JL, et al. A randomized single-blind pilot study of compensatory strategies in schizophrenia outpatients. Schizophr Bull 2002;28(2):283–92.

[44] Velligan DI, Diamond PM, Zeber J, et al. Cognition adaptation training improves adherence to medication and functional outcome in schizophrenia. [abstract to ICOSR]. Schizophr Bull 2007.

[45] Velligan DI, Mueller J, Wang M. Use of environmental supports among patients with schizophrenia. Psychiatr Serv 2006;57(2):219–24.

[46] Bellack AS. Skills traning for people with severe mental illness. Psychiatr Rehabil J 2004;27(4):375–91.

[47] Liberman RP, Wallace CJ, Blackwell G, et al. Skills training versus psychosocial occupational therapy for persons with persistent schizophrenia. Am J Psychiatry 1998;155: 1087–91.

[48] Heinssen RK, Liberman RP, Kopelowicz A. Psychosocial skills training for schizophrenia: lessons from the laboratory. Schizophr Bull 2000;26:21–46.

[49] Marder SR, Wirshing WC, Mintz J, et al. Two-year outcome for social skills training and group psychotherapy for outpatients with schizophrenia. Am J Psychiatry 1996;153: 1585–92.

[50] Benton MK, Schroeder HE. Social skills training with schizophrenics: a meta-analytic evaluation. J Consult Clin Psychol 1990;58:741–7.

[51] Corrigan PW, Wallace CJ, Green MF. Deficits in social schemata in schizophrenia. Schizophr Res 1992;8:129–35.

[52] Smith TE, Bellack AS, Liberman RP. Social skills training for schizophrenia: review and future directions. Clin Psychol Rev 1996;16(7):599–617.

[53] Kopelowicz A, Liberman RP, Zarate R. Recent advances in social skills training for schizophrenia. Schizophr Bull 2006;32(Suppl 1):S12–23.

[54] Mueser KT, Bellack AS, Blanchard J. Comorbidity of schizophrenia and substance abuse: implications for treatment. J Clin Psychol 1992;60:845–56.

[55] Tsuang J, Fong TW, Lesser I. Psychosocial treatment of patients with schizophrenia and substance abuse disorders. Addictive Disorders & Their Treatment 2006;5(2):53–66.

[56] Dixon LB, Postrado L, Delahanty J, et al. The association of medical comorbidity in schizophrenia with poor physical and mental health. J Nerv Ment Dis 1999;187(8): 496–502.

[57] Compton M, Weiss P, West J, et al. The associations between substance use disorders, schizophrenia-spectrum disorders, and axis IV psychosocial problems. Soc Psychiatry Psychiatr Epidemiol 2005;40(12):939–46.

[58] Margolese HC, Negrete JC, Tempier R, et al. A 12-month prospective follow-up study of patients with schizophrenia-spectrum disorders and substance abuse: changes in psychiatric symptoms and substance use. Schizophr Res 2006;83(1):65–75.

[59] Minkoff K. Developing standards of care for individuals with co-occurring psychiatric and substance use disorders. Psychiatr Serv 2001;52:597–9.

[60] Tsuang J, Ho A, Eckman TA, et al. Dual diagnosis treatment for patients with schizophrenia who are substance dependent. Psychiatr Serv 1997;48(7):887–9.

[61] Ho AP, Tsuang JW, Liberman RP, et al. Achieving effective treatment of patients with chronic psychotic illness and comorbid substance dependence. Am J Psychiatry 1999;156(11): 1765–70.

[62] Drake R, Essock SE, Shaner A. Implementing dual diagnosis services for clients with severe mental illness. Psychiatr Serv 2001;52:469–76.

[63] Bellack AS, Bennett ME, Gearon JS, et al. A randomized clinical trial of a new behavioral treatment for drug abuse in people with severe and persistant mental illness. Arch Gen Psychiatry 2006;63:426–32.

[64] Ziedonis D, D'Avanzo K. Schizophrenia and substance abuse, dual diagnosis & treatment: substance abuse and comorbid medical and psychiatric disorders. New York: Marcel & Dekker Inc.; 1998.

[65] Drake R, Wallach M, Alverson H, et al. Psychosocial aspects of substance abuse by clients with severe mental illness. J Nerv Ment Dis 2002;190:100–6.

[66] Ziedonis D, Smelson D, Rosenthal R, et al. Improving the care of individuals with schizophrenia and substance use disorders: consensus recommendations. J Psychiatr Pract 2005;11(5):315–39.

[67] Lehman AF, Goldberg R, Dixon LB, et al. Improving employment outcomes for persons with severe mental illnesses. Arch Gen Psychiatry 2002;59:165–72.

[68] Twamley EW, Jeste DV, Lehman AF. Vocational rehabilitation in schizophrenia and other psychotic disorders: a literature review and meta-analysis of randomized controlled trials. J Nerv Ment Dis 2003;191(8):515–23.

[69] McGurk SR, Mueser KT. Cognitive functioning, symptoms, and work in supported employment: a review and heuristic model. Schizophr Res 2004;70(2–3):147–73.

[70] Bond GR, Drake RE, Mueser KT, et al. An update on supported employment for people with severe mental illness. Psychiatr Serv 1997;48(3):335–46.

[71] Drake R, McHugo G, Bebout R, et al. A randomized clinical trial of supported employment for inner-city patients with severe mental disorders. Arch Gen Psychiatry 1999;56:627–33.

[72] Bond G, Dietzen L, McGrew J, et al. Accelerating entry into supported employment for persons with severe psychiatric disabilities. Rehabil Psychol 1995;40:91–111.

[73] Cook JA, Lehman AF, Drake R, et al. Integration of psychiatric and vocational services: a multisite randomized, controlled trial of supported employment. Am J Psychiatry 2005;162: 1948–56.

[74] Razzano LA, Cook JA, Burke-Miller JK, et al. Clinical factors associated with employment among people with severe mental illness. J Nerv Ment Dis 2005;193(11):705–13.

[75] Bustillo JR, Lauriello J, Horan WP, et al. The psychosocial treatment of schizophrenia: an update. Am J Psychiatry 2001;158(2):163–75.

[76] McFarlane WR, Dixon LB, Lukens E, et al. Family psychoeducation and schizophrenia: a review of the literature. J Marital Fam Ther 2003;29(2):223–45.

[77] Pilling S, Bebbington P, Kuipers E, et al. Psychological treatments in schizophrenia: I. Meta-analysis of family intervention and cognitive behaviour therapy. Psychol Med 2002;32:763–82.

[78] Hazel NA, McDonnell MG, Short RA, et al. Impact of multiple-family groups for outpatients with schizophrenia on caregivers' distress and resources. Psychiatr Serv 2004;55(1):35–41.

[79] Ganju V. Implementation of evidence-based practices in state mental health systems: implications for research and effectiveness studies. Schizophr Bull 2003;29(1):125–31.

[80] Lehman AF, Buchanan RW, Dickerson F, et al. Evidence-based treatment for schizophrenia. Psychiatr Clin North Am 2003;26(4):939–54.

Families and Schizophrenia: The View from Advocacy

Leighton Y. Huey, MD[a,b,]*, Harriet P. Lefley, PhD[b,c,d],
David L. Shern, PhD[b,e], Cynthia A. Wainscott, BA[b,f]

[a]Department of Psychiatry, University of Connecticut Health Center, School of Medicine, 263 Farmington Avenue, Farmington, CT 06030-1410, USA
[b]The Annapolis Coalition on the Behavioral Health Workforce, 222 Piedmont Avenue, Suite 8900, Cincinnati, OH 45219, USA
[c]National Alliance on Mental Illness, Colonial Place Three, 2107 Wilson Boulevard, Suite 300, Arlington, VA 22201, USA
[d]Department of Psychiatry and Behavioral Sciences, University of Miami Miller School of Medicine, D-29, PO Box 016960, Miami, FL 33101, USA
[e]Mental Health America (formerly The National Health Association), 2000 North Beauregard, 6th Floor, Alexandria, VA 22311, USA
[f]Mental Health America of Etowah Valley, 25 Waterside Drive, Cartersville, GA 30121, USA

The history of understanding and interpreting causality in any field is not necessarily a pretty picture with irreproachable logic in the discovery process, rationality in determining cause, clarity in delineating what should be done, and, in the end, the presentation of a definitive roadmap as to how one should think. The context of knowledge and beliefs at the time determine the state of an idea.

In the interpretation of human behaviors over the millennia, there are many examples of what would or should now be regarded as ranging from totally outlandish concepts to half-truths to plausible ideas that have some bearing on what is believed to be the case. In Psychiatry, similarly, has progressed from a purely descriptive and observational field in the nineteenth and much of the twentieth centuries to one that now seeks to link itself to the modern fields of neuroscience, genetics, pharmacology, psychology, medicine, sociology, and economics. It is not surprising, therefore, when viewing the history of the development of theories in psychiatry through the lens of hindsight, that the great thinkers sometimes made great blunders, shaped in good part by the limitations in knowledge of the time. Perhaps there is no more charged area in psychiatry historically than that involving families and schizophrenia. This article focuses on this topic from the perspective of national advocacy.

*Corresponding author. E-mail address: huey@psychiatry.uchc.edu (L.Y. Huey).

0193-953X/07/$ – see front matter
doi:10.1016/j.psc.2007.04.006
© 2007 Elsevier Inc. All rights reserved.
psych.theclinics.com

HISTORICAL CONCEPTS OF THE FAMILY AND ITS IMPACT ON THE INDIVIDUAL WITH SCHIZOPHRENIA
Where Does Vilification End and Fact Begin?

Early theorists in psychiatry and psychology, which initially were descriptive and observational fields, speculated that the association of schizophrenia running in families reflected disordered family relationships; indeed, a pathologic family environment and interpersonal family dynamics were believed to be causative in the development of schizophrenia [1,2]. In the array of etiologic theories of schizophrenia, poor parenting and family dysfunction prevailed as explanatory models from the 1940s to the 1970s. The effects of these theories are still felt by families who coped with illness during those years. Psychoanalytic theory attributed schizophrenia to early developmental failures and toxic maternal anxiety. In the textbooks of the day, schizophrenia was variously attributed to schizophrenogenic mothers, mutually contradictory directives of the double bind generating emotional paralysis; communication deviance in families; marital schism (producing sons who had schizophrenia) or skew (producing daughters who had schizophrenia); and other models of family dysfunction. In family systems theory, the person who had schizophrenia was viewed as the bearer and manifestation of the family pathology [3].

It was the concept of the "schizophrenogenic mother" postulated by Fromm-Reichmann [4] that ultimately catalyzed a deep and wounded response from families outraged by the blame for schizophrenia being affixed to mothers who were alleged to be rejecting, rigid, incapable of empathy, perfectionistic, and fearful of both sexual and interpersonal intimacy. Subsequently, with perhaps slightly more political correctness, the interpersonal machinations of the father were added as additional factors in the development of schizophrenia [5,6]. Nuance on this theme was posited by others who postulated that communication stress in the form of the "double-bind" hypothesis, in which the individual child or young adult could not fully and simultaneously satisfy the demands of both parents placed the individual who had incipient schizophrenia into the dilemma of a psychologic spread-eagle that accounted for the emergence of "schizophrenic symptoms" [7]. This proposal led, partly in response to these theories affixing blame to the family, along with general unhappiness about the quality and experience of care, and families' need and search for mutual support, to the emergence of the national family advocacy movement. This movement complemented the decades-old national advocacy movement founded by a mental health consumer, Beers [8]. For some, this development resulted in a period of anger and mistrust toward the psychiatric establishment, leading to an estrangement between families and providers that is still palpable among some despite the passage of time. Several factors diminished the power of those early theories, and they now are essentially outmoded. Numerous analyses showed that they could not be supported empirically [9]. Much more rigorous findings from twin, adoption, and high-risk studies were beginning to provide presumptive evidence of genetic linkages.

Proliferating findings from other areas of medicine, such as hematology, radiology, and neuroimaging, were demonstrating biologic parameters of schizophrenia. An added factor to what seems in retrospect to have been often free-wheeling speculation in the absence of data was the lack of a meaningful system of classification at the time many of these primarily descriptive hypotheses dominated the field.

A More Contemporary View

Although the diathesis-stress model prevails today, environmental stress is not usually defined as nurture. Rather, it is linked to intrauterine or neonatal insult from factors such as maternal starvation or type A influenza virus during gestation or to obstetric complications. These are the areas deemed most critical for prevention of schizophrenia [10].

As new drugs emerged to control psychotic symptoms, with concurrent acknowledgment of patients' rights to least-restrictive settings and the implementation of Medicaid and Federal disability programs, deinstitutionalization began to empty hospital beds. The community mental health center legislation to provide community care (PL 94-63) required crisis, inpatient, outpatient, day hospital, and community consultation services but lacked a mandate for housing. More than two thirds of hospitalized patients were returned to live with their families. Today this pattern varies greatly by ethnicity, with African Americans, Asians, and Hispanics more likely to have the ill person live at home [11]. Families, who in prior hospital practice had been systematically discouraged from seeing their loved ones and rarely had been given information about the disorder, were now the new caregivers of people who had schizophrenia.

The impact of home care giving emerged in new research on family burden. Objective burden consists of measurable effects in household disruptions, economic burden, caregivers' loss of work, social, and leisure roles, and time spent negotiating the mental health, medical, social welfare, and sometimes criminal justice systems. Subjective burden refers to the emotional effects on the caregiver and other household members. Findings of numerous studies across a range of psychiatric disorders indicate that 30% to 60% of caregivers suffer significant distress, with the negative impact highest in schizophrenia [12].

Instead of either or both parents being castigated as responsible for the emergence of schizophrenia, communication deviance was described within such families [13–16]. These early studies, with operational criteria and early research design, evolved into the concept of "expressed emotion." A high valence of emotional display characterized by hostility, negativism, criticism (ie, in "high expressed emotion" or "high-EE" families), was believed to create conflict and stress in the emotionally dependent individual who had schizophrenia. High expressed emotion was associated with relapse more often than low expressed emotion, leading to the interpretation that the nature of communication within families has a bearing on symptom development, relapse, and prognosis for a family member who has schizophrenia [16–18]. Although family pathogenesis theories have been discredited, the deleterious impact of illness and symptomatic behaviors can generate countertherapeutic responses in care-givers. This finding led to a new area of important research. As Barrowclough [12] notes, for at least 3 decades research on the family environment and schizophrenia has become almost synonymous with the work on. Caregivers' attitudes are assessed on the Camberwell Family Interview. Remarks indicating hostile criticism or emotional overinvolvement with the patient above a certain cutoff point characterize families with high expressed emotion; families whose communications rank below the cutoff point have low expressed emotion. In numerous studies, including international replications, the dichotomized ex-pressed emotion score is extremely reliable in predicting patient relapse after hospitalization. High expressed emotion in families is predictive of the course of illness in many psychiatric conditions, particularly depression [12]. Interna-tional schizophrenia research, however, shows that low expressed emotion is modal in families in traditional cultures, whereas high expressed emotion may be more typical of Anglo families in the United Kingdom, the United Sates, and Australia [19]. Leff and Vaughn [20] have linked the better prognosis for schizophrenia in the developing countries to the importance of low ex-pressed emotion in extended kinship networks, in contrast to the care-giving burden of nuclear families of the industrialized west. A number of studies have reported that prosocial factors in families with low expressed emotion, such as warmth and positive remarks, also tend to deter relapse [21,22].

The research in expressed emotion gave rise to early models of family psy-choeducation, replacing the older family therapies. Although family education originally focused on reducing high expressed emotion, it was soon realized that high expressed emotion could be modified easily by educating families about its negative effects,. Moreover, families with low expressed emotion also needed the education and support provided by an empirically derived in-tervention that had no preconceptions of family pathology. Psychoeducation presents schizophrenia as a biologically based, stress-related illness that leads to multiple problems in living. The generic components of psychoeducation are education about the illness, support for families, problem-solving strategies, and illness-management techniques. In addition to understanding patients' likely physiologic arousal to environmental stressors, learning to defuse crises, and recognizing prodromal cues of decompensation, families are taught to re-duce their own feelings of guilt, confusion, helplessness, and overresponsibility. They become less judgmental and learn appropriate limits and expectations. Psychoeducational interventions in the United Kingdom and the United States were developed as clinical research projects. In numerous rigorous studies, in-cluding international replications, they demonstrated their effectiveness in de-terring relapse and easing family burden [11,12]. Unfortunately, despite its being an evidence-based practice, family psychoeducation is not widely applied in mental health systems today [23]. The efficacy studies require a 9-month commitment, not always achievable. Applications of the basic model have been extended and modified in many countries in Europe and Asia [24]. In the United States, more compact, shorter models have developed, such as the 12-week Family-to-Family program of the National Alliance on Mental Illness (NAMI), which is supported by many public mental health authorities. Family support groups sponsored by NAMI are found in every state and in more than 1100 localities. Other groups sponsored by Mental Health America (MHA) (formerly, the National Mental Health Association) or local mental health authorities provide education and fellowship as well. Research by McFarlane [25] indicates that psychoeducation for multifamily groups provides better outcomes than single-family models. The multifamily group offers mutual support and help, shared experiences, resource information, exchange of coping strategies, and, in some cases, the hope of recovery.

Finally, in contrast to family burden, several investigators have attempted to focus on family satisfaction in living with a member with schizophrenia. A longitudinal study of 122 mother–adult child dyads found that maternal expressions of warmth and praise were associated with a better quality of life and higher life satisfaction in adults who had schizophrenia [26]. These authors note that "in the mental health field, the emphasis had been on fixing families … with relatively little emphasis on the families' strengths, particularly the families' role in enhancing the life satisfaction of their loved one by being there as a source of support." The authors suggest that prosocial family processes, like warmth in the research on expressed emotion, may enhance many clients' potential for recovery. With such an historical perspective, admittedly brief and incomplete, the authors now shift the focus to what would be considered a more contemporary perspective on the broad topic of families and schizophrenia.

HOW FAMILIES RESPOND TO SCHIZOPHRENIA

In the modern concept of illness, schizophrenia connotes many things to the individual unfortunate enough to be given a competent diagnosis of schizophrenia, to his or her family, and to society. Individuals who have schizophrenia and their families may share a range of understandable responses including fear, anger, grief, mourning, disbelief, demoralization, loneliness, desperation—and for some, hope, fortitude, resourcefulness, adaptability, perseverance, and political assertiveness. These responses are all part of contending with the common symptoms of schizophrenia, especially the fear that both the individual and their family must feel in experiencing and witnessing the onset of the disorder. It is important to have practical approaches to help families deal most effectively with the family member who has schizophrenia. Respected national advocacy organizations (eg, NAMI, MHA) play critical roles at multiple levels in helping individuals who have psychiatric disorders and their families.

Families differ in their understanding and acceptance of mental illnesses and in their coping strategies. Their responses depend on the duration of illness, symptom intensity, levels of burden, and relatives' attributions. Research shows that families with high expressed emotion, especially those that respond with hostile criticism, tend to attribute volition to patients for their disturbed behaviors. The same is true for high–expressed emotion professionals and line staff [12]. Families with low expressed emotion do not hold the patient responsible. They have been described as calm, warm, and accepting, despite coping with equally severe psychopathology [20]. Cultural differences are evident in the international literature and among ethnic groups in the United States. Comparative studies indicate that ethnic minority families show fewer causal attributions, more home care giving, lower family burden, and less psychologic distress than Anglo-American families [27].

Parents, siblings, spouses, and children may respond in different ways, but all suffer some level of grief. Because schizophrenia often strikes in late adolescence or early adulthood, parents mourn the loss of the premorbid personality, perhaps once bright with promise. There is a feeling of dual loss—of the person who was and of the person who might have been. They share the suffering of the loved one who has schizophrenia, who also mourns unfulfilled life aspirations. Siblings, too, grieve the loss of a playmate or older brother or sister, and some become involved caregivers later in life. Many siblings, however, report shame, anger, embarrassment, and inability to bring friends home. They resent the diversion of parental attention and later have unresolved conflicts and guilt. Spouses suffer the loss of a mate and often must bear sole or major responsibilities for childrearing and the economic life of the family. Children may live in an unpredictable world, bewildered by parental behaviors that can cycle from loving and nurturing to fear-inducing. They may endure long separations and brief visitations, sharing the grief of a parent aching for reunification with a beloved child. All these familial reactions and concerns are highly prevalent in the literature [11].

Most aging parents worry about who will care for a middle-aged child who has schizophrenia when they are gone. "Perceived family burden," a corollary concept to expressed emotion, is viewed by some as having more predictive value for relapse in schizophrenia then in controls. Other aging parents, however, report gratitude for the contributions of their loved one to the family welfare [26]. Perhaps this is why the term "burden" has been rejected and instead conceptualized as family care giving within a stress-appraisal-coping framework that accommodates positive as well as negative perceptions [28].

All families suffer the stigma of mental illness, on behalf of their loved one and sometimes by association. Stigma of course has adverse consequences in terms of availability of jobs, insurance, higher education, and possibilities for marriage. With advocacy groups working to change perceptions of mental illness in the popular media, and with increasing self-disclosure on the part of celebrities as well as the general public, there is beginning to be some reduction of stigma. Moreover, newer medications and psychosocial treatments, the recovery orientation in mental health services, and overt evidence of consumer strengths and talents are beginning to change the public face of mental illness.

WHAT FAMILIES WANT FOR THEIR LOVED ONES

Depending on the level of functioning of the person who has schizophrenia, families often are conflicted between wanting optimal protection for their loved ones and optimal opportunities for independent living. Family members often are the first to view psychotic episodes or suicide attempts. They need speedy access to crisis intervention, preferably in the home, that may avert the indignities of involuntary treatment. If inpatient care is indicated, both patients and families need relief from premature discharge that may recycle known patterns of rehospitalization, or, worse, homelessness or even jail.

Families want protections in terms of disability entitlements and more comprehensive, effective, and respectful services. NAMI, MHA, and others have advocated for protection and advocacy legislation and reduction of institutional seclusion and restraints. They have lobbied for equitable Federal benefits and insurance parity and have worked for greater use of the evidence-based Program of Assertive Community Treatment (PACT) programs that avoid hospitalization. Most recently, NAMI published a comprehensive report grading the states on mental health systems in terms of infrastructure, information access, services, and recovery supports. Some state administrations used their poor rating to receive additional funds for needed services [29]. MHA has launched *Dialog for Recovery* to provide specific help to consumers in navigating the recovery process as well as sponsoring successful, Medicaid-funded peer-specialist interventions around the nation. MHA's National Consumer Support Technical Assistance Centers and Self-Help Clearinghouses around the country strengthen consumer-run advocacy networks through grants and technical assistance to ensure that the consumer voice is always present in the planning, implementation, and evaluation of mental health delivery systems and their policies.

Above all, families share consumers' desires for greater autonomy and independent functioning of their loved ones. Despite areas of dispute, there is an inherent goodness-of-fit between the basic agendas of the consumer and family movements, a clear correlation between patient autonomy and caregiver relief. Families have the right to live their lives free from worry and pain. This right can be achieved only when patients have the right to achieve their fullest potential in a well-funded, evidence-based, peer-supported, and recovery-oriented mental health system.

WHAT FAMILIES WANT FROM THE HEALTH CARE SYSTEM

Given the evolution of knowledge regarding the origin and treatment of persons who have schizophrenia, families want a responsive and integrated health care system. They want a system that is safe and effective and that meaningfully engages the primary consumer and his/her family as partners in developing and implementing a treatment and support plan.

Above all else, the treatment system must focus on safety. Persons who have schizophrenia are at elevated risk of premature death both through suicide and from a large variety of physical causes [30,31]. Additionally, individuals who have psychotic disorders are at risk for involuntary care and restraint that present potential immediate health dangers as well as the longer-term effects of retraumatization for persons who are likely to have experienced trauma. For treatment to be safe, it must anticipate these risks and respond to them appropriately. At least three strategies seem critical to ensure safety. These strategies are related to the issues of effectiveness that are discussed later.

First, it is critical that a strong, continuous relationship be established between a person who has schizophrenia and a clinical team, probably a team in the specialty mental health sector. This relationship should be characterized by a true clinical alliance, one that is open, with shared decision making. Consumers sometimes report a reluctance to discuss how they might be feeling (eg, if they are feeling suicidal) with their therapist because they fear this revelation would invoke involuntary treatment (eg, hospitalization, medications against will, conservatorship). Shared decisions that are memorialized in advanced directives might allay some of these fears and increase the effectiveness with which suicidal thoughts and behaviors can be monitored and the individual who has schizophrenia can remain safe. To the degree that the primary consumer consents, family members clearly can be important partners in helping reduce the risk of suicidal behavior. A strong consumer/family/clinician partnership alliance may be among the most important suicide prevention strategies.

Second, it is essential that persons who have schizophrenia have a primary care home and a functioning partnership with their primary care provider. Although suicide is an important cause of premature mortality, persons who have schizophrenia are estimated to lose 25 years of life from a wide variety of causes including cardiovascular disease, endocrine disorders, hypertension, and other health problems. [30]. Although much needs to be known about how best to reduce this premature mortality, it generally is agreed that much stronger links should be formed with primary care [32]. Also, wellness programs that promote healthful behaviors and assist persons in managing the weight gain that is associated with many of the second-generation antipsychotic agents are thought to be an important part of an overall strategy to prolong life in persons who have schizophrenia.

Finally, it is important that that all care be trauma informed. A recent overview of the research on childhood trauma and schizophrenia states that although reported prevalence is relatively high, there are many methodologic problems, and evidence of a causal linkage is "controversial and contestable" [33]. Traumatic memories, however, may be severe and require sensitive interventions over and above the usual treatments. Any prior exposure may be exacerbated in institutional settings where retraumatization may occur. A survey of persons who had severe mental illness and a history of psychiatric hospitalization assessed the number and type of events that they experienced as harmful within a psychiatric setting. Forty-seven percent reported experiencing a *Diagnostic and Statistical Manual of Mental Disorders-IV*–defined traumatic event while in the hospital; 44% reported sexual or physical assault, and 23% reported intimidation or abuse from staff. Altogether, 86% reported traumatization from institutional events and procedures. Patients who experienced what the authors termed "sanctuary trauma" within the psychiatric setting had higher subjective distress scores, more recollections of fear, helplessness, or horror, and a longer period of feeling upset after discharge from the hospital

[34]. The use of restraints is a poignant example of treatment methods that may retraumatize persons who have a history of a trauma, reinforcing the psychologic damage attendant on traumatic experiences. Trauma experienced within a setting that is supposed to be protective and therapeutic is obviously outrageous and totally unacceptable. It is a complete refutation of the mandate to do no harm. These findings cry out for system reform.

Clearly, designing a health care system that promotes safety is essential. Additionally, families want health care systems that are effective. For a system to be effective, it must be accessible and provide evidence-informed, quality care. Accessibility involves temporal, financial, and psychologic dimensions. Given the chronic and recurrent nature of problems associated with schizophrenia, help must be available to consumers and their families continuously. Ideally this help involves a range of services that vary in intensity from emergency/inpatient care to drop-in centers, consumer self help, and mutual support groups. Care may involve face-to-face interaction or availability by telephone or the Internet.

For services to be accessible financially, the price of the services must allow them to be used when needed. Price involves both the out-of-pocket expenses for consumers and their families and reimbursement by insurers and other payers. Lack of adequate insurance coverage can be financially devastating for families and can leave individuals who have this chronic disease impoverished [35]. Affordability and availability—both importantly determined by the financing system—are critical to access.

Finally, services must by psychologically accessible. That is, services must be seen by the recipient of care and the family as personally relevant and responsive to their ideas regarding the nature of care needed. Helping an individual enter into a change process and a helping relationship through motivational interviewing [36], readiness preparation [37], or other engagement strategies is part of creating an accessible system. Understanding cultural and linguistic differences among individuals and having a strong focus on developing a genuine partnership that involves shared goals and strategies are keys to psychologic accessibility. As mentioned earlier, the fear of involuntary care (which may itself be retraumatizing) often makes care much less accessible. In fact, persons literally flee from helping relationships when they perceive the possibility of coercive interventions. Work by Monihan and colleagues [38,39] indicates that the perceived coercion in an intervention, rather than objective coerciveness, is critical in determining its detrimental effects. These findings underscore the importance of active engagement strategies to involve individuals in their care. Psychologic accessibility, therefore, implies dignity, respect, and hopefulness in the interactions between a consumer, the family, and the treatment system and is fundamental to implementing an effective program of care.

Effective care also must be science based and/or evidence informed. Results from the schizophrenia Patient Outcomes Research Team [40] indicate that the treatment of schizophrenia, like treatment in the general medical sector [41], does not comport with the best scientific evidence. Although an extensive review of this emerging literature is not presented here, it is critical that evidence-based approaches be available and delivered with fidelity in concept and design. The Substance Abuse and Mental Health Services Administration has developed a National Registry of Evidence-based Programs and Practices (http://modelprograms.samhsa.gov/template.cfm?page=nreppover) as a national resource for certifying programs as meeting systematic standards of scientific evidence. A toolkit for evidence-based family psychoeducation is available for mental health systems to use in involving families as educated partners in care.

Requiring a strong science base should not unnecessarily limit treatment or rehabilitation choices. When multiple approaches have been shown to be effective (eg, in improving community functioning), an array of program choices should be available. This array will support the match between an individual's needs, desires, and biology and the most effective treatments. These decisions should be informed by science but ultimately must be negotiated by a well-informed and informationally supported clinician in a meaningful partnership with a consumer and the consumer's family. Choice among evidence-based alternatives is essential.

Finally, as noted in the President's *New Freedom Commission on Mental Health* [42], recovery from severe mental illnesses should be the expected outcome of treatment and rehabilitation. Although each individual's specific outcomes are unique, a real life in the community is often a desired end point. Recovery-oriented services involve more than symptom management and must involve strategies to assure optimal community participation and recovery from illness. Rehabilitation, self-direction, development of natural supports, environmental accommodation, and support often are be key elements of recovery-oriented services.

In short, individuals who have schizophrenia and their families want the same features in their health care system that are desired by everyone: safety, effectiveness, and a real role in directing care resulting in optimal community participation. These qualities are not the legacy of the current system, which often has been inflicted on consumers who were assumed to be incompetent to participate in their care. Such alternatives never were acceptable and will not be tolerated by contemporary health care consumers and the people who care about them.

Although safety, effectiveness, and meaningful engagement seem like obvious characteristics of health care, they are not the rule for the current treatment environments. A poignant example involves the premature death of persons who have schizophrenia. There is nothing ambiguous about death as an outcome. These problems have been known for more than 50 years [43], but, instead of stimulating an effective response, the number of lost years of life has increased to about 25 years during the last 2 decades. The safety of the health care system has not been revised relative to this unambiguous outcome. There continues to be talk about better integration of health delivery systems, but very little real progress has been made in assuring that persons who have schizophrenia receive the health care they need. In fact, the problems are getting worse. When the history of this time is written, the inability or unwillingness to address this issue aggressively probably will be seen as shameful—much like custodial care in large institutions.

Similarly, although Harding and colleagues [44] did their seminal work on recovery in the late 1980s and Beers [8] and others who have mental illnesses have educated us about the hope and reality of recovery, many clinicians do not understand, embrace, or promote recovery. To clinicians, recovery often is defined in terms of symptom reduction and increased functional capacity. To consumers, recovery means moving beyond the constraints of the illness to achieve a positive self-concept and lead a satisfying life. Long-term studies suggest that as many as 50% of people diagnosed as having schizophrenia have good outcomes in terms of being able to live productive and satisfying lives [45]. Follow-up studies have shown that some patients who have schizophrenia can achieve recovery even without maintenance pharmacotherapy [46].

The President's *New Freedom Commission Report on Mental Health* [42] recommends a recovery-oriented mental health system that is consumer and family driven, based on the defined needs of service recipients rather than those of providers. The report's recommendations emphasize the importance of evidence-based psychiatric rehabilitative practices such as supported employment, skills training, assertive community treatment, and cognitive behavioral therapy to cope more effectively with symptoms. Also recommended are psychoeducation for families and ensuring a collaborative relationship between families and the treatment team.

Clinical staff still is not being trained adequately at all levels in the client-centered, rehabilitative techniques thought to speed recovery. Pharmacologic treatments probably have been overemphasized, and the role to the treating psychiatrist has been marginalized to focus almost exclusively on medication management and not on the overall management of health. Ironically, some of the most discriminatory attitudes toward persons who have mental illnesses that the authors have encountered have been expressed by clinical staff, many of whom provide little hope or optimism to persons who have schizophrenia or their families although it is known that hope is an essential ingredient for treatment engagement and recovery [37]. System barriers are discussed later, but it should be acknowledged here that the pace of change in clinician attitudes and skills has been embarrassingly slow. While psychiatrists have worked on the margins, thousands of years of productive lives have been lost. Psychiatrists must do more, and advocacy groups like MHA, NAMI, the Depression and Bipolar Support Alliance, and others must demand that the pace of change improve dramatically.

WHAT DO FAMILIES WANT FROM SOCIETY?

In support of a "real life in the community," families expect nondiscriminatory social policies that treat behavioral health no differently from general health. Families continue to suffer from the legacy of state hospital care in society's attitudes toward people who have schizophrenia and other severe mental illnesses. The state hospital era was characterized by a separate, state-funded system in which custodial care was the mode. The development of the community care system coextensive with the downsizing and occasional closure of state hospitals preserved this separately financed, separately administered, and separately regulated system. The separate community system was not comprehensive, however, and efforts to reform it highlighted the need for a broad range of services and supports to promote successful community living [47]. Given the state's traditional role and the general belief that persons who had schizophrenia had a progressively deteriorating course of illness requiring long-term institutional care, the development of health insurance largely omitted adequate coverage for the long-term treatment of mental illnesses. Results from the RAND Corporation's health insurance experiment regarding the price elasticity of demand for mental health services [48] and ongoing public ignorance regarding the legitimacy of less severe disorders perpetuated this unequal treatment of mental illnesses in health insurance. It now is understood that behavioral health conditions are legitimate health conditions in every respect and that their parity coverage in health insurance does not dramatically increase health care expenditures in a contemporary health insurance environment [49]. Therefore, discrimination against persons who have mental illnesses in both acute and long-term care is no longer sensible or tolerable. Families want this form of discrimination and all other discriminatory laws and policies to be eliminated.

Families also want society to adopt a public health model for the prevention and treatment of behavioral health conditions. Such a model would include surveillance systems to monitor population health status and systematic public health measures to improve the public's behavioral health and, ultimately, overall health status. Well- researched prevention programs exist and should become universally available, as should screening and early identification of mental illnesses. Rapid and effective services for persons who are identified as having mental health conditions could reduce the disability associated with these conditions and promote the full participation of persons who have mental illnesses in all aspects of society. For persons who develop disability associated with their conditions, rehabilitative services must be provided to promote the reacquisition of skills lost to illness. Social barriers to full participation that result in handicaps also must be identified and eliminated. Much as the development of ramps allowed wheelchair-bound persons greater mobility and subsequently greater participation in their environment, it is important to identify and eliminate restrictions that frustrate the full participation of persons who have behavioral health disorders in all aspects of society.

Similarly, families want society to realize that behavioral health conditions underlie social problems in every human service sector but generally are not the principal objective in any sector. School performance, for example, is affected dramatically by socioemotional functioning [50,51], but universal screening and treatment of these disorders still is not common and in some areas of the country is actively opposed. Most children in the juvenile and adult correctional system have behavioral health conditions that often are not identified or appropriately treated. Society must understand more fully the impact of these untreated or undertreated conditions on the health of the community.

Consistent with this broad, social perspective on health, families would like the total costs of inadequate prevention, treatment, and rehabilitation to be documented fully and understood. No longer should policies in one sector of society (eg, restriction of coverage for mental health conditions) be allowed to cause increased costs in other sectors of the economy (eg, correctional systems) [52] without the transparent recognition of the shift of expenses across sector. It is only with the adoption of a full societal-cost model that the inefficiencies in the present fragmented systems will become clearly apparent so that it will be possible to begin to develop integrated approaches to promoting public health.

Last, families of persons who have schizophrenia would like society to develop communities in which the family member can be welcomed fully and supported. Public attitudes that continue to stigmatize and shame persons who have schizophrenia significantly limit their ability to participate in all aspects of community life. Tolerance for differences among individuals is a core component of these attitudes that would benefit everyone in a community. Involvement rather than marginalization will contribute to community productivity and cohesion and will be related importantly to the recovery of individuals who have schizophrenia.

Families of persons who have schizophrenia, in short, want a society that supports these long-term disorders effectively and that promotes maximal community participation for all long-term disorders equitably. They want a society that responds humanely and quickly to persons who are becoming ill, a response that promotes well being and productivity. They want a society in which persons will have sufficient skills to succeed and where environments will be designed to prevent the development of illness or to minimize morbidity. As with their desires from the health care system, family desires for just and equitable treatment by society mirror those of everyone. When persons who have schizophrenia are welcomed into the community and can participate fully, everyone will benefit.

As in the overall health care system, the rate of change in society has been unacceptably slow. Psychiatrists, as advocates, have failed to make a compelling case to the general public and to marshal the political will to implement what they know is necessary. Advocacy organizations and concerned professionals must work together to develop the public and political pressure to address discrimination and to implement social policies that promote well being. Forming partnerships with other groups who do not have a parochial or guild interest in these issues (eg, sheriffs, public prosecutors and defenders, judges, school leaders, and others) is a promising strategy. It is in psychiatrists' enlightened self-interest to implement these policies, but, although they have made important progress in improving public attitudes, they have not yet convinced politicians and the public of the urgency and sensibility of these policies. More work is needed.

NEW MODELS

National advocacy in behavioral health reflects the shift to a consumer-oriented society and even more the dissatisfaction of patients and their families with the provider "field" (ie, psychiatrists, psychologists, social workers, nurses, counselors, hospitals and long-term care facilities, administrators, the government, and other entities). Additional unhappiness with the manner in which individuals who had psychiatric disorders were being treated by society in general extended the dissatisfaction to schools, businesses, housing, and politicians. As respected national advocacy organizations (eg, NAMI, MHA, the Depression and Bipolar Support Alliance, Children and Adults with Attention Deficit Disorder, and others) have become increasingly active with accompanying political clout, a number of initiatives have taken root within behavioral health. These initiatives translate into new models and concepts of care that transcend the power dynamic of the traditional provider–patient–family interaction. Here are some of the new models that reflect the process and outcomes that families want to experience in the treatment and support of persons who have schizophrenia:

1. Patients and families, trained as peer counselors, are formally incorporated into and reimbursed as members of the multidisciplinary treatment team assuring that patient and family perspectives are incorporated into all care systems.
2. Patients and families whose members are in care expect to be informed fully on all relevant information that has a bearing on assessment, treatment, and outcomes in the context of a shared decision-making paradigm.
3. Recovery and rehabilitation need to be central and functional concepts in the overall behavioral health care system. Clinicians and other caregivers should understand the importance of hope, skill-building, and supportive environments to maximize the fullest participation possible in society.
4. The separation of the traditional behavioral health care disciplines, promulgated primarily by the guilds, has no place in the framework of a comprehensive, integrated system of care. Although each of the disciplines has a unique set of skills, they are not substitutes for one another. Role differentiation within an integrated framework provides the comprehensive care needed by individuals who have schizophrenia. For example, psychiatrists must assume greater responsibility for the overall medical management with particular sensitivities to the management of comorbid illnesses; nurses must assume responsibility for ongoing medical support and patient education; social workers must assume responsibility for providing access to the full range of community supports and skills to manage community life; psychologists must assume responsibility for specific need and skill assessment required to craft treatment and rehabilitation plans. Other members of the professional team (eg, aides, assistants, and others), who often spend the most time with service recipients, must be involved fully in the treatment plan and supported to assure that the plan is delivered successfully. Fragmentation and poor role definition are not acceptable.
5. Preprofessional training across disciplines must reflect the characteristics of an integrated, interdependent system of care that involves patients and families explicitly and includes technologies to support recovery outcomes, so

that the next generation of providers will enter the workforce trained in these basic principles [53]. Funding should support innovative, cross-disciplinary training models that incorporate the principles articulated in this article.

6. Society, in general, and the individuals responsible for the distribution of public and private resources (eg, politicians, industry leaders) in particular must be educated regarding the prevalence of mental illness, the effects of not providing effective early recognition and intervention services, and the ultimate effects on both personal and community well being of untreated or ineffectively treated mental illnesses. Given the impact of psychiatric illness on the burden of disease and global economics, a reprioritization of resources is needed to address these issues properly, to a degree commensurate with their impact.

7. Information systems that support good practice must be designed, and payment systems that encourage such practice must be instituted. Practitioners must have information systems that support good clinical decision processes while appreciating the unique nature of every person's needs and circumstances. Health information systems also must be integrated so that the consumer and all the providers have access to a full range of information regarding the patient's care. Generally, the state of the health information infrastructure is very poor. It is hoped that someone reflecting on the state of health care in 2007 a decade from now will marvel that providers did as well as they did, given the inadequate support currently provided to clinicians in decision making and assessing the progress of care.

8. As with health in general, the present health care system concentrates more on medical care than on public health. Early identification and prevention can have major impact on reducing morbidity and, one hopes, on eliminating illness at some point in the future. In behavioral health, a more acute sense of public health concepts and methods must be developed. Advocates must insist on this framework in evaluating the effectiveness of science in impacting well being.

9. The meaningful integration of behavioral health into the general health care system is imperative to address the historically poor level of general health care received by individuals who have psychiatric disorders. The separate and unequal provision of health care to persons who have psychiatric disorders can no longer be tolerated.

10. Pay-For-Performance and similar concepts that reward good clinical behavior and punish poor clinical behavior in the form of differential reimbursement should become a standard of practice in behavioral health. Should accreditation and licensing of systems and individuals be linked to the concepts expressed herein? The need for improvement in all areas on behavioral health care, but in particular in the public sector where many individuals who have schizophrenia and their families initially or ultimately find themselves, is essential.

11. The collective political strength of national advocacy should have considerable influence on the funding of systems and practices from clinical, training, and research perspectives that reflect these principles and concepts.

SUMMARY

Historically, families of persons who have schizophrenia have been blamed for the development of the condition and subsequently have been excluded systematically from care. Now these notions, which never had much systematic empiric support, have been abandoned, and the importance of family involvement in the care of persons who have schizophrenia is becoming recognized. Family involvement often is critical to the recovery process and must be engaged actively whenever possible.

Although the engagement of the family in the care of the person who has schizophrenia is essential, it is not sufficient. Primary consumers and families realize that the entire care process needs to be redesigned. It must be explicitly collaborative in its orientation and must begin to include routinely evidence-based treatments that are informed by a vision of recovery. The inclusion of individuals in recovery and their families in the treatment and training process will help integrate these important perspectives into the core of the operation. The sobering data regarding early mortality among persons who have schizophrenia point out the need to work aggressively to assure full integration of behavioral and primary health care. This integration probably will be accomplished best through the development of integrated care settings, perhaps within the context of disease management programs, within primary care systems. The community mental health center may be an icon of the past representing the de facto segregation of individuals who have schizophrenia. Integration with primary care cannot be postponed any longer.

Finally, much work remains in changing public perceptions regarding the full inclusion of persons who have schizophrenia and in eliminating discriminatory laws, regulations, and practices within communities. This last point is probably the most fundamental challenge to society. At all levels, society must begin to embrace a vision of a meaningful life for the individual who has schizophrenia that, to the extent possible and despite the challenges, maximizes participation in a comprehensive program of identification, treatment, rehabilitation, and recovery. Early identification, early intervention, recovery, and rehabilitation have had limited impact in the current system of care. Such limitation marginalizes the quality of life of individuals who have schizophrenia and their families because of delays in accessing care that is proper, relevant, and compassionate. Only when this waste of human capital and the loss to communities through such marginalization is recognized fully will it be possible to move aggressively move to fix the broken approaches in the care for persons who have schizophrenia and other long-term, disabling illnesses.

References

[1] Sullivan HS. Peculiarity of thought in schizophrenia. Am J Psych 1925;82:21–86.
[2] Pollack HM, Malzberg B, Fuller RG. Heredity and environmental factors in the causation of manic-depressive psychosis and dementia praecox. Utica (NY): State Hospitals Press; 1939.
[3] Shaw S. Families and schizophrenia: repair and replacement in the treatment of families. Am J Soc Psych 1987;7:27–31.
[4] Fromm-Reichmann F. Notes on the development of treatment of schizophrenics by psychoanalysis and psychotherapy. Psychiatry 1948;11:263–73.
[5] Arieti S. Interpretation of schizophrenia. New York: Robert Brunner; 1955.

[6] Lidz T, Cornelison A, Fleck S, et al. The interfamilial environment of the schizophrenic patient. I: the father. Psychiatry 1957;20:329–42.

[7] Bateson G, Jackson D, Haley J, et al. Toward a theory of schizophrenia. Behav Sci 1956;1: 251–64.

[8] Beers CW. A mind that found itself. Pittsburgh (PA): University of Pittsburg Press; 1907.

[9] Howells JG, Guirguis WR. The family and schizophrenia. New York: International Universities Press; 1985.

[10] Warner R. The prevention of schizophrenia: what interventions are safe and effective? Schizophr Bull 2001;27:551–62.

[11] Lefley HP. Family caregiving in mental illness. Thousand Oaks (CA): Sage; 1996.

[12] Barrowclough C. Families of people with schizophrenia. In: Sartorius N, Leff J, Lopez-Ibor JJ, et al, editors. Families and mental disorders: from burden to empowerment. West Sussex (UK): Wiley; 2005. p. 1–24.

[13] Wynne LC, Singer MT. Thought disorder and family relations of schizophrenics I. A research study. Arch Gen Psychiatry 1963;9:191–8.

[14] Wynne LC, Singer MT. Thought disorder and family relations of schizophrenics II. A classification of forms of thinking. Arch Gen Psychiatry 1963;9:199–206.

[15] Wynne LC, Singer MT, Bartko JJ, et al. Schizophrenics and their families: research on parental communication. In: Tanner JM, editor. Developments in Psychiatric Research. London: Hodder & Stoughton; 1977. p. 254–86.

[16] Brown M, Bone M, Palison B, et al. Schizophrenia and social care. London: Oxford University Press; 1966.

[17] Leff J, Kuipers L, Berkowitz R, et al. A controlled trial of social intervention in the families of schizophrenic patients. Br J Psychiatry 1982;141:121–34.

[18] Leff J. Psychiatry around the globe. London: Gaskell; 1988.

[19] Lefley HP. Expressed emotion: conceptual, clinical, and social policy issues. Hosp Community Psychiatry 1992;43:591–8.

[20] Leff J, Vaughn C, editors. Expressed emotion in families. New York: Guilford; 1985.

[21] Lopez SR, Nelson HK, Polo AJ, et al. Ethnicity, expressed emotion, attributions, and course of schizophrenia: family warmth matters. J Abnorm Psychol 2004;113:428–9.

[22] Ivanic M, Vuletic Z, Bebbington P. Expressed emotion in the families of patients with schizophrenia and its influence on the course of illness. Soc Psychiatry Psychiatr Epidemiol 1994;29:61–5.

[23] Dixon L, McFarlane WR, Lefley H, et al. Evidence-based practices for services to families of people with psychiatric disabilities. Psychiatr Serv 2001;52:903–10.

[24] Lefley HP, Johnson DL, editors. Family interventions in mental illness: international perspectives. Westpo rt (CT): Praeger; 1996.

[25] McFarlane WR, editor. Multifamily groups in the treatment of severe psychiatric disorders. New York: Guilford Press; 2002.

[26] Greenberg JS, Knudsen KJ, Aschbrenner KA. Prosocial family processes and the quality of life of persons with schizophrenia. Psychiatr Serv 2006;57:1771–7.

[27] Lefley HP. The family experience in cultural context: Implications for further research and practice. New Dir Ment Health Serv 1998;77:97–106.

[28] Szmukler G. From family "burden" to caregiving. Psychiatr Bull 1996;20:449–51.

[29] National Alliance on Mental Illness. Grading the states: a report on America's health care system for serious mental illness. Arlington (VA): National Alliance on Mental Illness; 2006.

[30] Parks J, Svendsen D, Singer P, et al. Morbidity and mortality in people with serious mental illness. Alexandria (VA): National Association of State Mental Health Program Directors; 2006.

[31] Miller B, Paschall B, Svendsen DP. Mortality and medical comorbidity among patients with serious mental illness. Psychiatr Serv 2006;57:1482–7.

[32] Institute of Medicine. Quality chasm series. Washington, DC: The National Academies Press; 2005.

[33] Morgan C, Fisher H. Environment and schizophrenia: environmental factors in schizophrenia: childhood trauma-a critical review. Schizophr Bull 2007;33:3–10.

[34] Cusack KJ, Frueh BC, Hiers T, et al. Trauma within the psychiatric setting: a preliminary empirical report. Adm Policy Ment Health 2003;30:453–60.

[35] Himmelstein DU, Warren E, Thorne D, et al. Market watch: illness and injury as contributors to bankruptcy. Health Affairs Web Exclusive 2005. Available at: http://content. healthaffairs.org/cgi/content/full/hlthaff.w5.63/DC1. Accessed February 2, 2005.

[36] Miller W, Rollnick S. Motivational interviewing: preparing people for change. 2nd edition. New York: Guilford Press; 2002.

[37] Anthony WA. Recovery from mental illness: the guiding vision of the mental health service system in the 1990s. Psychosocial Rehabilitation Journal 1993;16:11–24.

[38] Dennis D, Monahan J, editors. Coercion and aggressive community treatment: a new frontier in mental health law. New York: Plenum Publishing Corporation; 1996.

[39] Monahan J, Hodge S, Lidz C. Coercion and commitment: understanding involuntary mental hospital admission. Int J Law Psychiatry 1995;18:249–63.

[40] Lehman AF, Steinwachs D. Translating research into practice: the schizophrenia Patient Outcomes Research Team (PORT). Schizophr Bull 1998;24(1):1–10.

[41] McGlynn E, Asch A, Adams SM, et al. The quality of health care delivered to adults in the United States. N Engl J Med 2003;348:2635–45.

[42] New Freedom Commission on Mental Health. Achieving the promise: transforming mental health care in America, final report. Rockville (MD), DHHS [Pub. No. SMA-03-3832], 2003.

[43] Felker B, Yazel JJ, Short D. Mortality and medical comorbidity among psychiatric patients: a review. Psychiatr Serv 1996;47(12):1356–63.

[44] Harding CM, Brooks GW, Ashikaga T, et al. Vermont longitudinal study of people with mental illness. Am J Psychiatry 1987;144:727–35.

[45] Bellack AS. Scientific and consumer models of recovery in schizophrenia. Schizophr Bull;32:432–42.

[46] Harrow M, Grossman L, Jobe TH, et al. Do patients with schizophrenia ever show periods of recovery? A 15 year multi-follow-up-study. Schizophr Bull 2005;31:723–34.

[47] Morrissey JP, Goldman HH. Cycles of reform in the care of the chronically mentally ill. Hosp Community Psychiatry 1984;35:785–93.

[48] Manning WG, Wells KB, Buchanan JL, et al. The effects of mental health insurance: evidence from the healthinsurance experiment. Santa Monica (CA): RAND Corporation; 1989 [Pub. no. R-3815-NIMH/HCFA].

[49] Goldman HH, Frank R, Burnam MA, et al. Behavioral health insurance parity for federal employees. N Engl J Med 2006;354:1378–86.

[50] Zins J, Weissberg R, Wang M, et al, editors. Building academic success on social and emotional learning: what does the research say? New York: Teachers College Press; 2004.

[51] Stoep AV, Weiss NS, Kuo ES, et al. What proportion of failure to complete secondary school in the US population is attributable to adolescent psychiatric disorder? J Behav Health Serv Res 2003;30(1):119–24.

[52] Domino ME, Norton EC, Morrissey JP, et al. Cost shifting to jails after a change to managed mental health care. Health Serv Res 2004;39:1379–402.

[53] A thousand voices: the national action plan on behavioral workforce development. The Annapolis Coalition. Rockville (MD): SAMHSA; 2006.

Recovery and Systems Transformation for Schizophrenia

Scott A. Peebles, PhD[a],*, P. Alex Mabe, PhD[a],
Larry Davidson, PhD[b], Larry Fricks[c], Peter F. Buckley, MD[a],
Gareth Fenley[a]

[a]Department of Psychiatry and Health Behavior, Medical College of Georgia,
1515 Pope Avenue, Augusta, GA 30912, USA
[b]Program for Recovery and Community Mental Health, Department of Psychiatry,
Yale University, Erector Square, Building 6 West, Suite 1C, 319 Pack Street, New Haven,
CT 06513, USA
[c]Appalachian Consulting Group, Incorporated, 1727 Turners Corner Road, Cleveland,
GA 30528, USA

B ecause of the convergence of several developments in the mental health field, the concept of recovery has emerged as a new and overarching consideration during the past 2 decades [1]. These recent developments include but are not limited to (1) the powerful impact of consumers' personal stories of recovery, (2) calls from mental health consumers to make services more consumer-driven, (3) the realization that consumers need more than symptom relief alone following the short-comings of deinstitutionalization [2], and (4) a growing body of empiric research by Bleuler and colleagues [3], Ciompi and colleagues [4], Harding and colleagues [5], and Strauss and colleagues [6,7], which demonstrated, contrary to the prevailing beliefs of many practitioners and consumers alike, that those diagnosed as having severe and persistent forms of mental illness (and schizophrenia in particular) are able to experience significant degrees of improvement over time.

The potential impact and strength of the recovery movement is reflected in the President's New Freedom Commission on Mental Health [8] making the reorientation of all mental health services to promoting recovery the core of its vision in transforming the nation's service delivery system. There has been much confusion in the field, however, as to precisely what "recovery" means within the context of serious mental illness. As Lehman [9] has pointed out, this new construct has the potential to be misunderstood and misapplied if not informed by empiric study and a commitment to ethical care. Lehman [9] argues that a lack of both of these important elements may lead to the use of treatment approaches that are not beneficial to the individuals obtaining care.

*Corresponding author. E-mail address: speebles@mcg.edu (S.A. Peebles).

0193-953X/07/$ – see front matter
doi:10.1016/j.psc.2007.04.009
© 2007 Elsevier Inc. All rights reserved.
psych.theclinics.com

Although consumers and practitioners alike would agree that individuals and families seeking mental health care have a basic human right to improved choices of care, recent efforts to link recovery concepts with empirically sound treatments for schizophrenia provide scientific legitimacy to the Recovery Movement. It is on the basis of this emerging empiric support that service providers should develop recovery-based service plans and training curricula for service providers as initial steps toward systems transformation. This article reviews the history of the recovery model, provides a conceptual framework for understanding the model, and discusses the innovative aspects of recovery-based service delivery (with a central focus on the integration of Certified Peer Specialists into patient care). This article also describes the targets of intervention for a recovery-based paradigm shift and discusses how these interventions might be best implemented (as informed by empiric research).

THE RECOVERY MODEL: AN HISTORICAL PERSPECTIVE

By far, the most influential and important contributions to the rise of the Recovery Movement came from the consumer movement and consumer leaders themselves, not from professionals. This article, however, focuses primarily on the professional and systemic developments that helped pave the way for the recovery movement to take hold. Elements of the recovery perspective have been evident in professional practice for decades (although emphasis on these elements has waxed and waned). The recovery model of service delivery also seems to incorporate (or be based in part on) characteristics of previous models (eg, Philippe Pinel's moral treatment approach [10]). The recovery perspective, however, promises innovations that these previous models did offer. In part, these innovations stem from the impact of the more recent historical events that were mentioned at the beginning of this article. The development of the recovery perspective is discussed in this historical context.

The creation of Alcoholics Anonymous in 1935 by Dr. Bob Smith and Bill Wilson was a watershed event for the future development of recovery-oriented models of care [11,12]. As White [12] pointed out, Alcoholics Anonymous was not the first mutual-assistance group for recovery from addiction (such groups existed in Native American communities in the late 1700s and early 1800s), but it was the first to provide a system of recovery and a solid organizational style to such efforts. Alcoholics Anonymous has remained an extremely influential and enduring force. It has spawned similar groups internationally, has led to the application of the Twelve Steps and Twelve Traditions to recovery from other addictions, has influenced professional treatment programs, and has maintained emphasis on the spiritual aspects of recovery and recovery processes [11,12]. The influence of Alcoholics Anonymous also has helped open the door to the acceptance of professionally incorporated peer-support and consumer-based services [11].

Geller [13] pointed out that, during the 1950s, a movement began within state hospitals in the United States that focused on preparing hospitalized individuals to return to the community. Unfortunately, this movement suffered from overcrowding in hospitals, a lack of hospital funding, and lack of uniformity in standards of care [13]. During the 1970s, however, this movement eventually developed into a service model now commonly referred to as "psychosocial rehabilitation."

Geller [13] reports that, as early as 1950, a group called "Friends of the Mentally Ill" was formed by current patients, former patients, and patients' family members to advocate for legislation to improve treatment and treatment domains. Furthermore, Geller [13] documents historical events during the past 50 years that probably contributed to the evolution of the recovery perspective, including job training, the inclusion of patient advocates in treatment, the formation of the influential National Alliance for the Mentally Ill in 1980, and the development of self-help groups and the production of self-help literature. Rosen [14] documents the rise of the self-help movement in the late 1960s and 1970s, recalling that this movement became so influential that the American Psychological Association formed a task force centered on investigating self-help interventions [15].

As a commentary on the extent of the unmet need of the mentally ill for services beyond medical care as currently provided, Kessler and colleagues [16] reported that many mentally ill individuals do not seek professional help because they wish to solve their problems independently (72.1%) or because they believe that their issues will resolve over time (60.6%). Norcross [17] asserts that "[a] massive, systemic, and yet largely silent revolution is occurring in mental health today and is gathering steam for tomorrow: self-help efforts without professional intervention."

Norcross [17] argues that psychologists and other mental health professionals would do well to involve themselves in the self-help revolution by

1. Valuing self-help more
2. Encouraging client self-change efforts that are based on empiric research
3. Researching self-help and self-change more effectively
4. Disseminating research findings
5. Better integrating psychotherapy (and other mental health interventions) with self-help strategies

At least one group of researchers has pursued this effort in earnest [18]. The Recovery Movement has the potential to assist in achieving these goals.

Finally, in the late 1990s, a group of psychologists led by former American Psychological Association President Martin Seligman began the Positive Psychology movement. This movement seems to have had a perspective similar to that of the Recovery Model in focusing on broader views of desired outcomes and thus targets for intervention. More specifically, Seligman and Csikszentmihalyi [19] urged that the study and practice of psychology shift its focus to concepts such as happiness, personal strengths, personality traits, or personal perspectives that predispose one toward happiness, fulfillment, and the pursuit of personal excellence. This introduction to a now extremely influential movement in the field was published in a special issue of the *American*

Psychologist, along with 15 articles supporting this shift in perspective. Five years later, Gable and Haidt [20] published a review article of this movement and defined Positive Psychology as "the study of the conditions and processes that contribute to the flourishing or optimal functioning of people, groups, and institutions." Gable and Haidt [20] report that this movement has led to important research regarding coping ability, optimism, locus of control, and the impact of positive emotional experiences on well-being and life satisfaction. These findings are consistent with a recovery-based call for greater optimism and hope for those who have chronic and persistent mental illness.

The aforementioned historical forces and events helped pave the way for the recent rise of the recovery perspective. Anthony [1] and Davidson and colleagues [21] have pointed out that mental health professionals have renewed their interest in incorporating elements of patient empowerment, fostering hope, and peer support in treatment models and service delivery systems. Because of more recent historical events and consumer movements, however, these elements are being incorporated in a different manner than previously considered. Recovery-based service delivery systems are innovative in three ways.

First, with the exception of the Positive Psychology model, previous models of treatment (eg, medical/disease models, psychosocial rehabilitation, and the bio-psycho-social perspective) emphasized symptom relief as the goal of treatment. Recovery-based service delivery systems define the goals of treatment more broadly. Although symptom management may be included as a key treatment goal, the emphasis is placed on outcomes such as increased life satisfaction, enhanced client empowerment, a greater sense of hope and commitment to recovery, and improved ability to seek and maintain social support.

Second, most of the previous models of treatment have tended to place clients or patients in a one-down relationship with practitioners [9,22]. The recovery perspective asserts that the relationship between mental health professional and client must change to become more collaborative [23]. Those following a recovery paradigm in treatment delivery seek to ensure that the client is a full partner in treatment efforts, with the right to ultimate choice of intervention [22,23].

Third, the identity of the patient/client has changed. No longer is the consumer of services on the outside looking in at the treatment team. Consumers, other individuals who have mental illness (not necessarily actively in treatment), and groups that advocate for individuals who have mental illness are now integral members of the treatment team [24]. Furthermore, the emergence of Certified Peer Specialists as providers of mental health services represents a further innovation in incorporating the consumers of services as integral members of a treatment team.

INTRODUCTION TO CONCEPTUALIZATION OF THE RECOVERY MODEL

Reisner [23] recently stated that "the Recovery Model is more an overarching philosophy of treatment than an empirically validated treatment in and of itself." This statement contains more than a grain of truth, although recent efforts to study the application of the recovery philosophy have lent empiric support to certain aspects of the model. Definitions of recovery abound, and the plethora of attempts to define this concept and treatment philosophy has led to much confusion [25]. In addition, the confusion in the field regarding what constitutes recovery has prevented, to an extent, progress in justifying the perspective from an empiric, scientific standpoint (although many would argue that such justification is not necessary, because the Recovery Movement is more a civil rights issue than one of scientific legitimacy) [25].

Confusion in defining recovery stems, in part, from inconsistencies in use of the term within psychiatry. For example, Davidson and colleagues [25] asserted that outcome studies centering on chronic and persistent mental illness have tended to define recovery as symptom relief and reduction of illness-related skill deficits [5,26,27]. The mental health consumers/survivors who have written about their recovery experiences define recovery in a very different manner. Instead of emphasizing symptom relief, deficit reduction, or return to a specific level of functioning, these consumers have defined recovery in terms of regaining their civil rights as members of the community, often while continuing to experience and be affected by mental illness [25]. In other words, for strictly medically oriented researchers and practitioners, recovery means relief of the mental condition so that a reasonable level of functioning can occur, whereas for consumers and their family members, recovery means an increased sense of hope, empowerment, social support, optimism, and personal responsibility despite the ongoing presence of a mental illness.

COMMONLY ACCEPTED DEFINITIONS OF RECOVERY

Two major summaries of the common elements of recovery have emerged recently. Following an extensive review of the recovery-based literature, Davidson and colleagues [25] asserted that recovery (as applied to chronic and persistent mental illness) is best defined as (1) the consumer's acceptance of mental illness and its potential effects/consequences, (2) development of a sense of hope regarding the future and the ability to cope with illness and its consequences, and (3) the creation and application of a new, changed sense of self (which usually entails a greater sense of empowerment, a view of mental illness as only one dimension of self, and a reclamation of personal responsibility for one's own life). These authors go on to state that, often, recovery in mental illness means searching for internal strengths and seeking external supports to strive for a more meaningful and fulfilling life, even in the face of symptoms that do not resolve or improve [25]. To illustrate and elucidate their definition of recovery further, Davidson and colleagues [25] also provided a list of nine common elements of recovery:

1. Renewing hope and commitment
2. Redefining self
3. Incorporating illness into life as a whole
4. Involvement in meaningful activities
5. Overcoming stigma

6. Assuming control
7. Becoming empowered and exercising citizenship
8. Managing symptoms
9. Finding social support

The second major summary of recovery and its essential components is contained in a recent statement released by the Substance Abuse and Mental Health Services Administration (SAMHSA) [28]. This summary lists 10 "Fundamental Components of Recovery":

1. Consumer self-direction
2. Individualized and person-centered treatment
3. Empowerment
4. An holistic treatment focus
5. A nonlinear perspective of change
6. Treatment focused on strengths instead of deficits
7. The inclusion of peer support in treatment
8. Respect for consumers and consumer self-respect
9. Consumer acceptance of personal responsibility
10. Hope in recovery

This definition of recovery was developed through the participation of more than 110 mental health consumers, their family members, mental health professionals, managed care representatives, accreditation body representatives, and political figures [28].

Farkas and colleagues [29] have described four key values in the recovery perspective that must guide clinical practice:

1. Person orientation (or, view of clients from a holistic perspective and with a full awareness of their strengths and weaknesses)
2. Person involvement (or, intimate consumer involvement in treatment planning and program development)
3. Self-determination/choice (or, emphasis on a partnership among consumers and those who provide interventions)
4. Growth potential (or, commitment to fostering hope and removing barriers to progress)

Although this conceptual framework is more parsimonious, it has not been studied empirically.

Others also have attempted to define the Recovery Model in a more parsimonious manner. One might argue that operationally defining nine or 10 different constructs might become unwieldy and unmanageable. Also, it would seem that some of the aforementioned common elements of recovery might be closely related (eg, individualized and person-centered treatment might include a holistic view, empowerment, and respect). Furthermore, some of the commonly cited recovery elements seem to be interventions (peer support) that follow from the philosophies of recovery. Although most of the attempts to condense the recovery perspective into a few key concepts have not been empirically based [22], at least one group of researchers has attempted to define recovery [30] empirically.

Resnick and colleagues [30] conducted an important study that provides empiric support for some oft-proposed dimensions of recovery. These researchers selected items that centered on aspects of the recovery orientation from the client survey used in the landmark Schizophrenia Patient Outcomes Research Team (PORT) study [31]. They then conducted principal component analyses and confirmatory factor analyses to pinpoint the crucial elements of recovery [30]. It is worth noting that Resnick and colleagues [30] chose to define recovery as a set of values that guide treatment rather than as a treatment outcome and that they chose to examine recovery from a consumer perspective. The statistical analyses suggested that four key factors comprised the Recovery Model from a consumer perspective: (1) knowledge (of the mental health system and how to obtain community assistance), (2) empowerment (a view of the self as an agent of change and ability to pursue needed services), (3) hope and optimism (including consumers' beliefs regarding their own mental health), and (4) life satisfaction (including family, social networking, living situations, community concerns, and sense of safety). Of these factors, empowerment explained the greatest proportion of the variance, followed by knowledge and hope and optimism, whereas life satisfaction explained the smallest proportion [30]. Although the authors were encouraged by their findings, they strongly advocated further research to define recovery better operationally.

SUMMARY AND SYNTHESIS OF THE RECOVERY MODEL

At its present stage of development the Recovery Model of service delivery is more a philosophical guide for providing treatment than an evidence-based model [23]. This model seems to be a recent development in mental health services that has been driven in large part by consumer concerns about the restoration of their civil rights, the quality of care being provided to persons who have chronic and serious mental illnesses, and the associated efforts to advocate for a more empowering and consumer-friendly model of care. As discussed previously, however, the historical roots of the model are older and deeper than most might expect. Also, despite being more a philosophy than circumscribed treatment, aspects of the Recovery Model have links with certain theoretical perspectives that have associated bodies of empiric literature [17,23,32].

Specifically, Recovery Models are linked to identified common factors in psychotherapy that include factors that include (but are not limited to) a highly collaborative relationship with the client, fostering self-efficacy (related to empowerment and client responsibility), fostering and promoting hope and expected improvement, and the social support of a therapeutic relationship. Recovery also incorporates individualized treatment planning, because consumers enter treatment at different levels of readiness or ability to change. The transtheoretical model of behavior change provides an underlying theory for Recovery Models that provide the basis for encouragement of self-change efforts (incorporating empowerment and social support), acceptance of a nonlinear process of change, and emphasis on levels of service based on consumer readiness to change. Also, the empirically supported multisystemic family therapy provides the theory and data to bolster Recovery Models' emphasis on empowerment and removal of social barriers, focus on the consumer's strengths, and use of a consumer-inclusive treatment team. Each of these theoretical underpinnings has garnered support from empiric research, and thus by extension these facets of the Recovery Model have some empiric support as well.

SYSTEMS TRANSFORMATION: EVIDENCE FOR PEER SUPPORT SERVICES

As mentioned previously, the recovery paradigm promises to lead to innovation and transformation of mental health delivery systems, despite its relative youth in the field of schizophrenia research. Although the work of transforming systems is still early in its own development, it has been described in the recently released Federal Action Agenda as requiring a "revolution" in mental health service delivery [33]. Such a revolution obviously will require substantial changes across many different levels and in many different components of the system, including funding and reimbursement mechanisms, policy changes, program and service structures, and workforce development strategies, to name only a few. For an example of the systemic approach required by transformation, interested readers are referred to an article providing an overview of the framework adopted by one state that has begun this process [34]. Perhaps the most important change to be introduced as part of the work of transformation, however, will be in reconceptualizing the role of the person who has serious mental illness. Recovery, rather than remaining the purview and responsibility of the practitioner, becomes the responsibility and area of expertise of the person who has the illness [35]. In addition to taking on the tasks associated with his or her own personal recovery, the person in recovery increasingly has a role in offering support, role modeling, mentoring, and other services to his or her peers. The remainder of this article focuses on this innovation as an example of the changes introduced by the transformation to a recovery orientation being promoted currently by the Federal government. After defining peer support and discussing possible peer support benefits and challenges, this article describes the initiatives in the State of Georgia regarding peer support as an example of this particular innovation, its aims, and its objectives.

DEFINING PEER SUPPORT

Solomon [36] defined peer support as social, emotional, and instrumental support offered or provided by individuals who share a common mental health condition to engender social or personal change. She noted that a peer in the context of peer support is an individual who was or is presently diagnosed as having a form of severe mental illness (ie, schizophrenia) and who has experience with obtaining mental health services [36]. In addition, the peer providing or offering services must be willing to self-identify as a current or past consumer of mental health services. Solomon [36] suggested that peer support might be provided in six categories of services:

1. Self-help groups (such as Schizophrenics Anonymous)
2. Internet support groups
3. Peer-delivered services
4. Peer-run or operated services
5. Peer partnerships (with those without psychiatric diagnoses)
6. Use of peer employees within an established mental health service unit

Davidson and colleagues [37] argued, however, that peer support is not the same conceptually as peer-involved services. These authors proposed that, although mutual support (such as a self-help or Internet support groups) and peer-run programs (such as Schizophrenics Anonymous) are valuable and worthy of study, these forms of peer intervention are not truly peer support [38]. In this context, peer support is defined as "involving one or more persons who have a history of mental illness and have experienced significant improvements in their psychiatric condition offering services and/or supports to other people with serious mental illness who are considered to be not as far along in their own recovery process" [37].

Also, Davidson and his colleagues [37] argue that peer support falls in the center between a one-directional treatment relationship (as in psychotherapy) and a reciprocal relationship (as in most consumer-run self-help programs), producing an asymmetrical relationship between peer provider and consumer. It is this conceptualization of peer support and its relationships that is considered in this article.

The specific tasks of the peer specialist providing peer support have yet to be defined completely, but initial attempts have been made to define what constitutes peer support. Davidson and colleagues [37] suggest that, based on their shared experiences and history with schizophrenia and other forms of mental illness, peer specialists can provide (1) acceptance, (2) understanding, (3) empathy, (4) a sense of community/social support (which may lead to greater hope, autonomy, efficacy, and increased sense of personal responsibility), (5) role modeling of a recovery journey, (6) coping and problem-solving skill development, and (7) reframing of consumers' views of the world and their place in it. It is conceivable that these interventions could be provided in individual, family, and/or group contexts.

POSSIBLE BENEFITS OF PEER SUPPORT

Empiric data regarding the possible benefits of peer support services are scant, although interest in this area of study is increasing among researchers in the field. Some consistent findings have emerged thus far. For instance, several studies have found that peer support and other peer interventions either reduced the use of hospitalization or crisis services by consumers, shortened hospital stays when hospitalization occurred, or promoted successful functioning in the community [38–43]. In addition, some evidence suggests that participants in peer-support services experience enhanced quality of life, reduced numbers of life problems, increased self-esteem, a more positive outlook on life, decreased substance abuse, and more satisfactory social support and functioning than those not participating [41,44].

Other benefits of peer-support services are beginning to emerge from the literature. Peer providers themselves have reported improved quality of life and have experienced fewer hospitalizations than peers who do not provide services [45–47]. Solomon [36] has noted that decreases in hospitalizations and shortened hospital stays led to great potential cost savings for the delivery system as a whole. Furthermore, Solomon [36] cites several studies that have demonstrated that use of peer providers often leads to a shift in provider attitudes toward consumers of mental health services that are less stigmatized and negative in nature [48].

CHALLENGES OF PEER SUPPORT SERVICES

Many providers and system administrators have expressed concern regarding the hiring and employment of peer specialists. Carlson and colleagues [49] have noted that many of these concerns fall into three particular categories: (1) dual-relationship issues, (2) role conflicts, and (3) confidentiality concerns. Dual-relationship issues generally arise when peer specialists are (1) hired by a system in which they were formerly or are presently obtaining services and (2) when the specific nature of the relationship between peer provider and individuals obtaining services must be spelled out [49]. Role conflicts inherent in provision of peer services include (1) power struggles between peer providers and traditional providers, and (2) the balancing of peer/consumer status with professional identity [49]. Finally, confidentiality concerns arise when the peer specialist obtains (or in the past has obtained) services from the organization for which he or she works and when the peer specialist becomes privy to information about a consumer of services of that the consumer does not want other providers to know.

Peer specialists and other peer providers also have expressed concerns about provision of peer interventions, although from a decidedly different perspective. Mowbray and colleagues [46] conducted a series of interviews with individuals who had served as peer providers. These providers expressed concerns ranging from more individual issues while on the job to suggested systemic changes within the mental health system. For example, individual concerns expressed by peer providers included reservations regarding limited hours on the job, inappropriate salary scales for responsibility and role, lack of a defined role or job description, and unstructured work hours or schedule. Peer providers' structural complaints involved the lack of available information regarding peer employment opportunities, a lack of opportunities to display valuable skills, and a lack of social programming or inclusion for peer providers [46]. The provision of supervision also was a major area of concern for peer providers. Problems mentioned included a lack of specific and constructive feedback, lack of support from professional staff, inadequate training for expected job tasks, too few hours in supervision, and conflicts with supervisors based on disparities in status and education [46].

Most telling, however, were peer providers' concerns about mental health systems in a general sense. These concerns included poor systemic/community resources for consumer assistance (transportation, occupational, and other resources), lack of systemic incentives to work rather than draw government benefits, a strong crisis orientation to services as opposed to a preventative structure, and the prevalence of stigma toward those diagnosed as having schizophrenia and other forms of persistent mental illness [46]. Some peer providers became so disillusioned with the mental health system that they chose to leave it with no plans to return.

Although the aforementioned concerns regarding peer support and other forms of peer intervention pose barriers to implementation and system transformation, they need not become prohibitive in nature. Ways of alleviating or preventing many of these issues from becoming unmanageable have been suggested. For example, Mowbray and colleagues [46] suggested four ways to foster system transformation. (1) Mental health system administrators should think ahead regarding structural matters pertaining to peer services (eg, the role of peer providers within the agency, recruitment strategies, defined job roles/responsibilities, career advancement opportunities, and integration of peer providers into care system) and plan accordingly. (2) Those providing supervision for peer providers must develop a defined structure and framework for their supervision. (3) The mental health system must rethink and retool professional roles and how these are defined (eg, licensure and credentialing standards, value of service equated with stature of degree obtained). (4) Persons who obtain services should understand clearly that the role of peer providers serve is different than friendship. Additionally, Carlson and colleagues [49] have suggested practical solutions to the issues related to dual relationships, role conflicts, and confidentiality that may arise.

AN EXAMPLE: PEER SUPPORT INITIATIVES IN THE STATE OF GEORGIA

Beginning in 1999, Georgia was the first state in the country to bill Medicaid for an independent service called "peer support" delivered by a trained workforce of Certified Peer Specialists [50]. According to Sabin [50], public sector officials and consumer leaders concluded that to achieve stable funding for peer-support services, the services would have to be developed in a way that made them eligible for Medicaid funding under Medicaid's psychiatric rehabilitation option. Accomplishing this objective required melding two cultures: the consumer Recovery Movement with its informality, vision, and energy and Medicaid, with its complex bureaucratic requirements. Sabin [50] further argued that the Certified Peer Specialist role is the fulcrum of Georgia's effort to manage its services for persons who have serious and persistent disorders in a manner that promotes consumer-friendly recovery values.

Sabin [50] points out that the primary responsibility of the Certified Peer Specialist is to provide direct services designed to assist consumers in regaining control over their own lives and control over their recovery processes. The aim of peer support is to provide an opportunity for consumers to direct their own recovery and advocacy process and to teach and support each other in the acquisition and exercise of skills needed for the management of symptoms and for the use of resources within the community. In addition to providing direct services, Certified Peer Specialist are trained to act as agents of change in the mental health system promoting strength-based recovery with their unique insight into self-directed recovery gained by their experience.

The Georgia training curriculum was designed by Ike Powell, Director of Training for the Appalachian Consulting Group (ACG) based in Georgia. The ACG, under contract from SAMHSA, has written a resource kit for national distribution in 2007 on how to bill Medicaid for peer-support services and train and certify a workforce of peers. The ACG has trained peers in Hawaii, South Carolina, Michigan, Iowa, Connecticut, Wyoming, Florida, Massachusetts, Washington, Illinois, and Texas. New training modules being developed by the ACG with the Benson-Henry Institute for Mind Body Medicine at Massachusetts General Hospital, Boston, Massachusetts will train peers in skills to reduce metabolic factors contributing to early death among consumers who have severe and persistent mental illness. The Georgia and ACG national training focus on the five stages in recovery designed by Ike Powell based on Dr. Pat Deegan's recovery from schizophrenia [51].

An overview of the training incorporates three things that contribute to the disabling power of a psychiatric disability—symptoms, stigma, and negative self-image. The five stages are five different ways that people relate to the disabling power of a psychiatric diagnosis at various times in their lives in regard to symptoms, stigma, and negative self-image. The stages, which are not necessarily sequential, are (1) being overwhelmed by the symptoms; (2) giving into the diagnosis, seeing no possibility of recovery, and becoming dependent on the system; (3) beginning to question how much their lives are really limited by the diagnosis and how much by their own belief system; (4) beginning to challenge what they had originally seen, or had been told, were limits; and (5) beginning the process of moving outside or beyond the system for their supports.

The Georgia/ACG national training helps the peers understand and identify each stage, how people get "stuck" at one stage, and interventions that enable people move on with their lives. After training for 2 weeks, peers must pass a written and oral examination that demonstrates they have a working knowledge of a set of core competencies. More than 300 peers have been trained and certified in Georgia, and the state now bills some $10 million annually for peer-support services. Notably, the Medical College of Georgia Department of Psychiatry and Health Behavior hired a Certified Peer Specialist to begin providing services and to assist with staff and trainee educational projects in November 2006.

Georgia's pioneering work in peer support was driven by a very well organized and outcomes-focused consumer movement. A statewide organization, the Georgia Mental Health Consumer Network with a membership of 3000 persons, holds an annual conference. At that conference five top priorities are determined by majority vote of the attendees. Almost every year the conference's highest priority has been employment. That vote resulted in a statewide effort that began in 1998 to move 20% of consumers in day treatment to community jobs with competitive pay by the end of 2000. The goal of putting 2500 consumers to work within 2 years was met 6 months ahead of schedule [52].

With an historic emphasis on employment that addresses the crushing poverty so many mental health consumers confront, it is no surprise that consumer leaders in Georgia were unanimous in advocating for a new workforce of Certified Peer Specialists to provide Medicaid-funded peer-support services when the state overhauled its Medicaid services under the rehabilitation option 8 years ago. Georgia's consumer leadership exemplifies Recommendation 2.2 of the report of the President's New Freedom Commission on Mental Health [8] regarding system transformation. Page 37 of that report [8] states:

> [Services must] involve consumers and families fully in orienting the mental health system toward recovery... recovery-oriented services and supports are often successfully provided by consumers through consumer-run organizations and by consumers who work as providers in a variety of settings, such as peer support and psychosocial rehabilitation programs.

The New Freedom Commission report goes on to say, on page 37 [8]:

> Consumers who work as providers help expand the range and availability of service and supports that professionals offer. Studies show that consumer-run services and consumer-providers can broaden access to peer support, engage more individuals in traditional mental health services, and serve as a resource in the recovery of people with a psychiatric diagnosis. Because of their experiences, consumer-providers bring different attitudes, motivations, insights and behavioral qualities to the treatment encounter.

Medicaid-billable consumer-operated services and consumer providers represent an emerging evidence base, demonstrating cost effectiveness and recovery outcomes that are transforming the system. Illness self-management and recovery is a SAMHSA-promoted evidence-based practice available for review at the SAMHSA Website, mentalhealth.samhsa.gov/cmhs/communitysupport/toolkits. Georgia's peer support services are part of a SAMHSA-funded randomized, controlled study underway by Dr. Judith Cook, Director, Mental Health Service Program, University of Chicago at Illinois that is now underway and that should be completed in the next 2 years.

Georgia's research of its Medicaid data shows that peer support is cost effective and efficient: the annual average per-person cost of day treatment is $6491, whereas the average annual per-person cost of peer support is $1000. Over a 260-day period, data from the treatment plans of more than 300 adult Medicaid recipients diagnosed as having schizophrenia, bipolar disorder, or severe depression showed a statistically significant improvement with peer-support services over day support services in three outcome measures: symptoms/behavior, skills, and needs/resources [53].

WHY PEER SUPPORT IS CRUCIAL TO THE TRANSFORMATION TO RECOVERY-ORIENTED SYSTEMS

Peer support should be a component in the transformation of any mental health system to a recovery-based orientation. The argument supporting this statement is drawn from the knowledge that the consumer advocacy movement is the primary catalyst for recovery and that peer support (as provided within the context of the existing mental health system) is the next logical step toward full inclusion of persons diagnosed as having schizophrenia and other forms of persistent mental illness in the treatment domain. Peer specialists (along with other peer providers) have a unique opportunity to advocate for changes in the mental health delivery system. These individuals may have the best opportunity to change provider attitudes and mental health systems internally, because they often are able to shift perspectives more readily than traditional practitioners (eg, from consumer to consumer-provider and to traditional provider).

SUMMARY

The recovery perspective in the care of individuals who have persistent forms of mental illness offers great promise for system administrators and providers of mental health services. Because the Recovery Movement began with the advent of organized consumer advocacy groups and their efforts to make their dissatisfaction with the current system heard (and not through academic study), the movement has been more a philosophical discussion than an empirically built model of care. In recent years, however, attempts have been made to reconcile the philosophical and empiric perspectives on recovery, and these attempts have had a significant degree of success. The recovery perspective offers specific innovations to mental health care for the chronically and persistently mentally ill individual: it requires practitioners to broaden their definition of improvement to encompass such concepts as life satisfaction, sense of life meaning/purpose, empowerment, and hope. It is crucial that administrators and practitioners adopt a broader view of patient care should they wish to provide recovery-oriented services.

Furthermore, recovery promises system transformation and innovations in care that will change the relationships among administrators, practitioners, and consumers of care. Everyone involved must now be a full partner in mental health care, rather than viewing the patient in a one-down status. As a corollary to this innovation, the identity of the consumer of mental health services also must change. As consumers become increasingly empowered, and their advocacy ability increases, partnership in deciding how service delivery will occur becomes a crucial component of systemic change. The advent of integration of certified peer specialists into delivery systems reflects this changed perspective, because those diagnosed as having persistent forms of mental illness are valued members of the treatment team.

Continued empiric support of the Recovery Model is necessary to document its effectiveness and efficacy. Despite the model's nascent stage of development, the empiric literature on interventions such as peer support is promising, indeed. The challenges inherent in recovery-based system shifts do not, at this stage, seem to outweigh the possible benefits for patients diagnosed as having schizophrenia and the like. Sound educational interventions regarding recovery are needed to foster further system transformations.

References

[1] Anthony WA. A recovery-oriented service system: setting some system level standards. Psychiatr Rehabil J 2000;24:159–68.

[2] Anthony WA. Recovery from mental illness: the guiding vision of the mental health service system in the 1990s. Psychiatr Rehabil J 1993;16:11–23.

[3] Bleuler M, Huber G, Gross G, et al. The long-term course of schizophrenic psychoses: the combined results of two research studies. Nervenarzt 1976;47:477–81.

[4] Ciompi L, Muller C. Life course and age of schizophrenics: long term follow-up study through old age. Monogr Gesamtgeb Psychiatr Psychiatry Ser, Mono 1976;12:1–242.

[5] Harding CM, Brooks GW, Ashikaga T, et al. The Vermont longitudinal study of persons with severe mental illness, I: methodology, study sample, and overall status 32 years later. Am J Psychiatry 1987;144:718–26.

[6] Strauss JS, Carpenter WT. The prediction of outcome in schizophrenia: I. Characteristics of outcome. Arch Gen Psychiatry 1972;27:739–46.

[7] Strauss JS, Carpenter WT. The prediction of outcome in schizophrenia: II. Relationships between predictor and outcome variables: a report from the WHO international pilot study of schizophrenia. Arch Gen Psychiatry 1974;31:37–42.

[8] President's New Freedom Commission on Mental Health. Achieving the promise: transforming mental health care in America. Publication # SMA 03-3832. Rockville (MD): Department of Health and Human Services; 2003.

[9] Lehman AF. Putting recovery into practice: a commentary on "What recovery means to us." Community Ment Health J 2000;36:329–31.

[10] Pinel P. Treatise on insanity. Delran (NJ): Gryphon Editions; 1988.

[11] Lile B. Twelve step programs: an update. Addictive Disorders and Their Treatment 2003;2: 19–24.

[12] White WL. Addiction recovery mutual aid groups: an enduring international phenomenon. Addiction 2004;99:532–8.

[13] Geller JL. The last half-century of psychiatric services as reflected in *Psychiatric Services*. Psychiatr Serv 2000;51:41–67.

[14] Rosen GM. Self-help or hype? Comments on psychology's failure to advance self-care. Prof Psychol Res Pr 1993;24:340–5.

[15] American Psychological Association Task Force on Self-Help Therapies. Task force report on self-help therapies. Washington, DC: American Psychological Association; 1978.

[16] Kessler RC, Soukup J, Davis RB, et al. The use of complementary and alternative therapies to treat anxiety and depression in the United States. Am J Psychiatry 2001;158:289–94.

[17] Norcross JC. Here comes the self-help revolution in mental health. Psychotherapy 2000;37: 370–7.

[18] Prochaska JO, DiClemente CC, Norcross JC. In search of how people change: applications to addictive behaviors. Am Psychol 1992;47:1102–14.

[19] Seligman MEP, Cskiszentmihalyi M. Positive psychology: an introduction. Am Psychol 2000;55:5–14.

[20] Gable SL, Haidt J. What (and why) is positive psychology? Review of General Psychology 2005;9:103–10.

[21] Davidson L, Chinman M, Kloos B, et al. Peer support among individuals with severe mental illness: a review of the evidence. Clinical Psychology: Science and Practice 1999;6: 165–87.

[22] Mead S, Copeland ME. What recovery means to us: consumers' perspectives. Community Ment Health J 2000;36:315–28.

[23] Reisner AD. The common factors, empirically validated treatments, and recovery models of therapeutic change. Psychol Rec 2005;55:377–99.

[24] Frese FJ, Stanley J, Kress K, et al. Integrating evidence-based practices and the recovery model. Psychiatr Serv 2001;52:1462–8.

[25] Davidson L, O'Connell MJ, Tondora J, et al. Recovery in serious mental illness: a new wine or just a new bottle? Prof Psychol Res Pr 2005;36:480–7.

[26] Carpenter WT, Kilpatrick B. The heterogeneity of the long-term course of schizophrenia. Schizophr Bull 1988;14:645–52.

[27] Davidson L, McGlashan TH. The varied outcomes of schizophrenia. Can J Psychiatry 1997;42:34–43.

[28] Substance Abuse and Mental Health Services Administration. National consensus statement on mental health recovery. Rockville (MD): US Department of Health and Human Services; 2006. Available at: http://download.ncadi.samhsa.gov/ken/pdf/SMA05-4129/ trifold.pdf. Accessed December 20, 2006.

[29] Farkas M, Gagne C, Anthony W, et al. Implementing recovery oriented evidence based programs: identifying the critical dimensions. Community Ment Health J 2005;41:141–58.

[30] Resnick SG, Fontana A, Lehman AF, et al. An empirical conceptualization of the recovery orientation. Schizophr Res 2005;75:119–28.

[31] Lehman AF, Steinwachs DM, Dixon LB, et al. Patterns of usual care for schizophrenia: initial results from the Schizophrenia Patient Outcomes Research Team (PORT) client survey. Schizophr Bull 1998;24:11–20.

[32] Henggeler SW, Borduin CM. Family therapy and beyond: a multisystemic approach to treating behavior problems of children and adolescents. Pacific Grove (CA): Brooks/Cole; 1990.

[33] Department of Health and Human Services. Achieving the promise: federal action agenda, first steps. Washington, DC: Substance Abuse and Mental Health Services Administration; 2005.

[34] Davidson L, Kirk T, Rockholz P, et al. Creating a recovery-oriented system of behavioral health care: moving from concept to reality. Psychiatr Rehabil J, in press.

[35] Davidson L, Flanagan E, Roe D, et al. Leading a horse to water: an action perspective on mental health policy. J Clin Psychol 2006;62(9):1141–55.

[36] Solomon P. Peer support/peer provided services: underlying processes, benefits, and critical ingredients. Psychiatr Rehabil J 2004;27:392–401.

[37] Davidson L, Chinman M, Sells D, et al. Peer support among adults with mental illness: a report from the field. Schizophr Bull 2006;32:443–50.

[38] Edmunson E, Bedell J, Archer R, et al. Integrating skill building and peer support in mental health treatment: the early intervention and community network development projects. In: Jeger M, Slotnick R, editors. Community mental health and behavioral ecology. New York: Plenum Press; 1982. p. 127–39.

[39] Chinman MJ, Weingarten R, Stayner D, et al. Chronicity reconsidered: improving person-environment fit through a consumer-run service. Community Ment Health J 2001;37: 215–29.

[40] Clarke GN, Herinckx HA, Kinney RF, et al. Psychiatric hospitalizations, arrests, emergency room visits and homelessness of clients with serious and persistent mental illness: findings

from a randomized trial of two ACT programs vs. usual care. Ment Health Serv Res 2000;2: 155–64.

[41] Klein A, Cnaan R, Whitecraft J. Significance of peer social support for dually diagnosed clients: findings from a pilot study. Res Soc Work Pract 1998;8:529–51.

[42] Nikkel R, Smith G, Edwards D. A consumer-operated case management project. Hosp Community Psychiatry 1992;43:577–9.

[43] Patrick V, Smith RC, Schleifer SJ, et al. Facilitating discharge in state psychiatric institutions: a group intervention strategy. Psychiatr Rehabil J 2006;29:183–8.

[44] Felton CJ, Stastny P, Shern DL, et al. Consumers as peer specialists on intensive case management teams: impact on client outcomes. Psychiatr Serv 1995;46:1037–44.

[45] Armstrong ML, Korba AM, Emard R. Mutual benefit: the reciprocal relationship between consumer volunteers and the clients they serve. Psychiatr Rehabil J 1995;19:45–9.

[46] Mowbray C, Moxley D, Collins M. Consumers as mental health providers: first-person accounts of benefits and limitations. J Behav Health Serv Res 1998;25:397–411.

[47] Sherman P, Porter R. Mental health consumers as case management aids. Hosp Community Psychiatry 1991;42:494–8.

[48] Cook J, Jonikas J, Razzano L. A randomized evaluation of consumer versus nonconsumer training of state mental health service providers. Community Ment Health J 1995;31: 220–38.

[49] Carlson LS, Rapp CA, McDiarmid D. Hiring consumer-providers: barriers and alternative solutions. Community Ment Health J 2001;37:199–213.

[50] Sabin J, Daniels N. Strengthening the consumer voice in managed care: VII. The Georgia Peer Specialist Program. Psychiatr Serv 2003;54:497–8.

[51] Deegan PE. Recovery: the lived experience of rehabilitation. Psychiatr Rehabil J 1988;9: 11–9.

[52] DelVecchio P, Fricks L, Johnson JR. Issues of daily living for persons with mental illness. Psychiatric Rehabilitation Skills 2000;4:410–23.

[53] Tiegreen WW. Employing consumers in mental health service delivery: What's in it for me? Presentation at the National Council for Community Behavioral Healthcare. Orlando, FL; April 8, 2006.

INDEX

Note: Page numbers of article titles are in **boldface** type.

0193-953X/07/$ – see front matter
doi:10.1016/S0193-953X(07)00087-1

© 2007 Elsevier Inc. All rights reserved.
psych.theclinics.com

Moving?

Make sure your subscription moves with you!

To notify us of your new address, find your **Clinics Account Number** (located on your mailing label above your name), and contact customer service at:

E-mail: elspcs@elsevier.com

800-654-2452 (subscribers in the U.S. & Canada)
407-345-4000 (subscribers outside of the U.S. & Canada)

Fax number: 407-363-9661

Elsevier Periodicals Customer Service
6277 Sea Harbor Drive
Orlando, FL 32887-4800

*To ensure uninterrupted delivery of your subscription, please notify us at least 4 weeks in advance of move.